Biomedical Informatics: Information Systems in Medicine and Health

Biomedical Informatics: Information Systems in Medicine and Health

Editor: Cole Webb

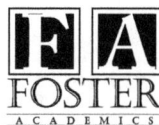

FA FOSTER ACADEMICS

www.fosteracademics.com

www.fosteracademics.com

FA
FOSTER
ACADEMICS

Cataloging-in-Publication Data

Biomedical informatics : information systems in medicine and health / edited by Cole Webb.
    p. cm.
Includes bibliographical references and index.
ISBN 978-1-63242-879-0
1. Medical informatics. 2. Bioinformatics. 3. Medicine--Data processing.
4. Health--Data processing. 5. Information storage and retrieval systems--Medicine.
6. Information storage and retrieval systems--Health. I. Webb, Cole.
R858 .B56 2020
610.28--dc23

Foster Academics,
118-35 Queens Blvd., Suite 400,
Forest Hills, NY 11375, USA

ISBN 978-1-63242-879-0 (Hardback)

Contents

Preface VII

Chapter 1   **Functionality of hospital information systems: results from a survey of quality directors at Turkish hospitals** 1
Mehmet Saluvan and Al Ozonoff

Chapter 2   **A computational application for multi-skill nurse staffing in hospital units** 12
Ana Respicio, Margarida Moz, Margarida Vaz Pato, Rute Somensi and
Cecília Dias Flores

Chapter 3   **A mobile phone based tool to identify symptoms of common childhood diseases in Ghana: development and evaluation of the integrated clinical algorithm** 21
Konstantin H. Franke, Ralf Krumkamp, Aliyu Mohammed,
Nimako Sarpong, Ellis Owusu-Dabo, Johanna Brinkel, Julius N. Fobil,
Axel Bonacic Marinovic, Philip Asihene, Mark Boots, Jürgen May and
Benno Kreuels

Chapter 4   **Information standards for recording alcohol use in electronic health records: findings from a national consultation** 30
Shamil Haroon, Darren Wooldridge, Jan Hoogewerf,
Krishnarajah Nirantharakumar, John Williams, Lina Martino and
Neeraj Bhala

Chapter 5   **Time series model for forecasting the number of new admission inpatients** 41
Lingling Zhou, Ping Zhao, Dongdong Wu, Cheng Cheng and Hao Huang

Chapter 6   **Developing a tablet computer-based application ('App') to measure self-reported alcohol consumption in Indigenous Australians** 52
KS Kylie Lee, Scott Wilson, Jimmy Perry, Robin Room, Sarah Callinan,
Robert Assan, Noel Hayman, Tanya Chikritzhs, Dennis Gray,
Edward Wilkes, Peter Jack and Katherine M. Conigrave

Chapter 7   **Development and validation of a model for the adoption of structured and standardised data recording among healthcare professionals** 63
Erik Joukes, Ronald Cornet, Martine C. de Bruijne, Nicolette F. de Keizer and
Ameen Abu-Hanna

Chapter 8   **Evidence-based usability design principles for medication alerting systems** 74
Romaric Marcilly, Elske Ammenwerth, Erin Roehrer, Julie Niès and
Marie-Catherine Beuscart-Zéphir

Chapter 9   **Using data-driven sublanguage pattern mining to induce knowledge models: application in medical image reports knowledge representation** 91
Yiqing Zhao, Nooshin J. Fesharaki, Hongfang Liu and Jake Luo

Chapter 10   **Effect of clinical decision rules, patient cost and malpractice information on
clinician brain CT image ordering**...104
Ronald W. Gimbel, Ronald G. Pirrallo, Steven C. Lowe, David W. Wright,
Lu Zhang, Min-Jae Woo, Paul Fontelo, Fang Liu and Zachary Connor

Chapter 11   **A pre-post study testing a lung cancer screening decision aid in primary care**...........112
Daniel S. Reuland, Laura Cubillos, Alison T. Brenner, Russell P. Harris,
Bailey Minish and Michael P. Pignone

Chapter 12   **A model for predicting utilization of mHealth interventions in low-resource
settings: case of maternal and newborn care**...121
Stephen Mburu and Robert Oboko

Chapter 13   **The relationship between hospital and ehr vendor market dynamics on
health information organization presence and participation** 137
Sunny C. Lin and Julia Adler-Milstein

Chapter 14   **Effective behavioral intervention strategies using mobile health applications
for chronic disease management**..146
Jung-Ah Lee, Mona Choi, Sang A Lee and Natalie Jiang

Chapter 15   **Using natural language processing methods to classify use status of dietary
supplements in clinical notes**..164
Yadan Fan and Rui Zhang

Chapter 16   **A bibliometric analysis of natural language processing in medical research** 171
Xieling Chen, Haoran Xie, Fu Lee Wang, Ziqing Liu, Juan Xu and
Tianyong Hao

Chapter 17   **Evaluating hospital websites in Kuwait to improve consumer engagement and
access to health information**..185
Dari Alhuwail, Zainab AlMeraj and Fatima Boujarwah

Chapter 18   **The QUEST for quality online health information: validation of a short
quantitative tool** 196
Julie M. Robillard, Jessica H. Jun, Jen-Ai Lai and Tanya L. Feng

Chapter 19   **What maximizes the effectiveness and implementation of technology-based
interventions to support healthcare professional practice?**...211
C Keyworth, J Hart, C J Armitage and M P Tully

Permissions

List of Contributors

Index

Preface

Over the recent decade, advancements and applications have progressed exponentially. This has led to the increased interest in this field and projects are being conducted to enhance knowledge. The main objective of this book is to present some of the critical challenges and provide insights into possible solutions. This book will answer the varied questions that arise in the field and also provide an increased scope for furthering studies.

Biomedical informatics is a field of information engineering that has applications in healthcare, particularly in the management and use of healthcare information. It is an interdisciplinary study that involves the design, adoption, development and IT-based innovations in healthcare services planning, delivery and management. Some of the tools of biomedical informatics are information and communication systems, computers, clinical guidelines, etc. It has applications in the areas of clinical medicine, pharmacy, nursing, public health, occupational therapy, biomedical research and physical therapy, among others. Some of the sub-fields of biomedical informatics are pathology informatics, imaging informatics, community health informatics, consumer health informatics, etc. Translational bioinformatics is an emerging field that integrates bio-statistics, molecular bioinformatics, clinical informatics and statistical genetics. It strives to identify the linkages between biological and clinical information, and enable better approaches to the study and treatment of diseases. This book explores all the important aspects of biomedical informatics in the present day scenario. The various studies that are constantly contributing towards advancing technologies and evolution of this field are examined in detail. The readers would gain knowledge that would broaden their perspective about the use of information systems in medicine and health.

I hope that this book, with its visionary approach, will be a valuable addition and will promote interest among readers. Each of the authors has provided their extraordinary competence in their specific fields by providing different perspectives as they come from diverse nations and regions. I thank them for their contributions.

Editor

Functionality of hospital information systems: results from a survey of quality directors at Turkish hospitals

Mehmet Saluvan[1]* (iD) and Al Ozonoff[1,2]

Abstract

Background: We aimed to determine availability of core Hospital Information Systems (HIS) functions implemented in Turkish hospitals and the perceived importance of these functions on quality and patient safety.

Methods: We surveyed quality directors (QDs) at civilian hospitals in the nation of Turkey. Data were collected via web survey using an instrument with 50 items describing core functionality of HIS. We calculated mean availability of each function, mean and median values of perceived impact on quality, and we investigated the relationship between availability and perceived importance.

Results: We received responses from 31% of eligible institutions, representing all major geographic regions of Turkey. Mean availability of 50 HIS functions was 65.6%, ranging from 19.6% to 97.4%. Mean importance score was 7.87 (on a 9-point scale) ranging from 7.13 to 8.41. Functions related to result management (89.3%) and decision support systems (52.2%) had the highest and lowest reported availability respectively. Availability and perceived importance were moderately correlated ($r = 0.52$).

Conclusion: QDs report high importance of the HIS functions surveyed as they relate to quality and patient safety. Availability and perceived importance of HIS functions are generally correlated, with some interesting exceptions. These findings may inform future investments and guide policy changes within the Turkish healthcare system. Financial incentives, regulations around certified HIS, revisions to accreditation manuals, and training interventions are all policies which will help integrate HIS functions to support quality and patient safety in Turkish hospitals.

Keywords: Hospital information systems, Electronic health records, Healthcare quality, Patient safety, Health information technology

Background

There have been steady efforts to improve quality in healthcare since the early 2000s, kickstarted by two reports released by the Institute of Medicine (IOM) [1]. The first report asserts that healthcare is not as safe as it should be and offers a substantial body of evidence pointing to medical errors as a leading cause of death and injury in the United States (U.S.). The second report focuses more broadly on how the healthcare delivery system can be redesigned to innovate and improve care [2]. Both reports suggest making effective use of information technologies as one of six necessary strategies for the redesign of healthcare systems [2, 3] and express concern over slow uptake of information technology in healthcare. Healthcare is an information-based science [4] and providers must have access to timely and accurate information to provide safe high-quality care [5]. Clearly, information management and health information technology (HIT) are fundamental to current and future healthcare delivery in the U.S., [6, 7] United Kingdom (U.K.), [8] and elsewhere [9–15].

Modern healthcare makes wide use of information technology [16, 17]. Most stakeholders agree that information technology such as electronic health records (EHRs) and computerized provider order entry (CPOE) will be critical to transforming the healthcare industry

* Correspondence: Mehmet.Saluvan@childrens.harvard.edu
[1]Center for Applied Pediatric Quality Analytics, Boston Children's Hospital, 300 Longwood Avenue, Boston, MA 02115, USA
Full list of author information is available at the end of the article

[6]. According to the IOM, HIT must play a central role in the redesign of the healthcare system if a substantial improvement in quality is to be achieved over the coming decade. Given the complexity of modern medicine, it is inevitable that HIT will play an ever increasing role in improving healthcare quality [18]. The imperatives of improving documentation, reducing error, and empowering patients will continue to use of information technology in healthcare. There is plenty of evidence that clinical informatics applications can address these imperatives to enhance patient outcomes, reduced costs, and provide access to knowledge [19].

Otherwise, healthcare costs are rising and all parties involved-government, insurers, hospitals and patients-are concerned. Costs must be reduced, but without major compromise of quality [20, 21]. The widespread adoption of HIT may reduce costs by way of improved efficiency and less duplication of effort in delivery of care services as well as a reduction in costly medical errors [22, 23]. Payment systems and provisions from payers have further incentivized the use of information systems in healthcare [24]. For example, the Centers for Medicare and Medicaid Services (CMS) provide up to $27B of incentive payments over 10 years to hospitals and healthcare providers that demonstrate meaningful use of certified electronic health record (EHR) systems in the U.S. [25, 26]. Simply put, "meaningful use" requires providers to demonstrate use of HIT to measure improvements in quality of care [27]. Similarly, England has invested at least £12.8 billion in a National Programme for Information Technology for the National Health Service in 2009 [15, 28].

Hospitals in particular are characterized by the high capacity of information and clinical data produced, and a new category of HIS now dominates in modern hospitals [16]. These systems aim to support high-quality, efficient, patient-centered care [29] with integrated support for the administrative and management tasks needed to support such care [30]. HIS systems have been shown to decrease the cost of quality care and the accessibility time to patient records [24]. The relevance of 'good' HIS for high-quality of care is obvious [29, 30]. Further advances of technology in healthcare include the use of information and communication technology (ICT) to support robust communications in an increasingly complex healthcare environment. ICT originally contributed to timely and efficient transmission of patient data, and its focus is now shifting to improve clinical data quality by using online clinical data acquisition and processing [31].

Implementation of HIS[1] systems has increased globally over the past 5 years, and higher-income countries are further in adoption and utilization of HIS systems compared to lower-income countries [32]. There are many competing HIS vendors each with their own products and different capabilities [33]. Most hospitals in higher-income countries are using comprehensive HIS, [12, 34–36] while in other parts of the world hospital orders for medications, laboratory tests, and other services are still paper-based [37]. This situation leads to a natural question: which core functions of HIS should be adopted for maximum impact on quality and patient safety?

This question was partially addressed in a 2003 IOM report which identified eight categories of core functionalities: health information and data; results management; computerized physician order entry; decision support system; electronic communication and connectivity; patient support; administrative processes; and reporting and population health management [38].

There is general consensus that the use of HIT should lead to more efficient, safer, and higher quality care [19, 39, 40]. There are few studies and data available on HIS implementation in countries with less mature healthcare systems. We hope to close this gap and provide new data on HIT implementation in Turkey.

Therefore the aim of this study is to determine availability of core HIS functions implemented in Turkish hospitals and their perceived importance on quality and patient safety.

Methods
Sampling frame
All licensed civilian hospitals in the nation of Turkey were eligible for this survey. Invitations to respond were sent to the Quality Director of each hospital from a listing of contact information maintained by the Turkish Ministry of Health (MoH). Military hospitals are not governed by the MoH and were excluded. In Turkish hospitals, QDs are responsible for planning and implementing quality and patient safety standards. Responsibilities of the QDs include: training and education of hospital staff; support and oversight of departmental quality committees; and coordination of internally and externally conducted audits [41]. We surveyed QDs since they are typically among the most knowledgeable staff about quality and patient safety aspects of hospital operations [42] (including use of HIS).

Survey instrument
We developed a survey instrument to collect data and perceptions on core functions of HIS implementation in Turkey. In order to develop the survey items, we began with national and international hospital quality standards maintained by the MoH and Joint Commission International. We reviewed features of HIS with supporting evidence to facilitate hospitals meeting these quality standards. We supplemented this initial list of

items with information from our review of the literature [38, 39, 41, 43, 44].

We note that two similar surveys have been conducted in the U.S. [39, 40]. Our instrument was developed independently for a specifically Turkish healthcare setting, but the items are derived from the same set of IOM documents and are broadly similar to the U.S. surveys. Davis and Thakkar delivered a brief 8-item survey to directors of Medical Informatics with three-level response scale (available/future implementation/no plans to implement) for each of the IOM-defined functionalities [40].We sought a more granular level of detail than that offered by this instrument. Jha et al. used a 32-item instrument, with each item reflecting one HIS function from 6 dimensions which approximate the IOM functionalities [39]. This instrument has been adapted for use in Japan, South Korea, and Spain [12, 14, 15]. Some items from the Jha survey are not appropriate for the Turkish setting, and we tailored the item selection to those most suitable to the Turkish healthcare system.

To assess the initial list of survey items, we performed a pilot study with a convenience sample of 17 QDs at hospitals across several provinces of Turkey. Staff roles in the pilot sample included physicians, nurses, computer engineers, healthcare administrators. The pilot survey was administered by email to the pilot study group and included 83 items. Each item described a core HIS function and used Likert scales to solicit opinions on the understandability and competency of each item to describe the intended HIS function. Many of these functions are either helpful or necessary to meet accreditation standards in the U.S. (e.g. by the Joint Commission), although there is no comparable national accreditation program implemented for hospitals in Turkey. Based on these pilot data, we updated the survey instrument by decreasing the number of items and revising some of the item descriptions. In particular, we removed or revised several items indicated as unclear or irrelevant based on free text comments from respondents.

The revised survey instrument includes 50 items, each of which describes a core functionality of HIS (see Additional file 1 for complete survey instrument translated from Turkish). Respondents are asked to provide two responses for each item. To reduce survey burden and complexity on respondents, we considered implementation to be 'all or nothing' and used binary responses to measure availability of core functions. The first scale measures availability of the HIS function with possible responses[2]: "available", "not available", or "unsure". Responses of 'unsure' were excluded and we treated availability as a binary response for all analyses. The second scale measures perceived importance of each item on the quality of healthcare provided by the hospital. This was measured on a 9-point Likert scale, with an available response of "unsure".

Item classification

Each of the 50 items was classified into one or more of the IOM domains described as follows:

1. Health Information and Data (HID): HID functions deliver critical information to providers to make clinical decisions e.g. medical and nursing diagnoses, drug allergies, problem lists, and clinical narratives. If this information is unavailable, low-quality and inefficient care may result [38, 40].
2. Results Management (RM): RM functions manage electronically results of all types including laboratory test results, radiology procedure results, and pathology reports. Computerized results are more accessible, timely, and accurate [38].
3. Computerized Physician Order Entry (CPOE): CPOE applications transmit physician orders electronically to the appropriate clinical service units [45]. The benefits of CPOE include elimination of lost or duplicate orders, improved accuracy, and reduced time to fill orders.
4. Decision Support System (DSS): DSS provides clinicians, staff, patients, or other individuals with knowledge and person-specific information to enhance health and health care. It encompasses a variety of tools and interventions such as computerized alerts and reminders, clinical guidelines, order sets, patient data reports and dashboards, documentation templates, diagnostic support, and clinical workflow tools [46]. DSS applications are embedded in the HIS and aim to detect critical situations or errors in care, and then notify the clinician perhaps with additional information to assist with clinical decisions [4, 47].
5. Electronic Communication and Connectivity (ECC): ECC functions include electronic communication tools such as e-mail and web messaging. These systems have been shown effective in facilitating provider communication with other providers and with patients, allowing for improved continuity of care and more timely interventions [38, 48, 49].
6. Patient Support (PS): Patient support functions involve the usage of HIT to encourage participation in patient care of patients, patient families, or third party caregivers. PS functions include patient portal, recording and monitoring patient education provided by hospital staff [38, 40].
7. Administrative Processes (AP): AP functions include electronic scheduling systems for admissions, inpatient and outpatient procedures, and visits. These systems increase the efficiency of hospital administration and improve the patient experience [38, 45].
8. Reporting and Population Health Management (RPHM): RPHM functions provide public and private sector reporting at the federal, state, and

local levels for safety, quality, and public health. This may include routine reporting of key quality indicators (sometimes referred to as clinical dashboards). This reduces the data collection and reporting burden, as well as the associated costs, and would likely increase the accuracy of the data reported [38, 50].

Data collection and analysis

The survey was administered by email invitation and all data collected by web survey. Information and an external link to the survey were available on the Turkish MoH web portal accessible by the quality director or delegate at each civilian hospital in Turkey. Hospital QDs were also informed about the survey via two e-mail reminders during a two-week period in March 2015. By design, only one respondent at each hospital was permitted to submit responses.

The survey instrument contained 50 items as described above. There was a section available to record opinions and recommendations as free text (general evaluation section), and additional items on institutional, demographic, and professional characteristics including: geographic province and sector; hospital type and bed size; gender, age, educational level; job title, tenure in current hospital role, and total years of professional experience.

We calculated frequencies and percentages of respondent demographic and professional characteristics. For each HIS function, we calculated percentage of respondents indicating the function was 'available' and calculated the mean and median values of perceived impact on quality. We examined the bivariate relationship between percentage availability of each HIS function and mean perceived importance of that function using scatterplots and Pearsonian correlation analysis. We calculated mean percentage availability and importance scores averaged across all hospitals for each of the survey items (Table 3), and also averaged across items within each of the 8 IOM categories (Table 4).

We managed and analyzed data using the R statistical package (v3.1.0 2015 R Institute).

Results

Institutional characteristics and response rates are reported in Table 1. 1486 hospitals were invited to participate, and we collected 464 responses (overall response rate 31.2% comparable to or greater than other similar national surveys [15, 40, 51]) representing all major geographic regions and 74 of 81 (91%) of provinces in Turkey. Response rates by section, hospital type, and bed size varied from 28.2% to 43.3%. Respondent hospital bed sizes ranged from 5 (minimum) to 1218 (maximum) beds (mean 157). The majority of responses came from general hospitals with fewer than 100 beds.

Table 1 Institutional characteristics and response rates

	Eligible Hospitals in Turkey	Number of responses (% of sample)	Response rate (%)
Hospital Sector			
Private	542	189 (40.7)	34.9
Ministry of Health	874	252 (54.3)	28.8
University	70	23 (5.0)	32.9
Hospital Type			
Training Hospital	144	53 (11.4)	36.8
Specialty Hospital	120	52 (11.2)	43.3
General Hospital	1222	359 (77.4)	29.4
Number of Beds			
99 and below	973	274 (59.1)	28.2
100–199	241	88 (19.0)	36.5
200–299	88	30 (6.5)	34.1
300–399	46	15 (3.2)	32.6
400 and above	138	57 (12.3)	41.3
TOTAL	1486	464 (100.0)	31.2

Our sample does not differ greatly on key characteristics from eligible hospitals in Turkey in terms of sector (chi-square $p = 0.22$) or number of beds ($p = 0.12$), although the sample slightly under-represents general hospitals (77% of sample, 82% of eligible hospitals, $p = 0.049$).

The demographics and professional characteristics of the participants are shown in Table 2. The majority of respondent QDs were female, college educated, trained as nurses, under the age of 40, with fewer than 10 years professional experience and hospital tenure.

Availability and mean perceived importance are reported for all 50 items (Table 3). Mean perceived importance was 7.87 (SD 1.71). Across all items, we observed lowest and highest means respectively of 7.13 (SD 2.25) (Item 2: predict time to examination on admission) and 8.41 (SD 1.81) (Item 50: data security). Availability of HIS functions, averaged across all 50 items and across all hospitals, was 65.6% (SD 20.0), with availability on particular functions ranging from 19.6% (SD 39.5) (item 15: telemedicine applications) to 97.4% (SD 16.0) (item 49: authorized access for staff). Respondent QDs reported that all HIS functions surveyed have an important effect on quality and patient safety (mean 7.87 on 9-point scale, SD 1.71).

We plotted the bivariate relationship between availability and perceived importance of HIS functions (Fig. 1). Availability and mean perceived importance are moderately correlated ($r = 0.52$, $p = 0.0001$). Functions with highest availability and perceived importance were those related to data security (items 49, 50) and laboratory services (items 8, 10), while those with lowest availability and perceived importance related to telemedicine (item 15) and patient education (items 28, 29). Functions

Table 2 Respondent demographics

Demographic features	Frequency (%)
Gender	
Female	314 (67.7)
Male	150 (32.3)
Education	
High school	18 (3.9)
Associate Degree	69 (14.9)
Bachelor Degree	211 (45.5)
Master	110 (23.7)
PhD	10 (2.2)
Medical Specialist	19 (4.1)
Missing	27 (5.8)
Job	
Physician	42 (9.1)
Nurse	235 (50.6)
Other Healthcare Staff	41 (8.8)
Engineer	11 (2.4)
Administrative Staff	101 (21.8)
Missing	34 (7.3)
Age Groups	
20–24	15 (3.2)
25–29	50 (10.8)
30–34	95 (20.5)
35–39	104 (22.4)
40–44	70 (15.1)
45–50	36 (7.8)
50 and above	22 (4.7)
Missing	72 (15.5)
Experience in current hospital work area/unit	
0–5 years	210 (45.3)
6–10 years	75 (16.2)
11–15 years	46 (9.9)
16–20 years	28 (6.0)
21–25 years	7 (1.5)
26 years and above	4 (0.9)
Missing	94 (20.3)
Experience in profession	
0–5 years	94 (20.3)
6–10 years	78 (16.8)
11–15 years	59 (12.7)
16–20 years	53 (11.4)
21–25 years	45 (9.7)
26 years and above	32 (6.9)
Missing	103 (22.2)

related to staff safety (items 34 and 44), medication safety (items 1, 24, 25, 26), and monitoring indicators (item 33) were less available than expected relative to their perceived importance. Conversely, functions related to patient access, comfort, and rights (items 2, 3, 5, 6) and operational activities (items 4, 12, 46) had lower perceived importance than we would expect based on availability.

We categorized all 50 items into eight non-exclusive IOM categories of HIT functionality (Additional file 1) and ranked the availability of functions within these domains from highest to lowest (Table 4). Functions related with result management (89.3%) and decision support systems (52.2%) had the highest and lowest reported availability score respectively. Respondent QDs reported functions related with CPOE to have the highest importance in terms of improving healthcare quality, while functions related with patient support were ranked as lowest.

Free text comments are classified and sorted by frequency (Table 5). Many respondents highlighted the importance of the study, their desire to review HIS from the perspective of quality and patient safety, and higher expectations of HIS functions to improve quality and patient safety.

Discussion

We investigated availability of HIS functions and their perceived importance on quality and patient safety by 50 items survey developed by authors, and received responses from hospital quality professionals from a broadly representative sample of Turkish hospitals in terms of geographic and institutional characteristics. Despite high levels of perceived importance across all 50 HIS functions which comprised our survey, on average only two-thirds of hospitals surveyed have adopted these functions and important functions like decision support systems are adopted at very low rates.

We focused on subgroups of HIS functions that are of special interest. First we considered the more highly available functions. Generally the most widely available functions are those related to data security, automation of laboratory processes, and administrative reporting. Reasons for this high adoption may include the importance of privacy and data security in the healthcare setting [52, 53]; pressure on laboratories to satisfy ongoing quality audits and maintain licensing or certification; or recommendations from MoH [54–56]. It is also worth noting that administrative functions are often highly valued by hospital leaders who are in a position to influence HIS purchasing decisions [6, 45, 57].

We examined more closely the relationship between availability and perceived importance of each item. We observed as expected that availability and perceived

Table 3 Average of availability and percieved importance [mean (SD)]

Item No	HIS functions	Availability (%)	Perceived importance (Over 9)
1	Display alerts for high risk medications (e.g. narcotics, sound-alike drugs, concentrated electrolytes) just prior to administration	47.7 (50.0)	8.07 (2.05)
2	Predict time to patient examination on admission	74.6 (43.6)	7.13 (2.25)
3	Record time to consultation after request from emergency department	82.4 (38.2)	7.66 (2.13)
4	Display real-time availability of patient beds	91.9 (27.4)	7.84 (1.99)
5	Flag and prioritize elderly and disabled patients	80.8 (39.4)	7.81 (1.99)
6	Provide electronic copy of patient records when requested (e.g. diagnosis list, lab test results, administered procedures, administered medications, discharge summary)	82.9 (37.7)	7.58 (2.02)
7	View all diagnostic test results including laboratory, radiology, pathology, nuclear medicine, endoscopy	92.4 (26.5)	8.12 (1.85)
8	Record times and performing staff of laboratory test samples throughout all laboratory phases i.e. sampling, accepting, analyzing, approving, and reporting	96.1 (19.4)	8.19 (1.79)
9	Display alerts for lab samples that do not meet acceptance criteria	72.4 (44.8)	7.96 (1.98)
10	Display alerts for laboratory tests that return panic values	96.5 (18.4)	8.33 (1.79)
11	Display reminders for internal and external lab quality control measures and keep their result for analyses	57.8 (49.4)	7.65 (2.12)
12	Record laboratory process problems (pre-analytic, analytic, and post-analytic)	71.0 (45.4)	7.76 (2.02)
13	Provide digital radiology images within internal network i.e. Picture Archiving and Communication System (PACS)	85.3 (35.5)	8.18 (1.89)
14	Monitor radiology appointment and reporting times	61.1 (48.8)	7.46 (2.13)
15	Support telemedicine applications	19.6 (39.5)	7.58 (2.28)
16	Monitor use of blood and blood products during order, preparation, acceptance, and implementation	74.3 (43.8)	8.11 (1.90)
17	Monitor blood and blood products stock and expiration date	78.1 (41.4)	8.16 (1.91)
18	Record disease severity as structured data (e.G. *apache* II, SAPS II, and PRISM)	50.7 (50.1)	7.64 (2.10)
19	Integrate nursing care plans into medical record	58.5 (49.3)	7.57 (2.26)
20	Record and integrate all clinical orders into medical record including laboratory test orders, medication orders, nursing care orders, nutrition therapy orders, rehabilitation therapy orders	84.2 (36.5)	7.94 (1.99)
21	Record and integrate all diagnostic, clinical, and surgical procedures into medical record including endoscopy, cardiac catheterization, radiotherapy, CT, and ultrasound	90.1 (29.9)	8.05 (1.95)
22	Record usage and monitor complications of anesthetic agents and sedatives administered outside of anesthesiology (e.g. endoscopy, cardiac catheterization, and IVF units)	52.2 (50.0)	7.81 (2.08)
23	Display clinical guidelines and provide alerts for deviations	50.2 (50.1)	7.53 (2.10)
24	Provide alerts for drug-drug interactions	45.5 (49.9)	7.98 (2.06)
25	Provide alerts for drug-food interactions	42.3 (49.5)	7.88 (2.12)
26	Provide alerts for drug-allergy interactions	41.9 (49.4)	8.07 (2.06)
27	Integrate Computerized Physician Order Entry	75.6 (43.0)	8.04 (1.98)
28	Provide alerts for patient education that is part of care plan or discharge plan	29.7 (45.8)	7.39 (2.23)
29	Record all patient education provided to patient	41.8 (49.4)	7.32 (2.18)
30	Record patient and staff safety events	57.0 (49.6)	7.86 (2.11)
31	Record emergency code alerts (e.g. Code Blue, Code White) and integrate with paging system	42.6 (49.5)	7.67 (2.22)
32	Record blood transfusion reactions as structured data	52.0 (50.0)	7.84 (2.17)
33	Monitor hospital key performance indicators automatically	62.6 (48.5)	7.96 (2.00)
34	Flag patients and warn staff of patients with risk of infection (e.g. HIV+, HepC+)	51.7 (50.0)	8.18 (2.04)

Table 3 Average of availability and percieved importance [mean (SD)] *(Continued)*

Item No	HIS functions	Availability (%)	Perceived importance (Over 9)
35	Monitor nosocomial infections and transmit surveillance data to national or international networks	44.8 (49.8)	7.83 (2.13)
36	Monitor and record sterilization processes including procedure date and time and material expiration date	32.8 (47.0)	7.76 (2.19)
37	Display real-time information necessary for unit managers including bed occupancy, waiting list, surgeries scheduled	88.9 (31.5)	7.85 (2.01)
38	Report periodically on operational statistics including monthly admissions, income-expenditure, services delivered	94.5 (22.8)	7.88 (1.94)
39	Provide alerts for devices that require periodic maintenance or calibration	29.5 (45.7)	7.76 (2.11)
40	Provide alerts for medications and medical supplies near expiration or at critically low stock levels	91.9 (27.3)	8.25 (1.85)
41	Provide inventory of all medical devices including location and responsible staff	57.4 (49.5)	7.65 (2.08)
42	Monitor and provide reminders for routine health screening of clinical staff	25.6 (43.7)	7.80 (2.13)
43	Identify, flag, and, prohibit duplicate patient records	83.0 (37.6)	8.14 (1.95)
44	Monitor occupational accidents and injuries	52.0 (50.5)	7.90 (2.10)
45	Display current organizational policies and procedures and provide alerts of updated documents	67.5 (46.9)	7.90 (2.09)
46	Record clinical staff certification and licensing information	78.8 (40.9)	7.80 (1.97)
47	Integrate and update information with hospital external website	56.1 (49.7)	7.73 (2.10)
48	Provide online patient portal to view, download, and transmit lab results	91.1 (28.5)	8.09 (1.86)
49	Provide access control management for different staff groupings	97.4 (16.0)	8.18 (1.85)
50	Provide data security and protection for electronic health information	93.6 (24.5)	8.41 (1.81)
	Average	65.6 (20.0)	7.87 (1.71)

importance are generally correlated (Fig. 1). However there were some functions that departed from the general pattern. For example, we identified three 'clusters' of items which were generally not as available as their perceived importance would suggest: staff safety, medication safety, and monitoring indicators. While focus has recently shifted to patient-centered care, it is also increasingly recognized that high quality care includes employee safety as well as patient safety. This change of emphasis is meant to ensure that a safety

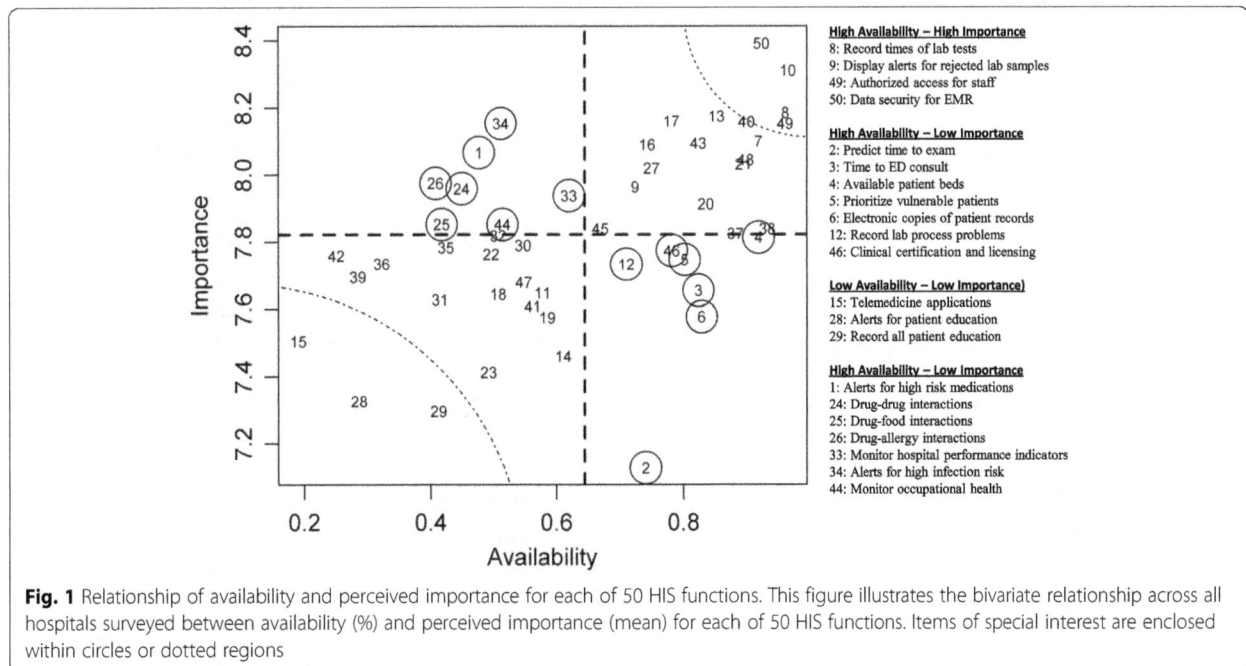

Fig. 1 Relationship of availability and perceived importance for each of 50 HIS functions. This figure illustrates the bivariate relationship across all hospitals surveyed between availability (%) and perceived importance (mean) for each of 50 HIS functions. Items of special interest are enclosed within circles or dotted regions

Table 4 Availability and perceived importance by IOM classification [mean (SD)]

	Availability (%)	Perceived importance
Result Management	89.3 (18.5)	7.87 (1.72)
Administrative Processes	71.7 (18.7)	7.86 (1.71)
Computerized Physician Order Entry	68.0 (25.1)	7.93 (1.80)
Electronic Communication and Connectivity	64.2 (21.3)	7.87 (1.72)
Reporting and Population Health Management	63.0 (24.5)	7.79 (1.78)
Health Information and Data	62.6 (24.0)	7.89 (1.75)
Patient Support	62.5 (27.1)	7.67 (1.76)
Decision Support Systems	52.2 (28.8)	7.88 (1.79)

culture pervades a healthcare organization, with the safety of the workforce and the work environment given equal standing as a safety priority [58]. Medication errors compose a sizable proportion of the total burden of medical errors, and information systems are an effective tool to prevent these errors [2, 3, 59, 60]. Monitoring indicators in real-time using HIS offers many advantages [61, 62]. This reflects discordance between hospital QDs and the hospital leaders who make decisions about HIS purchasing.

Table 5 Comments collected from the "general evaluation" section

Participant comments	Frequency
Thanks for the study and for the opportunity to evaluate HIS functionalities currently in use	33
Every HIS function in survey would positively affect quality of healthcare	22
Some functions are available as a part of our HIS, but they are not used	14
Turkish MoH should produce and share HIS for common use	12
HIT department support is insufficient, ineffective, or disregards users; technical problems lead to sub-optimal use	12
Every HIS function in survey should be mandatory for every HIS	10
Employees and managers lack training and experience to use HIS effectively	7
MoH should define certification standards for HIS and related products	5
Comments about specific functions (PACS, telemedicine, monitoring indicators, nursing care plans)	5
Suggested HIS functions related to quality and patient safety not included in survey	5
National integration of HIS and patient records available to all healthcare institutions	3
Integration problems between information systems used by MoH and hospitals	3
Total	**131**

Functions associated with patient access to services, patient comfort, patient rights, and hospital operations were evaluated as relatively less important than their availability. Indeed, QDs are expected to be more sensitive to patient satisfaction and patient experience. However our findings suggest that the administrator responsible for HIS selection might prioritize administrative needs and patient expectations driven by previously determined health policies [63] that might lead to diminished perceived importance among healthcare staff include quality directors.

Availability and perceived importance were concordant and generally high for features related to information security, patient safety, and laboratory services. Information security is a top priority for every institution and especially for hospitals, although there are no privacy laws in Turkey specific to healthcare such as the Health Information Portability Accountability Act (HIPAA). Moreover, patient safety and laboratory services standards were component of national quality standards from the first iteration, and hospitals have been surveyed against these standards several times [54, 64]. These findings are consistent with a positive effect from the quality survey process explained above.

Telemedicine applications and patient education functions had generally low availability and perceived importance. Although telemedicine has significant advantages for patients located in remote geographic regions far from qualified healthcare facilities [65–68], our finding is not surprising since many hospitals without remotely located patients may consider telemedicine a luxury. Patient empowerment via education is understood to be an important part of the healing process [69, 70]. We believe our findings have identified an important issue for further discussion among healthcare administrators and employees.

The IOM category reported most available was RM, with these functions present on average across 90% of respondent hospitals. Managing results electronically has substantial impact on unnecessarily ordered tests, and timeliness of reporting to providers. It is also significant to prevent medical errors [71–73]. The high level of RM function adoption among Turkish hospitals may accelerate future plans for electronic medical records shared throughout all Turkish healthcare providers, leading to eventual improvements in clinical care by increasing provider access to timely and accurate clinical data. Conversely, DSS is reported as the functional category least available in Turkish hospitals. DSS includes applications that combine clinical information with embedded medical knowledge to assist the human decision process [4]. These systems imply some higher level of information processing, or inference, by the computer [74]. Some respondents reported that both providers and hospital managers lacked the necessary knowledge for effective use of information systems (See Table 5). Thus general issues of staff training and expertise of management may explain lower availability of DSS in Turkish hospitals, as well as clinicians' willingness to ask, direct, and help vendors and hospital managers with the development and adoption of DSS. The literature supports the potential of DSS to improve patient safety and quality of care e.g. reminders for vital tasks, assistance with diagnoses, avoiding drug-drug interactions, enhancing clinical regulatory compliance, reducing unnecessary test orders, and identifying emerging disease outbreaks [6, 74–76]. Involving clinicians in DSS development, and increased awareness and investment in DSS will likely improve safety and quality across the Turkish hospital system.

Perceived importance was generally high across all items, and there were no substantial differences in across IOM categories. CPOE functions were perceived as most important and PS functions (e.g. patient portal) were generally perceived as less important. Similar research studying 89 U.S. healthcare facilities in 2005 rated categories 7.58 to 8.83 (out of 10) on importance, similar to our results. PS shows low in the U.S. as well as Turkey [40]. The same study showed 37% of respondents report current use of at least one component in all of the eight core HIS functionalities, while another study suggests that in 2009, only 1.5% of U.S. hospitals had comprehensive HIS i.e. present in all clinical units, and only an additional 7.6% have a basic system i.e. present in at least one clinical unit. Results from the U.S., Spain, and South Korea also show highest availability for RM functionality e.g. RM was available for 75% of U.S. hospitals [14, 15, 39]. There are broad parallels between the U.S. situation circa 2010 and the adoption of HIS in Turkey roughly 5 years later.

This study has several limitations. Although we examined reliability of individual items, we did not validate our survey using an independent sample nor did we validate against an existing instrument. We designed and piloted our survey with an aim of face validity, and our focus was on broad patterns of response rather than the psychometric properties of the survey instrument. The survey instrument does not include all HIS functions but rather 50 items to be most relevant to patient safety and quality as determined by researcher judgment and pilot testing. Although observed scores for perceived importance lie within a compressed range of values – mean responses across items range from 7.13 to 8.44 – our large sample allows for valid statistical comparison and correlation. Military hospitals were not included in the sample. Finally, promotion of the survey via the MoH e-mail and website may have induced a 'halo effect' of positive response bias.

Diverse HIS functions have been adopted at different rates in Turkey and across the world. This study, which supports previous research conducted in the U.S., presents potentially useful insight into the adoption of HIS functions to support patient safety and quality. Findings from this and similar surveys should be considered carefully by policymakers, software designers, clinicians, and hospital leaders. We recommend mandating certified software (or offering incentives) and surveying HIS functions during regular quality audits, two policy approaches which would support system-wide improvements. Another important issue that we identified is the training of hospital leaders and clinical staff. Technical support and training processes may be better defined by public regional authorities. Software designers may consider our results when developing HIS products and hospital leaders should make HIS purchasing decisions using information from QDs on which functions are perceived most important to patient safety and quality of care.

Conclusions

Our study corroborates previous work highlighting the perceived importance of HIT on quality and patient safety. After revision and tailoring to the specifics of other international settings, the expanded list of items in this study could be used elsewhere to increase awareness and to survey availability of HIS functions in other national healthcare systems. We believe that our survey is an important first step to understand the system-wide availability of specific HIS functions across hospitals in Turkey, and that similar surveys in other countries would yield valuable knowledge to guide policymakers and hospital leaders in many settings.

Our findings support the conclusion that HIS functions in Turkish hospitals are generally not as available as quality managers would like. Policymakers, hospital leaders, and software developers all have a potential role to address future improvements. Some policy levers include financial incentives to adopt specific HIS functions; government involvement in certification of software; regulations to encourage or enforce usage of certified HIS; and inclusion of desired functions into accreditation manuals. Each of these policies may help integrate HIS functions to support quality and patient safety in Turkish hospitals. Finally, further investment in training programs will be needed across organizational levels, including clinical employees, HIT support staff, and hospital leaders and managers.

Endnotes

[1]Terms such as Hospital Information System (HIS), Electronic Medical Record (EMR), Electronic Health Record (EHR), and Patient Health Record (PHR) are

used interchangeably in the literature. We have tried to use the term Hospital Information System (HIS) consistently throughout this paper unless it is necessary or relevant to differentiate terms.

[2]These terms are translated from Turkish responses "var", "yok", and "fikrim yok".

Abbreviations
AP: Administrative Processes; APACHE: Acute physiology and chronic health evaluation; CMS: Centers for Medicare and Medicaid Services; CPOE: Computerized physician order entry; CT: Computed tomography; DSS: Decision support system; ECC: Electronic communication and connectivity; EHR: Electronic health records; EMR: Electronic medical record; HepC: Hepatitis C; HID: Health information and data; HIPAA: Health Information Portability Accountability Act; HIS: Hospital information systems; HIT: Health information technology; HIV: Human immunodeficiency virus; ICT: Information and communication technology; IOM: Institute of Medicine; IVF: In vitro fertilization; MoH: Ministry of Health; PACS: Picture Archiving And Communication System; PRISM: Pediatric risk of mortality; PS: Patient support; QDs: Quality directors; RM: Result management; RPHM: Reporting and population health management; SAPS: Simplified acute physiology score; SD: Standard deviation; U.K.: United Kingdom; U.S.: United States

Acknowledgements
This research was supported by Turkish Ministry of Health, Department of Quality and Accreditation in Healthcare. We thank our colleagues from Department of Quality and Accreditation in Healthcare who provided assistance with collecting research data, although they may not agree with all of the interpretations and conclusions of this paper.

Funding
Not applicable

Authors' contributions
MS: conceived of and designed the study, performed the literature review, created and implemented the survey, analyzed the data, and drafted the manuscript text. AO: supervised the study, assisted with statistical analyses, contributed to the writing and editing of the manuscript text, and reviewed and approved its final version. Both the authors read and approved the final version of the manuscript.

Competing interests
The authors declare that they have no competing interests.

Author details
[1]Center for Applied Pediatric Quality Analytics, Boston Children's Hospital, 300 Longwood Avenue, Boston, MA 02115, USA. [2]Department of Pediatrics, Harvard Medical School, Boston, MA, USA.

References
1. IOM: The quality of health Care in America. 2013. http://www.nationalacademies.org/hmd/Activities/Quality/QualityHealthCareAmerica. Accessed 02 July 2014.
2. IOM. Crossing the quality chasm: a new health system for the 21st century. Washington (DC): National Academy Press; 2001.
3. IOM. To err is human: building a safer health system. Washington (DC): National Academy Press; 1999.
4. Hersh WR. Medical informatics: improving health care through information. JAMA. 2002;288:1955–8.
5. Abbott P, Taylor LA. The role of health information Technology in Improving Healthcare Quality and Patient Safety: Johns Hopkins University School of Nursing; 2007. p. 1–4.
6. Chaudhry B, Wang J, Wu S, Maglione M, Mojica W, Roth E, Morton SC, Shekelle PG. Systematic review: impact of health information technology on quality, efficiency, and costs of medical care. Ann Intern Med. 2006;144:742–52.
7. Chassin MR, Galvin RW. The urgent need to improve health care quality. Institute of Medicine National Roundtable on health care quality. JAMA. 1998;280:1000–5.
8. Luchenski SA, Reed JE, Marston C, Papoutsi C, Majeed A, Bell D. Patient and public views on electronic health records and their uses in the United kingdom: cross-sectional survey. J Med Internet Res. 2013; https://doi.org/10.2196/jmir.2701.
9. Nohr C, Andersen SK, Bernstein K, Bruun-Rasmussen M, Vingtoft S. Diffusion of electronic health records–six years of empirical data. Stud Health Technol Inform. 2007;129:963–7.
10. Urowitz S, Wiljer D, Apatu E, Eysenbach G, Delenardo C, Harth T, Pai H, Leonard KJI. Canada ready for patient accessible electronic health records? A national scan. BMC Med Inform Decis Mak. 2008;8:1472–6947.
11. Kaipio J, Laaveri T, Hypponen H, Vainiomaki S, Reponen J, Kushniruk A, Borycki E, Vanska J. Usability problems do not heal by themselves: national survey on physicians' experiences with EHRs in Finland. Int J Med Inform. 2017;97:266–81.
12. Inokuchi R, Sato H, Nakamura K, Aoki Y, Shinohara K, Gunshin M, Matsubara T, Kitsuta Y, Yahagi N, Nakajima S. Motivations and barriers to implementing electronic health records and ED information systems in Japan. Am J Emerg Med. 2014; https://doi.org/10.1016/j.ajem.2014.03.035.
13. Heimly V, Grimsmo A, Faxvaag A. Diffusion of electronic health records and electronic communication in Norway. Applied clinical informatics. 2011; https://doi.org/10.4338/ACI-2011-01-IE-0008.
14. Kim YG, Jung K, Park YT, Shin D, Cho SY, Yoon D, Park RW. Rate of electronic health record adoption in South Korea: a nation-wide survey. Int J Med Inform. 2017; https://doi.org/10.1016/j.ijmedinf.2017.02.009.
15. Marca G, Perez A, Blanco-Garcia MG, Miravalles E, Soley P, Ortiga B. The use of electronic health records in Spanish hospitals. Him J. 2014;43:37–44.
16. Vafaee A, Vahedian M, Esmaeily H, Kimiafar K. Views of users towards the quality of hospital information system in training hospitals. Journal of research in health sciences. 2010;10:47–53.
17. E.U. eHealth action plan 2012–2020-innovative healthcare for the 21st century. 2012.
18. Ortiz E, Clancy CM. Use of information technology to improve the quality of health care in the United States. Health Serv Res. 2003; https://doi.org/10.1111/1475-6773.00127.
19. Nguyen L, Bellucci E, Nguyen LT. Electronic health records implementation: an evaluation of information system impact and contingency factors. Int J Med Inform. 2014;83:779–96.
20. Bates DW, Pappius E, Kuperman GJ, Sittig D, Burstin H, Fairchild D, Brennan TA, Teich JM. Using information systems to measure and improve quality. Int J Med Inform. 1999; https://doi.org/10.1016/S1386-5056(98)00152-X.
21. Bates DW, Pappius EM, Kuperman GJ, Sittig D, Burstin H, Fairchild D, Brennan TA, Teich JM. Measuring and improving quality using information systems. Stud Health Technol Inform. 1998;2:814–8.
22. Nirel N, Rosen B, Sharon A, Blondheim O, Sherf M, Samuel H, Cohen AD. The impact of an integrated hospital-community medical information system on quality and service utilization in hospital departments. Int J Med Inform. 2010; https://doi.org/10.1016/j.ijmedinf.2010.06.005.
23. Hillestad R, Bigelow J, Bower A, Girosi F, Meili R, Scoville R, Taylor R. Can electronic medical record systems transform health care? Potential health benefits, savings, and costs. Health Aff. 2005;24:1103–17.
24. Sağıroğlu YÖ. Implementation difficulties of hospital information systems: a case study in a private Hospital in Turkey. İstanbul: Bogaziçi University; 2006.
25. HealthIT.gov: EHR Incentives & Certification. http://www.healthit.gov/providers-professionals/ehr-incentives-certification (2014). Accessed 16 Apr 2015.
26. David B, Tavenner M. The "meaningful use" regulation for electronic health records. N Engl J Med. 2010;363:501–4.
27. HRSA: What is "meaningful use". 2015. https://www.cms.gov/Regulations-and-Guidance/Legislation/EHRIncentivePrograms/downloads/MU_Stage1_ReqOverview.pdf. Accessed 16 Apr 2015.

28. Black AD, Car J, Pagliari C, Anandan C, Cresswell K, Bokun T, McKinstry B, Procter R, Majeed A, Sheikh A. The impact of eHealth on the quality and safety of health care: a systematic overview. PLoS Med. 2011; https://doi.org/10.1371/journal.pmed.1000387.

29. Haux R, Winter A, Ammenwerth E, Brigl B. Strategic information Management in Hospitals. An introduction to hospital information systems. New York: Springer; 2004.

30. Haux R. Health information systems- past, present, future. Int J Med Inform. 2006;75:268–81.

31. Takeda H, Matsumura Y, Nakajima K, Kuwata S, Zhenjun Y, Shanmai J, Qiyan Z, Yufen C, Kusuoka H, Inoue M. Health care quality management by means of an incident report system and an electronic patient record system. Int J Med Inform. 2003;69:285–93.

32. WHO. Global diffusion of eHealth: making universal health coverage achievable. Report of the third global survey on eHealth. Genova: world health. Organization. 2016;

33. Anderson JG. Social, ethical and legal barriers to e-health. Int J Med Inform. 2007;76:480–3.

34. HealthITDashboard: Quick Stats. https://dashboard.healthit.gov/quickstats/quickstats.php (2017). Accessed 5 Jan 2017.

35. Borycki EM, Newsham D, Bates DW. eHealth in North America. Yearb Med Inform. 2013;8:103–6.

36. Hyppönen H, Kangas M, Reponen J, Nøhr C, Villumsen S, Koch S, Hardardottir GA, Gilstad H, Jerlvall L, Pehrsson T. Nordic eHealth benchmarking: Nordic Council of Ministers; 2015.

37. WHO. Atlas of eHealth country profiles: the use of eHealth in support of universal health coverage: based on the findings of the third global survey on eHealth 2015. Geneva, Switzerland: World Health Organization. p. 2016.

38. IOM. Key Capabilities of an electronic health record system letter report. USA: National Academy of Sciences; 2003.

39. Jha AK, DesRoches CM, Campbell EG, Donelan K, Rao SR, Ferris TG, Shields A, Rosenbaum S, Blumenthal D. Use of electronic health records in U.S. hospitals. N Engl J Med. 2009;360:1628–38.

40. Davis DC, Thakkar M. Perceived level of benefits and risk Core functionalities of an EHR system. In: Joseph T, editor. Healthcare information systems and informatics: research and practices. New York: Information Science Publishing; 2008. p. 297–312.

41. TurkeyMoH. Healthcare quality standards-hospital. Ankara: Pozitif Matbaa; 2016.

42. Taylan G, EB Bİ, Naldöken Ü. Determination of profiles of quality directors who work for Turkey Ministry of Health hospitals. In: Ünal D, Okumuş N, editors. VI International conference on healthcare performance and quality. Antalya, Turkey: Miki Matbaacılık San. ve Tic. Ltd. şti; 2016.

43. CMS: Medicare & Medicaid EHR incentive program meaningful use stage 1 requirements overview. http://www.cms.gov/Regulations-and-Guidance/Legislation/EHRIncentivePrograms/downloads/MU_Stage1_ReqOverview.pdf 2010. Accessed 18 Apr 2015.

44. International JC. Joint commission international accreditation standards for hospitals. 5th ed: Joint Commission Resources; 2013.

45. Glandon GL, Smaltz DH, Slovensky JD. Austin and Boxerman's İnformation systems for healthcare. Chicago: AUPHA Health Administration Press; 2008.

46. Osheroff JA, Teich JM, Middleton B, Steen EB, Wright A, Detmer DE. A roadmap for National Action on clinical decision support. J Am Med Inform Assoc. 2007; https://doi.org/10.1197/jamia.M2334.

47. Bright TJ, Wong A, Dhurjati R, et al. Effect of clinical decision-support systems: a systematic review. Ann Intern Med. 2012; https://doi.org/10.7326/0003-4819-157-1-201207030-00450.

48. Ammenwerth E, Buchauer A, Bludau B, Haux R. Mobile information and communication tools in the hospital. Int J Med Inform. 2000;57:21–40.

49. Haun JN, Lind JD, Shimada SL, Martin TL, Gosline RM, Antinori N, Stewart M, Simon SR. Evaluating user experiences of the secure messaging tool on the veterans affairs' patient portal system. J Med Internet Res. 2014;16

50. Birkhead GS, Klompas M, Shah NR. Uses of electronic health records for public health surveillance to advance public health. Annu Rev Public Health. 2015;36:345–59.

51. Fox BI, Pedersen CA, Gumpper KF. ASHP national survey on informatics: assessment of the adoption and use of pharmacy informatics in U.S. hospitals-2013. Am J Health Syst Pharm. 2015;72:636–55.

52. Fernandez-Aleman JL, Senor IC, Lozoya PA, Toval A. Security and privacy in electronic health records: a systematic literature review. J Biomed Inform. 2013;46:541–62.

53. Papoutsi C, Reed JE, Marston C, Lewis R, Majeed A, Bell D. Patient and public views about the security and privacy of electronic health records (EHRs) in the UK: results from a mixed methods study. BMC Medical Informatics and Decision Making. 2015; https://doi.org/10.1186/s12911-015-0202-2.

54. TurkeyMoH. Standards of accreditation in health, hospital kit – v1.1/2015. Ankara: Pozitif Printing Press Ltd. Co.; 2015.

55. MoH. Tibbi Laboratuvarlar Yönetmeligi, vol. 28790: Resmi Gazete; 2013.

56. MoH. Hastane Bilgi Yönetim Sistemleri Alim Kilavuzu. In: İvMİD B, editor. 5.1 ; 2010.

57. Esatoğlu AE, Köksal A. Hastanelerde Bilgisayar Teknolojisinin Kullanımı. Ankara Üniversitesi. Tıp Fakültesi Mecmuası. 2002;55:29–40.

58. Reid JH. Patient safety: staff safety – hand in hand? Journal of Perioperative Practice 2011;21:363.

59. Hughes RG, Blegen MA. Medication administration safety. In: Hughes RG, editor. Patient safety and quality: an evidence-based handbook for nurses. Rockville (MD); 2008.

60. IOM. Preventing medication errors. Washington, DC: National Academy Press; 2007.

61. Backman C, Vanderloo S, Momtahan K, d'Entremont B, Freeman L, Kachuik L, Rossy D, Mille T, Mojaverian N, Lemire-Rodger G, et al. Implementation of an electronic data collection tool to monitor nursing-sensitive indicators in a large academic health sciences Centre. Nurs Leadersh. 2015;28:77–91.

62. Silow-Carroll S, Edwards JN, Rodin D. Using electronic health records to improve quality and efficiency: the experiences of leading hospitals.: the Commonwealth Fund; 2012.

63. TurkeyMoH. Transformation in health. 2003.

64. TurkeyMoH. Institutional performance and quality applications in healthcare. Ankara: Lazer Ofset; 2009.

65. Gualano MR, Bert F, Andriolo V, Grosso M, Minniti D, Siliquini R. Use of telemedicine in the European penitentiaries: current scenario and best practices. Eur J Pub Health. 2016; https://doi.org/10.1093/eurpub/ckw145.

66. Mehrotra A, Jena AB, Busch AB, Souza J, Uscher-Pines L, Landon BE. Utilization of telemedicine among rural Medicare beneficiaries. JAMA. 2016; https://doi.org/10.1001/jama.2016.2186.

67. Zhang XY, Zhang P. Telemedicine in clinical setting. Experimental and therapeutic medicine. 2016; https://doi.org/10.3892/etm.2016.3656.

68. Douglas MD, Xu J, Heggs A, Wrenn G, Mack DH, Rust G. Assessing telemedicine utilization by using Medicaid claims data. Psychiatr Serv. 2016; https://doi.org/10.1176/appi.ps.201500518.

69. Te Boveldt N, Vernooij-Dassen M, Leppink I, Samwel H, Vissers K, Engels Y. Patient empowerment in cancer pain management: an integrative literature review. Psycho-Oncology. 2014; https://doi.org/10.1002/pon.3573.

70. Jotterand F, Amodio A, Elger BS. Patient education as empowerment and self-rebiasing. Medicine, health care, and philosophy; 2016. https://doi.org/10.1007/s11019-016-9702-9.

71. King J, Patel V, Jamoom EW, Furukawa MF. Clinical benefits of electronic health record use: national findings. Health Serv Res. 2014;49:392–404.

72. Petrides AK, Bixho I, Goonan EM, Bates DW, Shaykevich S, Lipsitz SR, Landman AB, Tanasijevic MJ, Melanson SE. The benefits and challenges of an interfaced electronic health record and laboratory information system: effects on laboratory processes. Arch Pathol Lab Med. 2017;141:410–7.

73. Kruse CS, DeShazo J, Kim F, Fulton L. Factors associated with adoption of health information technology: a conceptual model based on a systematic review. JMIR Med Inform. 2014;2

74. Berner ES. Clinical decision support systems: state of the art. AHRQ publication. 2009;90069

75. Garg AX, Adhikari NJ, McDonald H, et al. Effects of computerized clinical decision support systems on practitioner performance and patient outcomes: a systematic review. JAMA. 2005; https://doi.org/10.1001/jama.293.10.1223.

76. Levick DL, Stern G, Meyerhoefer CD, Levick A, Pucklavage D. Reducing unnecessary testing in a CPOE system through implementation of a targeted CDS intervention. BMC Med Inform Decis Mak. 2013;13:1472–6947.

A computational application for multi-skill nurse staffing in hospital units

Ana Respicio[1,5]* , Margarida Moz[2], Margarida Vaz Pato[2], Rute Somensi[3] and Cecília Dias Flores[4]

Abstract

Background: Approaches to nurse staffing are commonly concerned with determining the minimum number of care hours according to the illness severity of patients. However, there is a gap in the literature considering multi-skill and multi-shift nurse staffing. This study addresses nurse staffing per skill category, at a strategical decision level, by considering the organization of work in shifts and coping with variability in demand.

Methods: We developed a method to determine the nursing staff levels in a hospital, given the required patient assistance. This method relies on a new mathematical model for complying with the legislation and guidelines while minimizing salary costs. A spreadsheet-based tool was developed to embed the model and to allow simulating different scenarios and evaluating the impact of demand fluctuations, thus supporting decision-making on staff dimensioning.

Results: Experiments were carried out considering real data from a Brazilian hospital unit. The results obtained by the model support the current total staff level in the unit under study. However, the distribution of staff among different skill categories revealed that the current real situation can be improved.

Conclusions: The method allows the determining of staff level per shift and skill depending on the mix of patients' illness severity. Hospital management is offered the possibility of optimizing the staff level using a spreadsheet, a tool most managers are familiar with. In addition, it is possible to evaluate the implications of decisions on workforce dimensioning by simulating different demand scenarios. This tool can be easily adapted to other hospitals, using local rules and legislation.

Keywords: Nurse staffing, Multi-skill staffing, Shift work, Spreadsheet staffing model, Decision support

Background

Healthcare institutions must be well equipped with efficient and effective resources to provide healthcare to a more and more demanding population. As service must meet population needs, and costs with human resources represent a large amount of the operational costs in those institutions, accurate workforce planning is a very important task.

In the healthcare sector, nurses represent the main workforce to plan. The special kind of service they provide is to look after people in different severity conditions and the care cannot be postponed. To determine the nurse staff levels, decision makers must take into account not only the variable demand for nursing care, but also the need to safeguard the health and goodwill of the nurses themselves, beyond the guidelines and legislation in force.

This section continues with a review of studies related to nurse workforce planning in general, and nurse staffing problems, in particular, highlighting some aspects that still deserve research. The definition of the multi-skill nurse staffing problem under study is then presented. Section Methods presents a two-phase methodology and describes the optimization model. An application using real-world data from a Brazilian hospital is described in Section Results, illustrated with the spreadsheet implementation of the model. Besides, a sensitivity analysis is conducted. A discussion of the experimental

* Correspondence: alrespicio@fc.ul.pt
[1]CMAF-CIO, Faculdade de Ciências, Universidade de Lisboa, Lisbon, Portugal
[5]Departamento de Informática, Faculdade de Ciências, Universidade de Lisboa, Bloco C6, Piso 3, 1749-016 Lisboa, Portugal
Full list of author information is available at the end of the article

results follows in the corresponding section. The paper ends with the Section Conclusions.

Nurse workforce planning

In hospitals that work around the clock every day, the daily nurse work must be organized in shifts, and for each nurse a schedule must be posted in advance, indicating the sequence of days off and daily work shifts for the next planning period. Therefore, hospital administration needs to solve three interrelated problems, as stated in the seminal paper of Warner [1]. At the strategic decision level, the staffing problem consists of determining the dimension of the workforce required to provide the healthcare needed in all hospital units over a long-term planning horizon [2]. In the medium-term, at the tactical level, the scheduling/rostering problem is solved, so as to determine the set of schedules for all nurses of each unit that meets the variable demand per shift during a planning period, typically of one month, or 28 days, while respecting labour agreements [1, 3]. In the short-term, at the operational decision level, the rerostering problem determines the necessary changes in the current roster when daily disruptions occur [4, 5].

These different types of decision have associated models that have been widely studied, however in the majority of the cases to tackle specific situations, as surveyed for human resources in general [6, 7]. In the nurses' work planning context there are also some surveys revealing the considerable amount of research work in this area, which is mainly due to the specific legislation of each country and specific norms of the institutions [8–10]. Therefore, it is hard to conceive a general system for nurse staffing, scheduling/rostering and rerostering suitable for addressing all cases.

In the current study, we focus on the staffing problem with the purpose of determining the multi-skill nursing staff level per shift, derived from nurse-to-patient indicators applied to the demand for healthcare. We also take into account the further need of assigning nurses to shifts, complying with the labour legislation in force. Adequate nursing care is forced by hard constraints because it is the primary goal, while the minimization of salary costs is set as objective function.

We propose a new model to this problem and, relying on the model, we developed a spreadsheet-based tool that can be easily used in hospital units.

Nurse staffing

The nurse staffing problem must take into account nurses' workload measures and, in some cases, the allocation of nurses to the different daily shifts, considering the particular working environment, patient safety ratios and labour rules. Many authors highlight the positive correlation between the decrease of staffing levels and the decrease in quality of nurse care [11–13] as well as with the decrease in financial performance of hospitals [14]. Other authors also stress the negative impact of nurse turnover and the use of temporary nurses on patient care and nurse satisfaction [11, 15–17].

Hence, defining accurate nurse staffing levels is an important objective of every hospital administration, under pressure to reduce costs, while providing high quality health services. Approaches to nurse staff dimensioning are commonly concerned with determining the minimum number of nursing care hours per patient. Hurst [18] classified the methods to measure nursing workload into five categories: (1) professional judgement, based on the experience and knowledge of professionals; (2) average number of nurses per occupied bed; (3) the acuity-quality method, based on patient dependency; (4) regression analysis; and (5) the timed-task/activity method, based on the type and frequency of nursing interventions. Nursing workload naturally depends on the condition of patients, and several scoring systems to determine nurse-to-patient ratios have been proposed [19, 20]. Therefore, hospitals and healthcare public administrations frequently lay down specific instructions to guide hospital managers and head nurses in staffing and scheduling tasks. That is the case of the "Resolução COFEN-293/2004" from the Brazilian Nurse Federal Council, which sets the nursing hours per patient for inpatient units according to four categories of illness severity [21].

Elkhuizen et al. [22] propose a general model that determines multi-shift nurse staff levels. The model does not consider different nursing skills and works for 24-h cover. It calls for computing average bed occupation on a daily basis, using calendar work days. Legal minima for nurse-to-patient ratios, set by international guidelines (USA and Australia), were used to establish the corresponding different ratios for three shifts (early, late and night). These ratios, together with the bed occupation and some coefficients to include absences, led to the advised number of nurses per shift. An application to a real setting is presented along with a what-if analysis. Kortbeek et al. [23] propose stochastic models for nurse staffing per shift with demand based on nurse-to-patient ratios. One of the models simultaneously staffs permanent nurses per hospital unit and floating nurses that may work at any hospital unit. The authors do not consider different nurse skills. They apply their models to a hospital in Amsterdam. To the best of our knowledge, the first work that explicitly models multi-skill multi-shift nurse staffing is that of Bordoloi and Weatherby [24], specifically developed for one hospital unit in Alaska. These authors present a linear programming model considering three skill categories and three shifts of equal length, thus defining nine decision variables. The demand per day (in hours) was estimated from historical data and divided per shifts according to the nurses' experience. The model minimizes salary costs and considers ratio constraints on work provided by differently-skilled staff and demand constraints per shift. These authors also perform a linear programming sensitivity analysis. More recently, Harper et al. [2] present a comprehensive study for multi-skill multi-shift nurse staffing in United Kingdom hospitals. The model proposed is a stochastic linear programming model that considers the minimization of costs aggregated over one year, subject to demand-fulfilment constraints per day and for different skills. The proposed computational tool is applied with user-defined parameters to obtain an aggregate level of staff.

Other authors integrate staffing and scheduling. Venkataraman and Brusco [25] propose a stochastic methodology that starts by solving a mixed integer linear programming model for a six-month period. This model has two integer variables (number of full-time and part-time nurses) and six continuous variables (overtime hours per month) and its solution is given as input to another mixed integer linear programming model for the scheduling problem. Different shifts and different skills are considered. More recently, Maenhout and Vanhoucke [26] also integrate nurse staffing and scheduling, applied to a hospital in Ghent. This study proposes a mixed integer linear programming model where the staffing decisions are represented by surplus and slack variables that account for under or over staffing of multi-skilled nurses per shift, with respect to the required number of nurses per ward, skill, day and shift.

No research work was found that addresses the nurse staffing problem by simultaneously considering the multi-skill staff levels required for different length shifts; respecting the scores of a scoring system as well as labour legislation, guidelines and internal institution rules; and balancing the number of employees per skill and per shift. Moreover, the literature lacks computational tools to dimension differently-skilled nursing staff, that are easy for practitioners to use, and adaptable to different hospital environments.

Problem definition

The study reported in this paper concerns a nurse staffing problem that aims to determine the size of nursing teams in a Brazilian hospital context. Personnel are grouped into two categories according to healthcare nursing skills: nurses – the group of the more skilled personnel; and nursing technicians – those who perform the auxiliary and basic care tasks, although professionally certified. In the hospital, apart from this permanent pool, dimensioned at the strategic decision level, there is also a floating pool of nurses and technicians, dimensioned at the tactical level, outside the scope of this study. The number of nurses should be at least a given

proportion of the total staff, depending on the patient mix. Once assigned to a shift, nurses and technicians of this pool do not switch to another shift during the long-term planning horizon. Personnel assigned to night shift cannot work on consecutive days, due to labour legislation. Therefore, these personnel are grouped into odd night shift and even night shift workers. Moreover, the staff level in these two shifts must be equal, due to hospital rules.

The main objective of the nurse staffing problem is to determine the number of nurses and of nursing technicians to be assigned to the permanent pool of a hospital unit, complying with the demand for healthcare per shift and minimizing salary costs. The needs for healthcare service must be continuously satisfied by workers who are entitled to a specific number of days off and holidays, as well as absences. In this context, all types of absences are taken into account by the application of a Technical Safety Index (TSI) [21].

Methods

To determine the dimension of the permanent pool of nurses and nursing technicians for a hospital, the proposed methodology follows two phases, as illustrated by Fig. 1. The staffing is solved per hospital unit because each unit has different requirements in terms of nursing work, due to the different patient illness severity. For instance, the Intensive Care Unit (ICU), the Neurosurgery Unit, and the Cerebrovascular Accident Unit (CVA) typically treat high severity illness patients. In addition, the personnel of the permanent pool are assigned per hospital unit. The method considers the demand for a day since the guidelines stipulate the amount of daily nursing care.

Phase I

Phase I computes the required number of nursing care hours per day, according to the specific guidelines in use. For this computation, the necessary data are the estimated number of patients and their respective illness severity. For instance, the Brazilian COFEN guidelines [21] recommend a minimum number of nursing hours per patient, per day for each category of illness severity (minimal, intermediary, semi-intensive, or intensive care). In addition, the minimum ratio of nurses to nursing workers is also computed (as proposed by COFEN).

The output of *Phase I* is given as input to *Phase II*.

Phase II

Phase II proceeds with the dimensioning of personnel, additionally considering the following data from the institutional rules: the hourly salary costs per level of skill (nurses and technicians) and shift (morning, afternoon, odd and even nights), the shifts lengths, lower bounds for the staff per skill and shift, and parameters to

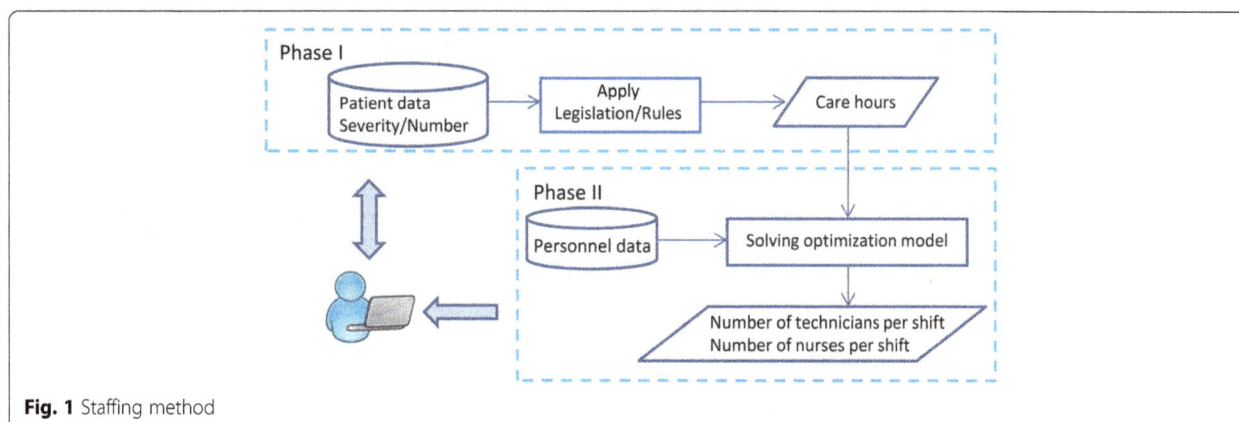

Fig. 1 Staffing method

balance the staff between shifts and per skill. Other data come from COFEN guidelines: the TSI, acting as a buffer to cover all types of personnel absences, and the ratio of nurses to total staff.

The problem consists of determining the number of nurses and technicians required per shift, respecting the following conditions:

- the total number of hours of nurse and technician work assigned to all shifts cannot be less than the required nursing care hours per day (*hours*) [Constraints (1)];
- the percentage over the minimum staff level required to cover all types of personnel absences must be satisfied, corresponding to the application of the TSI (represented by the parameter *p*) [Constraint (2)];
- the number of nurses must be at least a given percentage-ratio (*prop*) of the total number of nursing-workers, i.e. nurses plus technicians [Constraint (3)];
- the number of workers, of each skill, assigned to morning and afternoon shifts do not differ more than a specified parameter, so to balance the workload among these shifts (represented by parameters α_i, $i = n, t$) [Constraints (4)];
- two groups of night shifts are considered – odd nights (night 1) and even nights (night 2), because staff cannot work on consecutive nights, according to labour legislation [Constraints (5)];
- a minimum staff level per shift for each of nurses and technicians must be respected [Constraints (6)].

Adequate nursing care is enforced by the above hard constraints, while control of costs is achieved through the objective function of the model [Function (7)], where costs of both types of night shift are considered.

An optimization model is proposed and its mathematical formulation is presented in [Additional file 1]. It corresponds to an integer linear programming problem, insofar as it involves optimization of a linear function depending on non-negative integer variables subject to linear (in)equalities that express the constraints of the model. The solution for this model is obtained using a standard optimization solver.

The minimum imposed by Constraints (6) ensures that the demand to be immediately satisfied is covered, while Constraints (1) guarantee that these and other nursing activities, which do not need immediate execution in a given shift, are performed during the day. The minimum staff levels per shift can be adapted to accommodate different requirements for care per shift.

The decision maker can execute *Phase I* followed by *Phase II* repeatedly, with different demand scenarios to extract managerial indicators, thus supporting the decision making process regarding the staffing of the permanent pool. This allows him/her to evaluate the impact on staff level due to fluctuations in demand for healthcare. Complementarily, other constraints imposed by hospital management rules, sector guidelines, and legislation can be considered.

The results of *Phase II* – solution of the staffing problem – will be inputs for scheduling/rostering. In this hospital context, nursing-workers do not change shifts.

Results

The methodology is illustrated with the case of Hospital São José (HSJ). HSJ is part of Irmandade Santa Casa de Misericórdia de Porto Alegre, Brazil, and its units are characterized by the type of healthcare service provided: Emergency, Inpatient Units (ICU, CVA, PRT/CNV, and Neurosurgery), Intensive Care, Diagnosis and Treatment Units, and Outpatient and Surgical Center [27].

Experiment description

For the experiment, we considered real data from five HSJ units. Figure 2 displays the data used for model application. For each unit, data concerning the demand of

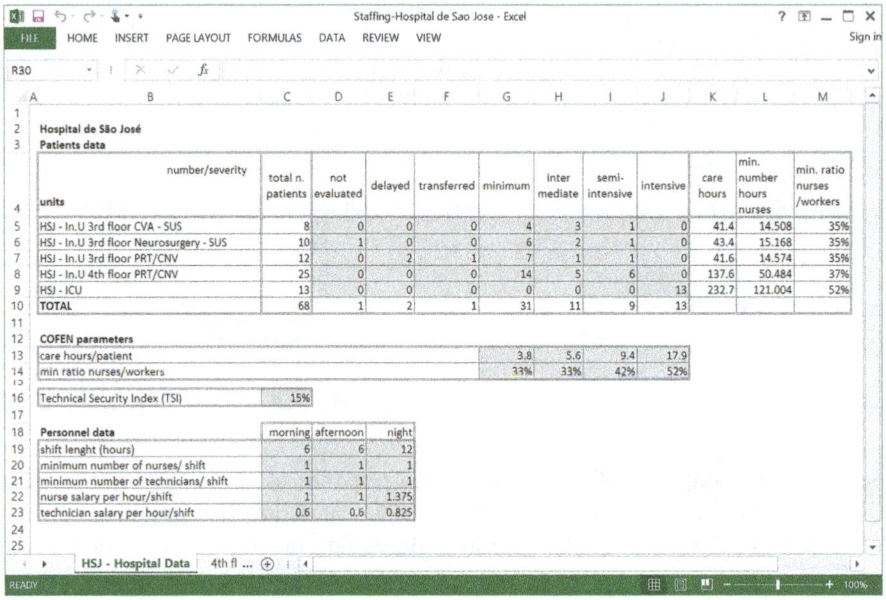

Hospital de São José

Patients data

units \ number/severity	total n. patients	not evaluated	delayed	transferred	minimum	inter mediate	semi-intensive	intensive	care hours	min. number hours nurses	min. ratio nurses /workers
HSJ - In.U 3rd floor CVA - SUS	8	0	0	0	4	3	1	0	41.4	14.508	35%
HSJ - In.U 3rd floor Neurosurgery - SUS	10	1	0	0	6	2	1	0	43.4	15.168	35%
HSJ - In.U 3rd floor PRT/CNV	12	0	2	1	7	1	1	0	41.6	14.574	35%
HSJ - In.U 4th floor PRT/CNV	25	0	0	0	14	5	6	0	137.6	50.484	37%
HSJ - ICU	13	0	0	0	0	0	0	13	232.7	121.004	52%
TOTAL	68	1	2	1	31	11	9	13			

COFEN parameters

care hours/patient	3.8	5.6	9.4	17.9
min ratio nurses/workers	33%	33%	42%	52%

Technical Security Index (TSI)	15%

Personnel data	morning	afternoon	night
shift lenght (hours)	6	6	12
minimum number of nurses/ shift	1	1	1
minimum number of technicians/ shift	1	1	1
nurse salary per hour/shift	1	1	1.375
technician salary per hour/shift	0.6	0.6	0.825

Fig. 2 Data used for model application

one day was considered, and the following numbers were compiled: number of inpatients requiring minimal care, intermediary care, semi-intensive care and intensive care. The unclassified inpatients were counted as needing intermediary care.

The Brazilian guidelines for nursing professional practice, COFEN [21], define the minimum number of nursing care hours per patient per 24 h (Art. 4th): 3.8 h per patient requiring minimal care, 5.6 h for intermediary care, 9.4 h for semi-intensive care and, 17.9 h for intensive care, respectively. COFEN also specifies a minimum ratio of nurses to the total workforce which is set according to the category with the largest number of inpatients. This proportion is set to 33% for the minimal and intermediary care, 42% for the semi-intensive care, and 52% for the intensive care. In addition, the TSI is set to 15%, according to COFEN.

The method is applied using a Microsoft Excel spreadsheet [28]. The data in spreadsheet "HSJ – Hospital Data" are organized in three tables (Fig. 2). The first table, "Patients data", contains the number of patients and their corresponding illness severity for the different hospital units on a specific day. The second table, "COFEN parameters", contains the model's parameters. Finally, the table "Personnel data" is used in *Phase II*. The shifts' lengths, which are not all equal, are consistent with the hospital operating rules. The minimum number of nurses and technicians per shift (*lines 20* and *21*) are set to one. Due to confidentiality reasons, the labour costs are omitted, and we assume a labour cost of 1 monetary unit per hour per nurse, and that the labour cost for technicians is 60% of that value. Work in the night shift receives an increase of 37.5% in salary.

The output of *Phase I*, for each unit, is in column "care hours" and is given by summing up the product of the number of patients in the unit (*columns G* to *J*) by the required care hours per patient severity (*line 13*), and also in *column M*, the ratio of nurses with respect to the total of nursing-workers.

Spreadsheet implementation of the model

The model for *Phase II* was implemented using the Solver from Excel [28] as shown in Fig. 3 for the unit "In. U 4th floor PRT/CNV". The spreadsheet "4th floor – Mathematical Model" is organized into four main areas including all data, variables and formulae of the mathematical model in [Additional file 1].

The "nurses" area comprises *columns C* to *E* which include parameters (*lines 3* to *11*) and variables (*line 12*). *Line 3*, "hours constraint", contains the shifts lengths (in this case equal for all shifts and skills) taken from sheet "HSJ – Hospital Data". *Line 5* "minimum percentage" contains the parameters needed for Constraint (3) of the problem by setting *prop* equal to the value in *cell S5*, which is equal to the minimum ratio of nurses to workers for this unit, in *cell M8* of "HSJ – Hospital Data" sheet (Fig. 2). *Line 10* contains the minimum staff level in each shift which, in this case, is set equal to 1 in Constraints (6) for all shifts. *Line 11* has the salary costs per shift, which are computed by multiplying the value of labour cost per hour by the shift length in hours, using the data in spreadsheet "HSJ – Hospital Data". As

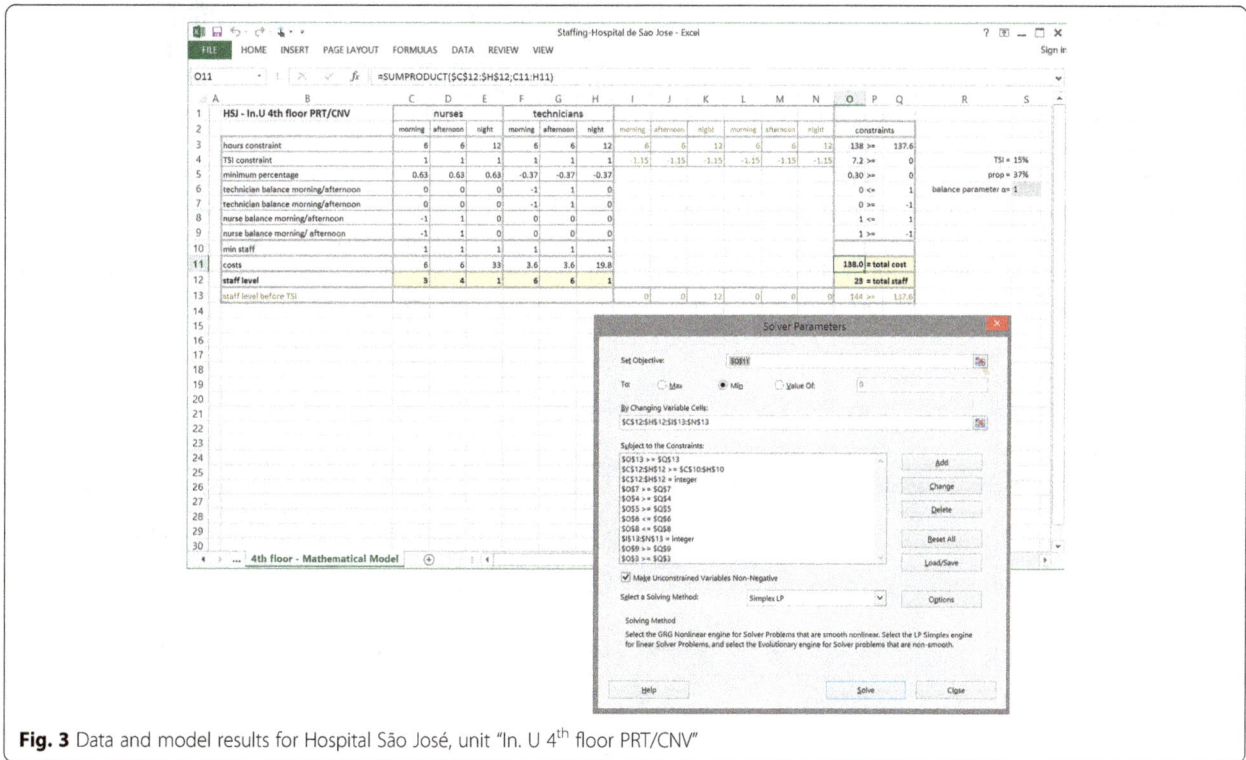

Fig. 3 Data and model results for Hospital São José, unit "In. U 4th floor PRT/CNV"

the model in the solver just refers to a single day, to take into account the staff for the two types of night shift, "night 1" and "night 2", the cost for the night shift is counted twice (Constraints (5)). *Line 12* is reserved for the variables' values. For "technicians", the corresponding information is given in *columns F to H*.

Columns I to N include data for auxiliary variables to respect staff levels before TSI application, which are used in Constraints (1) and (2): *line 3* contains the shifts length to be included in the first inequalities of Constraints (1); *line 4* implements Constraint (2), with TSI from "HSJ – Hospital Data", and *line 13* contains the values of these variables.

Finally, *columns O to Q* include information for solving the problem: constraints and the objective function. *Column O* (from *lines 3* to 9) contains the excel formulae to be used in Solver, while *column Q* contains the constant terms related to Constraints (1) to (4).

To balance the number of nurses and technicians between morning and afternoon shifts, a single parameter is set by the user in *cell S6*. In this application, we consider the balance parameter to be equal both for nurses and technicians.

The mathematical model is formulated for Solver software, in the window "Solver Parameters": in the field "Set Objective" *cell O11* must be inserted. The respective value

Table 1 Impact of changes in parameters

parameters		staff level for nurses					staff level for technicians					total staff	total cost
min. staff	balance $a_n = a_t$	morning	afternoon	night 1	night 2	total	mor-ning	afternoon	night 1	night 2	total		
1	1	3	4	1	1	9	6	6	1	1	14	23	138.0
1	2	4	3	1	1	9	5	7	1	1	14	23	138.0
1	3	2	5	1	1	9	5	7	1	1	14	23	138.0
2	1	2	3	2	2	9	5	5	2	2	14	23	171.6
2	2	2	3	2	2	9	4	6	2	2	14	23	171.6
2	3	2	3	2	2	9	4	6	2	2	14	23	171.6
3	1	3	3	3	3	12	3	3	3	3	12	24	216.0
3	2	3	3	3	3	12	3	3	3	3	12	24	216.0
3	3	3	3	3	3	12	3	3	3	3	12	24	216.0

is the objective function value to be minimized through the variables in *C12:H12* and *I13:N13*. Constraints are added in the constraints section, all variables are set to nonnegative values and the method selected is "Simplex LP" (a simplex based branch-and-bound algorithm).

By clicking button "Solve", the algorithm runs and determines the model output, which is also shown in Fig. 3. The solution obtained, in *cells C12 to H12*, indicates the number of nurses and technicians for the three daily shifts. In this case, the solution gives 3

nurses for the morning, 4 for the afternoon and 1 for the night shifts; for technicians the numbers are 6, 6 and 1, respectively. The total salary cost for this solution is 138.0 monetary units, as shown in *cell O11*.

Sensitivity of the model to parameter variation

To assess the sensitivity of the model solutions regarding variations of the parameters, we analysed the impact of changes in the minimum staff level per

Table 2 Real data and model results for Hospital São José, in unit "In. U 4th floor PRT/CNV"

date	weekday	data						results of *Phase I*	
		number of patients by illness severity level						care hours COFEN	minimum ratio nurses/workers COFEN (%)
		total		minimal	intermediary	semi-intensive	intensive		
07–09–2016	Wednesday	34		21	10	3	0	164.0	35
08–09–2016	Thursday	25		15	8	2	0	120.6	34
09–09–2016	Friday	26		16	8	2	0	124.4	34
10–09–2016	Saturday	21		13	7	1	0	98.0	34
11–09–2016	Sunday	23		15	6	2	0	109.4	35
12–09–2016	Monday	25		17	7	1	0	113.2	34
13–09–2016	Tuesday	34		24	8	2	0	154.8	34
14–09–2016	Wednesday	35		22	11	2	0	164.0	34

staff levels

date	results of *Phase II*										real situation	
	number of nurses per shift				number of technicians per shift				number of nurses	number of technicians	number of nurses	number of technicians
	morning	afternoon	night 1	night 2	morning	afternoon	night 1	night 2				
07–09–2016	3	4	2	2	7	8	1	1	11	17	4	22
08–09–2016	3	3	1	1	5	6	1	1	8	13	4	22
09–09–2016	3	3	1	1	5	6	1	1	8	13	4	22
10–09–2016	2	2	2	2	3	4	1	1	8	9	4	22
11–09–2016	2	3	2	2	4	5	1	1	9	11	4	22
12–09–2016	2	3	1	1	5	5	1	1	7	12	4	22
13–09–2016	4	4	1	1	7	7	1	1	10	16	4	22
14–09–2016	3	4	2	2	7	8	1	1	11	17	4	22

shift along with variations of the balance parameter ($\alpha_n = \alpha_t$). Table 1 presents the results of this analysis.

Increasing the minimum staff level required per shift increases the total cost because it forces the assignment of extra staff to more expensive shifts. Increasing the balance parameter provides more flexibility to distribute workers among shifts, and consequently the cost decreases. For instance, a solution for balance parameter $\alpha_n = 2$, requiring a maximum difference of 2 nurses between the morning and afternoon shifts, is also a solution when $\alpha_n = 3$ which requires a maximum difference of 3 workers between the morning and afternoon shifts, while a solution for $\alpha_n = 3$ may not satisfy a balance parameter of $\alpha_n = 2$. This can be observed in Table 1, when minimum staff is 1, the solution for $\alpha_n = 2$ includes 4 nurses in the morning and 3 in the afternoon, also satisfying $\alpha_n = 3$; while the solution for $\alpha_n = 3$ considers 2 nurses in the morning and 5 in the afternoon, and thus does not satisfy $\alpha_n = 2$.

When the minimum number of staff is fixed, variations of the balance parameter value do not have an impact on the total cost or total number of staff. In fact, when the minimum number of staff is fixed to 1, different solutions with the same cost were obtained for different values of the balance parameter (from 1 to 3). When the minimum staff level is set to 2, the total cost increases by 24.2% and the staff levels remain equal to 9 for nurses and 14 for technicians. Increasing the minimum staff level from 2 to 3 increases the total cost by 25.8%, leading to a solution where at least 12 nurses and 12 technicians must be assigned, which sum up to 24 (3 workers of each skill and shift).

Discussion

The methodology proposed was applied to data related with bed occupation and type of nursing care required by patients in several units of HSJ. In particular, a study was undertaken for the unit "In. U 4th floor PRT/CNV", for a duration of eight consecutive days, from Wednesday, September 7, 2016. The first part of Table 2 displays the data relating to the number of patients by illness severity level, the number of nursing care hours according to COFEN (as explained in subsection "Hospital data") and the corresponding minimum ratio of nurses to workers (*prop* parameter in the model). The second part of the table presents the results obtained from *Phase II* of the method.

The results show that total staff required varies between 17 and 28 workers. The total staff in the real situation is constant and equal to 26. This number of workers is greater than or equal to the staff levels obtained by the method for all days except for Wednesdays, for which two

additional workers are needed. Regarding the number of nurses, the results reveal that in the real situation there is a lack of nurses if the COFEN guidelines are applied, while the number of technicians is greater than the one obtained by the model. This reveals that in the current real situation the minimum ratio of nurses to the total workforce, which depends on the mix of patients' illness severity (subsection "Hospital data") is not covered by the permanent pool of nurses. In these cases, nurses from the floating pool may be assigned.

As a result of this experiment, we may observe that the proposed methodology was conceived to support the hospital management decision making process, so to improve the personnel dimensioning, and better agree with the COFEN guidelines.

Conclusions

A new methodology was developed to determine the multi-skill nursing staff level to be assigned per shift during a long-term planning horizon, in a hospital, complying with legislation, nurse work guidelines, and rules in force, while minimizing hospital costs. This complex staff dimensioning problem was adapted to the Brazilian context, considering a real world hospital, with two skill categories – nurses and technicians – and three work shifts of different durations. The proposed method applies to a single unit and allows the hospital management to determine the staff level per shift and per skill category as a function of the mix of severity. The workforce for a hospital can be obtained by executing the method for all its units.

The staff dimensioning method, at the strategic decision level, will provide input for lower level decision stages concerning personnel planning.

Another contribution of this study is a decision support tool, embedding the staffing method and implemented in a Microsoft Excel spreadsheet. [Additional file 2] contains the tool described in this manuscript. Most managers are familiar with usage of this software, therefore, the spreadsheet model is designed in an intelligible way to allow for an easy utilization. The tool also provides support to analyse scenarios with different mix of severity. Moreover, the decision maker can modify different parameters, such as shift lengths, salary costs, minimum staff level required per shift and skill, and the parameter to balance workforce, and evaluate their impact on results. The model and the tool developed are easily customizable to integrate the working rules of different hospital contexts.

As future work we intend to apply and evaluate the developed methodology in other healthcare contexts, namely in Portuguese public hospital units.

Abbreviations

CVA: Cerebrovascular Accident Unit; HSJ: Hospital São José; ICU: Intensive Care Unit; PRT/CNV: Unit for Patients with Health Plan; SUS: Unified Health System (in Brazil)

Acknowledgements

We would like to thank the Hospital São José of the Irmandade Santa Casa de Misericórdia de Porto Alegre, Brazil for contributing with real data for the experiment. We acknowledge the reviewers for their helpful comments on a previous version of the manuscript. We thank Dr. Rob Mills for the English language review.

Funding

This work was partially supported by Portuguese funding from Fundação para a Ciência e a Tecnologia (FCT), under project UID/MAT/04561/2013 and Brazilian funding through project 442780/2014-1 - Edital MCTI/CNPq/Universal 14/2014. The funding body had no role in the design of the study and collection, analysis, and interpretation of data and in writing the manuscript.

Authors' contributions

AR, MM, MVP are responsible for the methodology conception, implementation and design of the experiment. RS and CDF are responsible for problem definition, real data gathering and discussion. All authors contributed for the background section, read and approved the final manuscript.

Competing interests

The authors declare that they have no competing interests.

Author details

[1]CMAF-CIO, Faculdade de Ciências, Universidade de Lisboa, Lisbon, Portugal. [2]ISEG and CMAF-CIO, Universidade de Lisboa, Lisbon, Portugal. [3]Pavilhão Pereira Filho, Santa Casa de Misericórdia Porto Alegre and Universidade Federal de Ciências da Saúde de Porto Alegre, Hospital São José, Porto Alegre, Brazil. [4]Universidade Federal de Ciências da Saúde de Porto Alegre, Porto Alegre, Brazil. [5]Departamento de Informática, Faculdade de Ciências, Universidade de Lisboa, Bloco C6, Piso 3, 1749-016 Lisboa, Portugal.

References

1. Warner DM. Scheduling nursing personnel according to nursing preference: a mathematical programming approach. Oper Res. 1976;24(5):842–56.
2. Harper PR, Powell NH, Williams JE. Modelling the size and skill-mix of hospital nursing teams. J Oper Res Soc. 2010;61:768–79.
3. Smet P, Bilgin B, De Causmaecker P, Vanden Berghe G. Modelling and evaluation issues in nurse rostering. Ann Oper Res. 2014;218:303–26.
4. Moz M, Pato MV. A genetic algorithm approach to a nurse Rerostering problem. Computers OR. 2007;34:667–91.
5. Clark A, Moule P, Topping A, Serpell M. Rescheduling nursing shifts: scoping the challenge and examining the potential of mathematical model based tools. J Nursing Manag. 2015;23:411–20.
6. Van den Bergh J, Belien J, De Bruecker P, Demeulemeester E, De Boeck L. Personnel scheduling: a literature review. EJOR. 2013;226(3):367–85.
7. Defraeye M, Van Nieuwenhuyse I. Staffing and scheduling under nonstationary demand for service: a literature review. Omega. 2016;58:4–25.
8. Cheang B, Li H, Lim A, Rodrigues B. Nurse rostering problems - a bibliographic survey. EJOR. 2003;151(3):447–60.
9. Burke EK, De Causmaecker P, Berghe GV, Van Landeghem H. The state of the art of nurse rostering. J Scheduling. 2004;7(6):441–99.
10. Kellogg DL, Walczak S. Nurse scheduling: from academia to implementation or not? Interfaces. 2007;37(4):355–69.
11. Kash BA, Castle NG, Naufal GS, Hawes C. Effect of staff turnover on staffing: a closer look at registered nurses, licensed vocational nurses, and certified nursing assistants. The Gerontologist. 2006;46(5):609–19.
12. Rochefort CM, Buckeridge DL, Abrahamowicz M. Improving patient safety by optimizing the use of nursing human resources. Implement Sci. 2015;10:89.
13. Giuliano KK, Danesh V, Funk M. The relationship between nurse staffing and 30-day readmission for adults with heart failure. J Nursing Admin. 2016; 46(1):25–9.
14. Everhart D, Neff D, Al-Amin M, Nogle J, Weech-Maldonado R. The effects of nurse staffing on hospital financial performance: competitive versus less competitive markets. Health Care Manag Rev. 2013;38(2):146–55.
15. Flynn M, Mckeown M. Nurse staffing levels revisited: a consideration of key issues in nurse staffing levels and skill mix research. J Nursing Manag. 2009;17(6):759–66.
16. O'Brien-Pallas L, Murphy GT, Shamian J, Li X, Hayes LJ. Impact and determinants of nurse turnover: a pan-Canadian study. J Nursing Manag. 2010;18:1073–86.
17. Chana N, Kennedy P, Chessell ZJ. Nursing staffs' emotional well-being and caring behaviours. J Clinical Nursing. 2015;24:2835–48.
18. Hurst K. Selecting and applying methods for estimating the size and mix of nursing teams: a systematic review of the literature commissioned by the Department of Health. Leeds: Nuffield Institute for Health, University of Leeds; 2003.
19. Cullen DJ, Civetta JM, Briggs BA, Ferrara LC. Therapeutic intervention scoring system: a method for quantitative comparison of patient care. Crit Care Med. 1974;2(2):57–112.
20. Miranda DR, Nap R, de Rijk A, Schaufeli W, Iapichino G, et al. Nursing activities score. Crit Care Med. 2003;31(2):374–82.
21. COFEN. Resolução COFEN-293/2004. 2004. http://www.cofen.gov.br/resoluo-cofen-2932004_4329.html. Accessed 26 Feb 2016.
22. Elkhuizen SG, Bor G, Smeenk M, Klazinga NS, Bakker PJ. Capacity management of nursing staff as a vehicle for organizational improvement. BMC Health Serv Res. 2007;7(1):1.
23. Kortbeek N, Braaksma A, Burger CA, Bakker PJ, Boucherie RJ. Flexible nurse staffing based on hourly bed census predictions. Int J Prod Econ. 2015;161:167–80.
24. Bordoloi SK, Weatherby EJ. Managerial implications of calculating optimum nurse staffing in medical units. Health Care Man Rev. 1999;24(4):35–44.
25. Venkataraman R, Brusco MJ. An integrated analysis of nurse staffing and scheduling policies. Omega. 1996;24(1):57–71.
26. Maenhout B, Vanhoucke M. An integrated nurse staffing and scheduling analysis for longer-term nursing staff allocation problems. Omega. 2013; 41(2):485–99.
27. ISCMPA. Hospital São José - Neurosurgery, Irmandade da Santa Casa da Misericórdia de Porto Alegre. 2017. http://www.santacasa.org.br/en/sao-jose. Accessed 10 Feb 2017.
28. Microsoft. Microsoft Office Professional Plus 2013. 2017. https://technet. microsoft.com/ en-us/office/. Accessed 10 Feb 2017.

A mobile phone based tool to identify symptoms of common childhood diseases in Ghana: development and evaluation of the integrated clinical algorithm

Konstantin H. Franke[1,2], Ralf Krumkamp[2], Aliyu Mohammed[3], Nimako Sarpong[3], Ellis Owusu-Dabo[3], Johanna Brinkel[4], Julius N. Fobil[5], Axel Bonacic Marinovic[6], Philip Asihene[7], Mark Boots[7], Jürgen May[2] and Benno Kreuels[1,2*] [iD]

Abstract

Background: The aim of this study was the development and evaluation of an algorithm-based diagnosis-tool, applicable on mobile phones, to support guardians in providing appropriate care to sick children.

Methods: The algorithm was developed on the basis of the Integrated Management of Childhood Illness (IMCI) guidelines and evaluated at a hospital in Ghana. Two hundred and thirty-seven guardians applied the tool to assess their child's symptoms. Data recorded by the tool and health records completed by a physician were compared in terms of symptom detection, disease assessment and treatment recommendation. To compare both assessments, Kappa statistics and predictive values were calculated.

Results: The tool detected the symptoms of cough, fever, diarrhoea and vomiting with good agreement to the physicians' findings (kappa = 0.64; 0.59; 0.57 and 0.42 respectively). The disease assessment barely coincided with the physicians' findings. The tool's treatment recommendation correlated with the physicians' assessments in 93 out of 237 cases (39.2% agreement, kappa = 0.11), but underestimated a child's condition in only seven cases (3.0%).

Conclusions: The algorithm-based tool achieved reliable symptom detection and treatment recommendations were administered conformably to the physicians' assessment. Testing in domestic environment is envisaged.

Keywords: mHealth, Algorithm, Symptom assessment, Decision making, computer assisted, Interactive voice response, Africa, Children

Background

Despite a reduction of childhood mortality by 53% since 1990, almost six million children under 5-years died in 2015 [1]. High child mortality rates are observed especially in sub-Saharan Africa, where 83 out of 1000 live births die, mostly due to acute respiratory infections, diarrhoeal disease and malaria [2]. Timely diagnosis and treatment of diseases are life-saving, yet provision and access to health-care services are still limited in many areas of sub-Saharan Africa [3]. Long distances to health care facilities have a strong influence on health-seeking behaviour and many deaths could be prevented if adequate treatment was initiated earlier [4, 5].

To improve diagnosis and treatment for children living in rural and remote areas, innovative strategies are needed. mHealth (mobile Health), the use of mobile devices to support public health measures, offers great potential to enhance communication between patients

* Correspondence: b.kreuels@uke.de
[1]Division of Tropical Medicine, First Department of Medicine, University Medical Center Hamburg-Eppendorf (UKE), Hamburg, Germany
[2]Infectious Disease Epidemiology, Bernhard Nocht Institute for Tropical Medicine (BNITM), Hamburg, Germany
Full list of author information is available at the end of the article

and the professional health care system [6, 7]. Mobile phone targeted health interventions have increasing potential in many developing countries, since the number of mobile phone subscriptions is constantly growing and the mobile phone network is also expanding to rural areas [8].

The idea of this study was the development of an mHealth tool to support guardians of children living in areas with limited access to health care. To achieve this goal, the Integrated Management of Childhood Illnesses (IMCI) guidelines [9] were used to develop a clinical algorithm to assess disease symptoms in sick children that could be implemented into an interactive voice response (IVR)-system applicable in automated health hotlines. The transfer of information would rely on audio files - rather than on text messages - which could be useful for the multitude of illiterates in sub-Saharan Africa [10]. At the beginning of the development and repeatedly every 6 months during the consecutive process of testing, data analysis and writing of the manuscript (last search on 13.09.2017) we conducted a systematic literature search on PubMed to identify studies that had evaluated mHealth tools in African settings.

So far, the systematic literature research has not revealed any studies using algorithm based IVR-systems for disease detection in children [7, 11, 12]. Some studies have been conducted in which the IMCI guidelines were translated into mHealth interventions to assist health care workers. In one study by Ginsburg et al. a mHealth application, integrating a digital version of the IMCI guidelines with a breath counter and a pulse oximeter, was developed to support health care workers in the diagnosis of pneumonia in children in Ghana [13]. The authors concluded that their tool had "the potential to facilitate prompt diagnosis and assessment" [14]. In another study by Rambaud-Althaus et al. the authors developed a new algorithm for the management of children under 5 years of age living in resource poor settings. It included point-of-care tests and clinical predictors for acute illnesses to improve the rational use of antimicrobials [15]. In a subsequent controlled non-inferiority study in Tanzania they concluded that the use of their algorithm "improved clinical outcome and reduced antibiotic prescription" [16]. However, these studies aimed at health care workers, whereas our study directly targets guardians of sick children.

This study was part of the electronic Health Information and Surveillance System project (eHISS) that aimed at conceptualizing and piloting a mobile phone based tool to collect individual disease information and to provide corresponding treatment recommendations. Health information from participating populations and the simultaneous collection of spatio-temporal data on the incidence of fever, diarrhoea and respiratory distress were envisaged for monitoring potential disease outbreaks. This manuscript presents the development and evaluation of an algorithm based tool to identify symptoms of common childhood diseases and to provide basic treatment recommendations, focussing on testing its medical correctness. User experiences with the finalized tool were evaluated in another study [17].

Methods
Decision making process
An expert panel consisting of clinicians, epidemiologists/biostatisticians, public health experts and communication researchers was involved in the development of the clinical algorithm and its translation into an IVR-system. The panel met three times over a period of 2 years to discuss the draft versions of the system and to decide on necessary adjustments using a Delphi method-like approach. A detailed description of the panel's composition and the methods how the clinical algorithm and IVR-system were developed, amended and evaluated (further evaluation results are also published elsewhere [18]) is given in the supplementary files (see Additional file 1).

Development of the algorithm
The IMCI guidelines served as a template representing the standard of care for diagnosis and management of childhood illnesses in primary health care in resource poor settings. Furthermore, they give concise instructions on how to manage the most common childhood diseases. After assessing a child's condition ("ask, look, feel"), the IMCI's flowchart will guide the user to a disease, assign it to a respective triage level (immediate referral, management in the outpatient facility or home management) and give instructions for treatment [9]. To apply the IMCI guidelines to the target population (lay people vs. medical personnel) and the field of application (home use in IVR-system vs. health care setting), it was necessary to make some changes in the IMCI flowchart. As the IMCI guidelines were developed for medical personnel, they needed to be amended to ensure comprehension by lay people while gaining the maximum possible amount of information about a child's health status. Therefore, we used only questions that could be answered without pre-existing medical knowledge and did not require a clinical inspection and examination. The panel excluded questions that included physical examination (e.g. counting the breaths or identifying oedema), since we could not expect to get reliable results from untrained people. It allowed asking for symptoms (i.e. fever, cough, diarrhoea, vomiting), the existence of dangerous symptoms ("danger signs") and further questions to assess the level of respiratory infection

and dehydration. Diseases and their respective symptoms were included and excluded based on the prevalence of symptoms as determined by a survey of the hospital's record-book that was analysed for a year preceding the study and with data on diagnoses from ongoing studies on disease aetiology. The main diagnoses made in the study hospital (multiple diagnoses possible) are *Plasmodium falciparum* malaria (59%), pneumonia and other respiratory tract infections (33%), gastrointestinal infection (17%), and bloodstream infections (5%) (unpublished data). The IMCI's three triage levels for respective diseases remained the same, only the advice was refocused for home use (e.g. presentation to a hospital immediately/in 24 h (algorithm) vs. referral or management in the outpatient facility (IMCI)). After this modification process the panel determined the order of questions. The IMCI guidelines' hierarchic structure was kept by assessing the severity of a confirmed symptom with additional questions.

The algorithm's tasks were to identify symptoms of common childhood illnesses (symptom detection), to detect an illness (disease assessment) as well as to estimate the severity of the symptoms and give suitable advice (treatment recommendation). These three tasks were to be compared to the physicians' findings and recommendations.

The finalized clinical algorithm was based on dichotomous questions asked successively as shown in Fig. 1. The first questions referred to the child's age and the existence of "danger signs" such as inability to drink or breastfeed and neurological emergencies (e.g., convulsions and unconsciousness). The following questions aimed at identifying the symptoms fever, cough, diarrhoea and vomiting. Whenever the guardians responded that their child suffered from one of these symptoms, more specific questions (highlighted with grey background) were asked to assess symptom severity. Based on the symptom severity, calls were assigned to a treatment recommendation: A = requiring emergency treatment, B = requiring causal treatment or C = requiring home care. Additional advice was given on how to manage the child on the way to the hospital (e.g., "offer enough to drink") or on how to treat the child at home (e.g., advise on the use of oral rehydration salts, if applicable). The algorithm was designed to register information on multiple symptoms for one participant but assigned calls to only one treatment recommendation according to the most life-threatening condition.

The following disease assessments with different severity levels were included in the algorithm: *inability to drink or breastfeed*; *neurological emergency*; *severe febrile disease*; *febrile disease*; *respiratory tract infection* (RTI) categorized as *severe*, *moderate* or *mild*; *gastrointestinal infection* (GI-infection) with *severe*, *moderate* or *no dehydration*; and *dysentery*.

Development of the IVR-system

The users' requirements concerning the application of a mobile phone based IVR-system for seeking health care were investigated by ascertaining the caregivers' attitudes, their motivations for adoption and the barriers to its implementation in focus group discussions [18]. Data from this analysis was used to implement the clinical algorithm in an IVR-system (the IVR-system incorporating the clinical algorithm will be referred to as the "tool"). Based on their experience in working with mothers in the area, clinicians translated the questions and recommendations into the commonly spoken language Twi in the manner they would ask these questions during medical consultations and recorded them as audio files. VOTO Mobile (now called Viamo [19]), a Ghana-based company specializing in interactive SMS (short message service) or voice calls [19], developed and operated the IVR-system. Users started consulting the tool by calling a hotline. After hearing the audio files, users answered the questions by pressing number codes and were thereby (navigated) guided through the algorithm's questions. Subsequently, the tool was tested by participants and challenges in the usage of the tool were assessed in further focus group discussions. The usability (System Usability Scare median: 79.3; range: 65.0–97.5) was rated acceptable [17]. Additionally, the tool was piloted with 50 target users to make sure that the audio files and the respective questions are really understood. All participants could understand the questions and were able to use the tool via mobile phone.

Study area and participants

This cross-sectional study was conducted at the Agogo Presbyterian Hospital (APH) in Ghana between October 2014 and January 2015. APH is a district hospital and provides beds for about 250 patients. The study was conducted in the children's outpatient department that is frequently visited by families for both emergency and follow-up treatment.

Guardians were recruited to the study if they were ≥18 years old, accompanying a sick child (≥1 month and < 15 years), fluent in the local language Twi and if they had not come for referral treatment or review. Ethical approval for this study was obtained from the Kwame Nkrumah University of Science and Technology (KNUST) in Kumasi, Ghana (Reference number: CHRPE/AP/278/14).

Study procedures

Guardians were recruited in the OPD before seeing the attending physician. Study procedures were explained and written informed consent was obtained from the guardians. Study personnel instructed the participant on how to use the tool before the participant conducted the phone call and completed the tool's questions. After

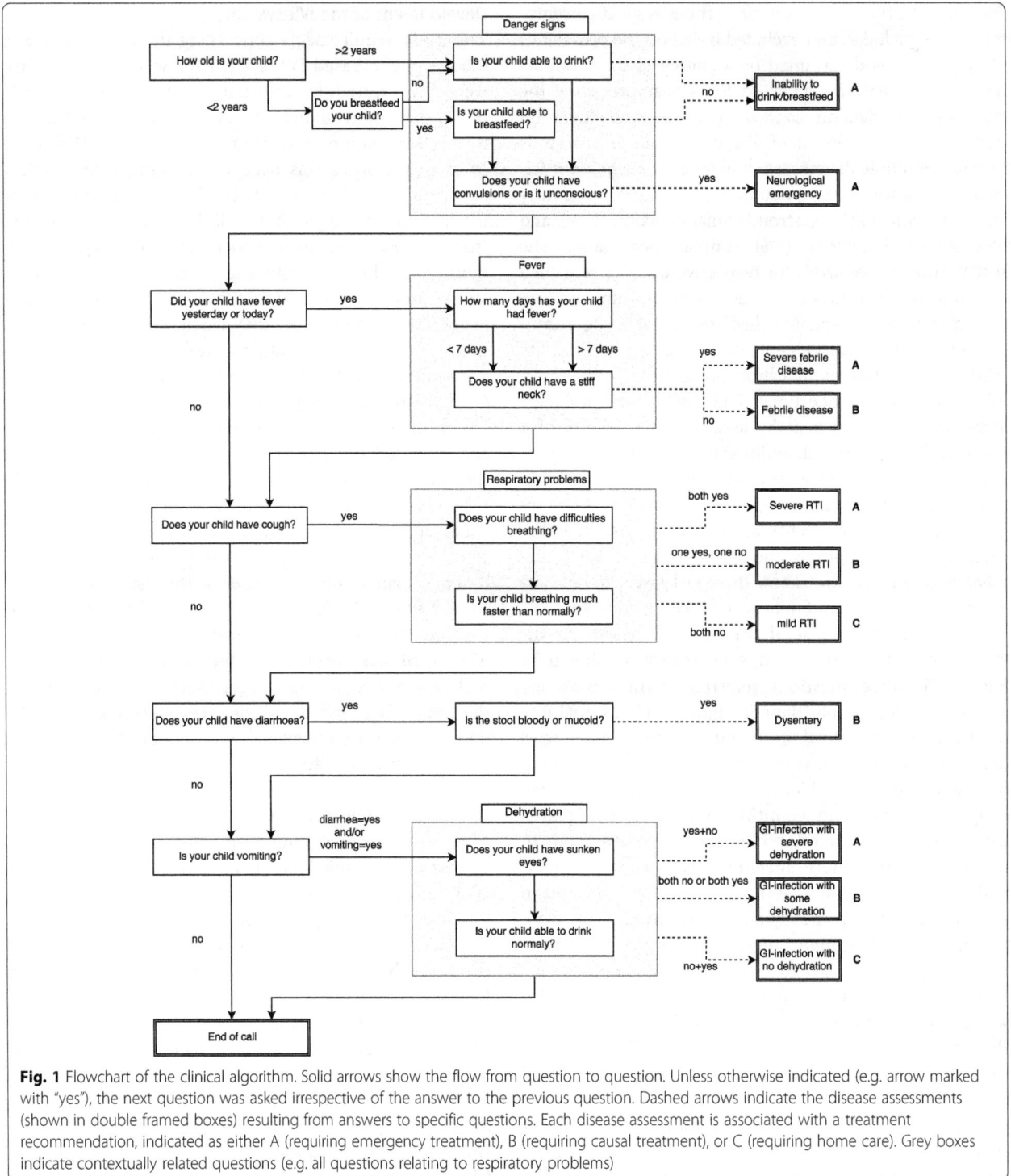

Fig. 1 Flowchart of the clinical algorithm. Solid arrows show the flow from question to question. Unless otherwise indicated (e.g. arrow marked with "yes"), the next question was asked irrespective of the answer to the previous question. Dashed arrows indicate the disease assessments (shown in double framed boxes) resulting from answers to specific questions. Each disease assessment is associated with a treatment recommendation, indicated as either A (requiring emergency treatment), B (requiring causal treatment), or C (requiring home care). Grey boxes indicate contextually related questions (e.g. all questions relating to respiratory problems)

finishing the phone call, the participant consulted the physician, who wrote a report into the patient file. The patient file was reviewed and a member of the study team, who was blinded to the results from the tool assessment, transcribed symptoms, diagnoses, treatment procedures and possible reassessment recommendations on a questionnaire.

Data analysis

The tool's performance against the medical records was evaluated by measuring the inter-rater agreement using Cohen's Kappa and corresponding *p*-value. The Kappa values were interpreted as suggested by Landis and Koch [20]. Other calculated values were sensitivity, specificity, positive predictive value (PPV) and negative predictive value (NPV). As this was an explorative study, sample size was not based on a formal calculation, but determined by the number of participants that could be recruited within the planned recruitment period of 3 months. To achieve reliable results it was intended to recruit at least 200 participants.

The tool's outcome was compared to the physicians' findings (used as gold standard) in three categories: symptom detection, disease assessment and treatment recommendation. While the detected symptoms could be compared directly to the respective physicians' notes, variables had to be created to evaluate disease assessment and treatment recommendation. Concerning disease assessment, the tool's findings (e.g., *severe RTI*) were compared to variables composed of physicians' assessment (e.g., tachypnoea) or diagnoses (e.g., pneumonia). Concerning treatment recommendations, three variables were defined, composed of the physicians' assessment, treatment or advice for re-evaluation. These three variables allowed comparison to the tool's treatment recommendations (A1–3), determining the need for emergency, causal or home treatment, as shown in Table 1. Data were analysed using Stata 14 (College Station, TX: StataCorp LP).

Results
Study participants
A total of 294 participants were recruited for this study. Of these, 57 (19.4%) were excluded from the analysis as they did not complete the algorithm ($n = 27$, 9.2%), contained missing data in their hospital files ($n = 20$, 6.8%) or did not show any symptoms considered by the tool ($n = 10$, 3.4%), namely conjunctivitis, constipation, polydactyly, seborrheic dermatitis, pruritus and vaginal bleeding. Finally, data from 237 participants were included into the study.

Table 1 Comparing the tool's treatment recommendation to the physicians' assessment

Triaged as	Tool	Physicians' notes
A	Requiring emergency treatment: "Take your child to the nearest hospital immediately!"	Emergency treatment (e.g. i.v. fluids, i.v. antibiotics, i.m./i.v. antimalarial drugs) or hospitalization for further investigation
B	Requiring etiologic treatment: "Take your child to the nearest hospital within 24 h!"	Etiologic treatment (e.g. antibiotics, antimalarial drugs in oral form etc.) or follow-up
C	Requiring home care: "Treat your child at home and assess disease progression carefully!"	Symptomatic treatment (e.g. nasal drops or paracetamol) or follow-up was not expected to be needed

The median age of the guardians was 31 years (range: 18–71, interquartile range: 24–36) and the vast majority was female ($n = 227$, 95.8%). The median age of the children was 3 years (range: 0–14, interquartile range: 1–4). Most children ($n = 213$, 89.9%) were accompanied by their biological parents. In total, 192 (81.0%) participants reported to use a mobile phone regularly.

Evaluation of the tool
Symptom detection
The highest agreement between the findings of the tool and the physician was observed for cough (percentage agreement 82.3%, kappa = 0.64, $p < 0.01$, sensitivity = 91.5%, NPV = 87.4%). Good agreement was also seen for fever (83.5%, kappa = 0.59, $p < 0.01$, sensitivity = 90.4%, NPV = 74.6%) and diarrhoea (84.4%, kappa = 0.57, $p < 0.01$, sensitivity = 86.1%, NPV = 96.5%), while vomiting showed reasonable agreement (76.4%, kappa = 0.42, $p < 0.01$, sensitivity = 67.2%, NPV = 88.2%, Table 2).

Disease assessment
As shown above, the algorithm derived 11 disease assessments for the most common childhood diseases. The physicians neither diagnosed inability to drink/breastfeed and stiff neck, nor symptoms determining severe febrile disease in any of the patients. Thus, nine out of 11 disease assessments were available for data analysis. The results are displayed in Table 3.

The five most common physicians' diagnoses were *febrile disease* ($n = 167$, 70.5%), *moderate RTI* ($n = 66$, 27.9%), *GI-infection with no dehydration* ($n = 62$, 26.2%), *mild RTI* ($n = 53$, 22.4%) and *severe RTI* ($n = 22$, 9.3%). *GI-infection with some dehydration* ($n = 15$, 6.3%), *dysentery* ($n = 7$, 3.0%), *GI-infection with severe dehydration* (n = 6, 2.5%) and *neurological emergency* (n = 1, 0.4%) were less often diagnosed.

Good agreement was observed *for febrile disease* (78.9%, kappa = 0.51, $p < 0.01$, sensitivity = 83.2%, NPV = 63.2%), while fair agreement was seen for *severe RTI* (84.0%, kappa = 0.3, $p < 0.01$, sensitivity = 54.6%, NPV = 94.9%) and *GI-infection with some dehydration* (81.9%, kappa = 0.25, $p < 0.01$, sensitivity = 66.7%, NPV = 97.4%). *GI-infection with no dehydration* (73.4%, kappa = 0.2, $p < 0.01$, sensitivity = 27.4%, NPV = 77.7%) showed slight agreement. The highest percentage-agreement was noted for *GI-infection with severe dehydration*, even though with a low kappa, as this condition was diagnosed by the physicians very rarely (93.3%, kappa = 0.08, $p = 0.1$, sensitivity = 16.7%, NPV = 97.8%). The algorithm detected five out of seven cases of *dysentery* entailing fair agreement

Table 2 Comparison of the tool and the physicians in terms of symptom detection

Symptom	Agreement (%)	Cohen's kappa	p-value [a]	Sensitivity (%)	Specificity (%)	PPV [b]	NPV [c]	Prevalence (%)
Fever	83.5	0.59	< 0.01	90.4	67.1	86.8	74.6	70.5
Cough	82.3	0.64	< 0.01	91.5	71.0	79.3	87.4	54.9
Diarrhoea	84.4	0.57	< 0.01	86.1	84.0	54.4	96.5	18.1
Vomiting	76.4	0.42	< 0.01	67.2	79.3	51.3	88.2	24.5

[a] p-value for Cohen's Kappa
[b] PPV = positive predictive value
[c] NPV = negative predictive value

(84.0%, kappa = 0.17, p < 0.01, sensitivity = 71.4%, NPV = 99.0%).

The physicians noted one case of convulsions, which was not detected by the tool. Nevertheless, 53 participants misdiagnosed their children with convulsions or unconsciousness resulting in a poor agreement for *neurological emergency* (77.2%, kappa = − 0.01, p = 0.71, sensitivity = 0%, NPV = 99.5%).

Treatment recommendation

As shown in Table 4, the physicians ranked most of the children as B (requiring causal treatment [n = 175, 73.8%]), followed by A (requiring emergency treatment [n = 48, 20.3%]) and C (requiring home care [n = 14, 5.9%]), while the tool assessed the majority of patients as

A (n = 171, 72.2%), followed by B (n = 55, 23.2%) and C (n = 11, 4.6%). The tool detected 42 out of 48 cases that were assessed as A by the physician (87.5%) and ranked the six (12.5%) remaining cases as B. These six cases were severe forms of malaria and sepsis requiring hospitalization. The tool ranked them as B due to the disease assessment *febrile disease*.

Out of the 175 physician-ranked B-cases, 47 cases (26.9%) were correctly identified as B by the tool, 121 patients (69.1%) were ranked as A and 7 (4.0%) as C. The tool underestimated the latter cases as *mild RTI* or *GI-infection with no dehydration*, but these patients received causal treatment (e.g., with antibiotics) by the physicians or were asked to present for reassessment on the following days. Among the 14 physician-ranked C-

Table 3 Accordance of the tool's disease assessments and the physicians' findings ordered to the respective treatment recommendation

	Agreement (%)	Cohen's kappa	p-value [a]	Sensitivity (%)	Specificity (%)	PPV [b]	NPV [c]	Prevalence [d] (%)
A								
Neurological emergency	77.2	− 0.01	0.71	0	77.5	0	99.5	0.4
Severe RTI [e]	84.0	0.3	< 0.01	54.6	87.0	30.0	94.9	9.3
GI-infection [f] with severe dehydration	93.3	0.08	0.09	16.7	95.2	8.3	97.8	2.5
Inability to drink/breastfeed	n/a	n/a	n/a	n/a	n/a	n/a	n/a	n/a
Severe febrile disease	n/a	n/a	n/a	n/a	n/a	n/a	n/a	n/a
B								
Febrile disease	78.9	0.51	< 0.01	83.2	68.6	86.3	63.2	70.5
Moderate RTI [e]	63.7	0.05	0.21	27.3	77.8	32.1	73.5	27.9
GI-infection [f] with some dehydration	81.9	0.25	< 0.01	66.7	82.9	20.8	97.4	6.3
Dysentery	84.0	0.17	< 0.01	71.4	84.3	12.2	99.0	3.0
C								
Mild RTI [e]	62.5	−0.07	0.87	17.0	75.5	16.7	76.0	22.4
GI-infection [f] with no dehydration	73.4	0.2	< 0.01	27.4	89.7	48.6	77.7	26.2

A = requiring emergency treatment
B = requiring causal treatment
C = requiring home care
[a] p-value for Cohen's Kappa
[b] PPV = positive predictive value
[c] NPV = negative predictive value
[d] Prevalence of the disease assessments made by the physicians
[e] RTI = respiratory tract infection
[f] GI-infection = gastrointestinal infection

Table 4 Accordance of the tool and the physicians in terms of treatment recommendation

Tool's treatment recommendation	Physicians' assessment			Total
	A	B	C	
A	42	121	8	171
B	6	47	2	55
C	0	7	4	11
Total	48	175	14	237

A = requiring emergency treatment
B = requiring causal treatment
C = requiring home care

cases, four were correctly assessed, (28.6%) correctly, however two (14.3%) were declared as B and eight (57.1%) as A.

Overall, data analysis indicated a weak agreement (39.2%, kappa = 0.11, $p < 0.01$) between the tool's treatment recommendation and the physicians' assessment. Nevertheless, as described above, underestimation of disease severity was low. Only seven out of 237 cases (3.0%) would have been ranked as C although they needed to be examined by a physician (either A or B by the physician). Furthermore, the accordance of tool and physicians' assessment, whether a child should be presented at a hospital (A or B) or not (C), showed strong agreement (92.8%) with fair kappa values (0.28).

Discussion

This study describes the development and evaluation of an algorithm-based IVR-tool for guardians of sick children in sub-Saharan Africa. It was shown that, compared to the subsequent examination by attending physicians, the tool performed well in identifying the three leading disease symptoms fever (agreement = 83.5%, kappa = 0.59), cough (agreement = 82.3%, kappa = 0.64), and diarrhoea (agreement = 84.4%, kappa = 0.57). The detection of vomiting was moderate (agreement = 76.4%, kappa = 0.42). Additionally, the tool was able to give out appropriate treatment recommendations. Merely seven out of 237 patients (3.0%) were not sent to the hospital by the tool, although physicians applied causal treatment for specific illnesses (e.g. prescribed antibiotics). These results indicate that the tool can provide basic treatment recommendations without a medical health care professional nearby, although disease assessment was not achieved in a reliable way. The discrepancy between adequate treatment recommendations and inadequate disease assessment may be explained by the registration of multiple disease assessments but only one treatment recommendation. Guardians were not able to answer the more specific questions correctly after confirming a symptom, but they seemed to be able to estimate the need for treatment. This was shown by the tool's good performance in deciding whether or not a child has

to be presented at a hospital (agreement = 92.8%, kappa = 0.28). Thus, this tool could contribute to timely diagnosis and treatment and may be effective in lowering childhood mortality in areas with limited access to health care services.

Success and failure of this tool are strongly dependent on the guardians' ability to correctly assess their children's health status. A systematic review by Geldsetzer et al. evaluated the guardians' recognition of childhood illnesses in developing countries. Due to low values of sensitivity for the recognition of fever, diarrhoea and pneumonia, the authors concluded that "survey data based on these reports should not be used for disease burden estimations" [21]. In comparison our results show considerably higher values of sensitivity for fever and diarrhoea, but slightly lower values of specificity. Generally, guardians detected symptoms of common childhood illnesses with higher sensitivity but lower specificity compared to other studies [21]. Our results indicate that guardians of sick children can contribute to disease surveillance, at least by identifying their children's symptoms.

In contrast, the results for disease assessment generally revealed inadequate performance of the tool. A possible reason may be that questions were too imprecise to achieve reliable assessment corresponding to the physicians' findings. It was considered whether more questions could improve the assessment, but concluded that more than 15 possible items would only protract the questioning and, thus, lower user satisfaction. Moreover, one has to acknowledge the structural difference in the diagnostic process of a machine vs. a human being. The tool heavily depended on the data which were only received by asking questions; finally, data were collected in a binary yes/no form. In contrast, the physician can get additional specific clues by examining the patient and can put information into perspective.

A systematic literature search was conducted to identify mHealth studies that aimed at improving child health before the development of the algorithm. None of the reviewed publications used an algorithm-based IVR-tool for the detection of symptoms or the assessment of a child's health status. Most of the mHealth interventions focused on improving patient follow-up and medication adherence as well as data collection/transfer and reporting [11, 22–25]. The targeted group for decision-support-systems was medical personnel [12, 16, 26–28]. The communication channels primarily used were short messaging services (SMS) [29–31], whereas IVR-systems were not used at all [7, 11, 32].

Given that this is the first study using an IVR-tool operating on a medical algorithm to receive health information and process them into a health assessment, it had several limitations that should be considered in future studies. First, the IMCI guidelines proved to be difficult when compared to the physicians' notes so that some questions, especially the danger signs, could not be measured adequately. Reasons might be the low prevalence (e.g., for convulsions and unconsciousness, which were fast-tracked through the OPD), the lack of the guardians' medical knowledge of danger signs (as reported in other studies [16]) or the fact that the physicians assessed a child's health status in a different way than the IMCI. Future studies should use structured questionnaires to be filled out by the physicians during consultation to record clinical assessment and improve comparisons between the findings made by the tool and the physician.

Second, not all characteristics of the IMCI guidelines could be implemented into the algorithm. One of its key components is the assessment by the community health worker: inspecting the child (e.g., for chest indrawing), measuring the body temperature and counting the breaths ("ask, look, feel"). We could not transfer these tasks onto guardians without medical experience or otherwise the data would be unreliable and result in biased information. Thus we had to reduce the complexity of the IMCI guidelines in such a way that they could be understood by the guardians and correct data could be obtained. Naturally, this happened at the expense of the diagnostic performance, which was anticipated during the development of the algorithm. However, since we wanted to avoid recommending home care in severe illnesses, we designed the algorithm to detect symptoms as sensitive as possible and accepted the compromise between symptom detection with high sensitivity on the one hand and "overestimating" a child's condition on the other hand.

Third, the study was conducted in a children's OPD of a well-equipped district hospital, which implicated a higher prevalence and severity of diseases compared with everyday life. Due to this instance, the tool's performance could be appropriately evaluated for the treatment recommendations A and B, but the prevalence of C-cases was too low. Therefore, our research group initiated another study in fieldwork to evaluate our tool in the domestic setting, where more C-cases were suspected.

The study results indicate the ability of the tool to detect symptoms of common childhood diseases and to give suitable treatment recommendations. Our research group further found that our tool was applicable and accepted by Ghanaians in focus group discussions [17]. Furthermore, the project group developed a software application for space-time surveillance and model-based analysis within the eHISS system. Provided its adequate performance in the domestic setting, the panel of clinicians and epidemiologists could use the gathered information to update and optimize the tool. In its final version, the eHISS tool is envisaged to provide people with health information and give health authorities and health policy makers reliable data on prevailing disease syndromes.

Conclusions

This study reports the applicability of an algorithm-based IVR-tool to correctly identify symptoms of the most common childhood diseases in sub-Saharan Africa and to deliver appropriate health advice via mobile phone. While disease assessment did not work sufficiently, it was shown that symptom detection was feasible and comparable to the physicians' findings. By providing appropriate treatment recommendations, the tool could support decision making for indecisive guardians of sick children. It could serve as a second opinion and turn the balance in favour of presenting at a hospital, while reducing the number of unnecessary journeys. Especially with distant and time-consuming trips to the closest health care facility early presentation could prevent complicated courses of disease. These study results could also be applied to enhance disease surveillance initiatives, e.g. obtaining direct information by calling people from a distinct area instead of dispatching health care personnel.

Additional file

Additional file 1 Detailed description of the expert panel's composition and function. This file contains detailed information about the composition of the expert panel, division of responsibilities and decision making process during the development of the algorithm and IVR-system. Additionally, the results of the panel meetings are displayed. The list of the panel members, their respective expertise and role in the project is summarized in a table. (DOCX 33 kb)

Abbreviations
APH: Agogo Presbyterian Hospital; eHISS: electronic Health Information and Surveillance System; GI-infection: Gastrointestinal infection; IMCI: Integrated Management of Childhood Illnesses; IVR: Interactive voice response; KNUST: Kwame Nkrumah University of Science and Technology; mHealth: mobile Health; NPV: Negative predictive value; OPD: Outpatient department; PPV: Positive predictive value; RTI: Respiratory tract infection; SMS: Short message service; WHO: World Health Organization

Acknowledgements
We would like to thank all study participants and the staff of the Agogo Presbyterian Hospital.

Funding
The "Electronic Health Information and Surveillance System for sub-Saharan Africa" project, was supported by the German Federal Ministry of Education and Research: Grant number 01DG13019A and 01DG13019B. The funding body had no influence on the design of the study, collection, analysis, and interpretation of data and in writing the manuscript.

Authors' contributions

KF, RK and BK developed the algorithm, analysed the data and wrote the first draft of the manuscript. KF and AM conducted the study in Ghana and collected the data under the supervision of NS and BK. NS and EOD translated the algorithm into Twi. EOD JF and JM created the eHISS project had input on both the design of the study and the final version of the algorithm,. PA and MB integrated the algorithm into the IVR-system hosted on servers by VOTO Mobile and ran the IVR-System during the study. JB and EOD evaluated the acceptance of the IVR-tool in the local population and influenced the design of the algorithm based on these data. ABM formed a concept for a real-time mapping technology for spatio-temporal data and influenced the design of the algorithm to make it suitable for data collection. All authors gave substantial input on the development and evaluation of the tool during 3 meetings in Hamburg (January 2014), Accra (October 2014) and Kumasi (November 2015). All authors have revised the manuscript and read and approved the final version.

Competing interests

The authors declare that they have no competing interests.

Author details

[1]Division of Tropical Medicine, First Department of Medicine, University Medical Center Hamburg-Eppendorf (UKE), Hamburg, Germany. [2]Infectious Disease Epidemiology, Bernhard Nocht Institute for Tropical Medicine (BNITM), Hamburg, Germany. [3]Kumasi Center for Collaborative Research in Tropical Medicine (KCCR), College of Health Sciences, Kwame Nkrumah University of Science and Technology (KNUST), Kumasi, Ghana. [4]Department of Public Health Medicine, School of Public Health, University of Bielefeld, Bielefeld, Germany. [5]School of Public Health, University of Ghana, Accra, Ghana. [6]National Institute for Public Health and the Environment (RIVM), Bilthoven, The Netherlands. [7]Viamo, Accra, Ghana.

References

1. Bocquenet G, Chaiban T, Cook S, Escudero P, Franco A, Romo CG, et al. The state of the World's children 2016: United Nations; 2016.
2. Liu L, Oza S, Hogan D, Chu Y, Perin J, Zhu J, et al. Global, regional, and national causes of under-5 mortality in 2000–15: an updated systematic analysis with implications for the sustainable development goals. Lancet. 2016;388:3027–35.
3. Bhutta ZA, Black RE. Global maternal, newborn, and child health — so near and yet so far. N Engl J Med. 2013;369:2226–35.
4. Kadobera D, Sartorius B, Masanja H, Mathew A, Waiswa P. The effect of distance to formal health facility on childhood mortality in rural Tanzania, 2005-2007. Glob Health Action. 2012;5:1–9.
5. Krumkamp R, Sarpong N, Kreuels B, Ehlkes L, Loag W, Schwarz NG, et al. Health care utilization and symptom severity in Ghanaian children – a cross-sectional study. Fernandez-Reyes D, editor. PLoS One 2013;8:e80598.
6. Howitt P, Darzi A, Yang G-Z, Ashrafian H, Atun R, Barlow J, et al. Technologies for global health. Lancet. 2012;380:507–35.
7. Hurt K, Walker RJ, Campbell JA, Egede LE. mHealth interventions in low and middle-income countries: a systematic review. Glob J Health Sci. 2016;8:183.
8. International Telecommunication Union. ICT Facts and Figures 2016. 2016;
9. WHO. Integrated Management of Childhood Illness Chart Booklet; 2014. p. 1–76.
10. UNESCO-UIS. Adult and youth literacy: national, regional and global trends, 1985–2015. UIS information paper: UNESCO Institute for Statistics; 2013.
11. Brinkel J, Krämer A, Krumkamp R, May J, Fobil J. Mobile phone-based mHealth approaches for public health surveillance in sub-Saharan Africa: a systematic review. Int J Environ Res Public Health. 2014;11:11559–82.
12. Bediang G, Bagayoko CO, Geissbuhler A. Medical decision support systems in Africa. Yearb Med Inf. 2010:47–54.
13. Ginsburg AS, Delarosa J, Brunette W, Levari S, Sundt M, Larson C, et al. mPneumonia: development of an innovative mHealth application for diagnosing and treating childhood pneumonia and other childhood illnesses in low-resource settings. PLoS One. 2015;10: e0139625.
14. Ginsburg AS, Agyemang CT, Ambler G, Delarosa J, Brunette W, Levari S, et al. MPneumonia, an innovation for diagnosing and treating childhood pneumonia in low-resource settings: a feasibility, usability and acceptability study in Ghana. PLoS One. 2016;11:1–14.
15. Rambaud-Althaus C, Shao AF, Kahama-Maro J, Genton B, D'Acremont V. Managing the sick child in the era of declining malaria transmission: development of ALMANACH, an electronic algorithm for appropriate use of antimicrobials. PLoS One. 2015;10:e0127674.
16. Tuhebwe D, Tumushabe E, Leontsini E, Wanyenze R. Pneumonia among children under five in Uganda: symptom recognition and actions taken by caretakers. Afr Health Sci. 2015;14:993.
17. Brinkel J, May J, Krumkamp R, Lamshöft M, Kreuels B, Owusu-Dabo E, et al. Mobile phone-based interactive voice response as a tool for improving access to healthcare in remote areas in Ghana - an evaluation of user experiences. Tropical Med Int Health. 2017;22:622–30.
18. Brinkel J, Dako-Gyeke P, Krämer A, May J, Fobil JN. An investigation of users' attitudes, requirements and willingness to use mobile phone-based interactive voice response systems for seeking healthcare in Ghana: a qualitative study. Public Health. 2017;144:125–33.
19. Viamo – About Us. [cited 2016 May 13]. Available from: https://viamo.io/about-viamo/. https://viamo.io/press-releases/voto-now-viamo/
20. Landis JR, Koch GG. The measurement of observer agreement for categorical data. Biometrics. 1977;33:159–74.
21. Geldsetzer P, Williams TC, Kirolos A, Mitchell S, Ratcliffe LA, Kohli-Lynch MK, et al. The recognition of and care seeking behaviour for childhood illness in developing countries: a systematic review. PLoS One. 2014;9:e93427.
22. Aranda-Jan CB, Mohutsiwa-Dibe N, Loukanova S. Systematic review on what works, what does not work and why of implementation of mobile health (mHealth) projects in Africa. BMC Public Health. 2014;14:188.
23. Tomasi E, Facchini LA, Maia MDFS. Health information technology in primary health care in developing countries: a literature review. Bull World Health Organ. 2004;82:867–74.
24. Hamainza B, Killeen GF, Kamuliwo M, Bennett A, Yukich JO. Comparison of a mobile phone-based malaria reporting system with source participant register data for capturing spatial and temporal trends in epidemiological indicators of malaria transmission collected by community health workers in rural Zambia; 2014. p. 1–13.
25. Lee SH, Nurmatov UB, Nwaru BI, Mukherjee M, Grant L, Pagliari C. Effectiveness of mHealth interventions for maternal, newborn and child health in low- and middle-income countries: systematic review and meta-analysis. J Glob Health. 2016;6:10401.
26. Källander K, Tibenderana JK, Akpogheneta OJ, Strachan DL, Hill Z, ten Asbroek AHA, et al. Mobile health (mHealth) approaches and lessons for increased performance and retention of community health Workers in low- and Middle-Income Countries: a review. J Med Internet Res. 2013;15:e17.
27. Blank A, Prytherch H, Kaltschmidt J, Krings A, Sukums F, Mensah N, et al. "Quality of prenatal and maternal care: bridging the know-do gap" (QUALMAT study): an electronic clinical decision support system for rural sub-Saharan Africa. BMC Med Inform Decis Mak. 2013;13:44.
28. Agarwal S, Perry HB, Long L-A, Labrique AB. Evidence on feasibility and effective use of mHealth strategies by frontline health workers in developing countries: systematic review. Tropical Med Int Health. 2015;20:1003–14.
29. Githinji S, Kigen S, Memusi D, Nyandigisi A, Wamari A, Muturi A, et al. Using mobile phone text messaging for malaria surveillance in rural Kenya. Malar J. 2014;13:107.
30. Ngabo F, Nguimfack J, Nwaigwe F, Mugeni C, Muhoza D, Wilson DR, et al. Designing and implementing an innovative SMS-based alert system (RapidSMS-MCH) to monitor pregnancy and reduce maternal and child deaths in Rwanda. Pan Afr Med J. 2012;13:31.
31. Stockwell MS, Kharbanda EO, Martinez RA, Lara M, Vawdrey D, Natarajan K, et al. Text4Health: impact of text message reminder-recalls for pediatric and adolescent immunizations. Am J Public Health. 2012;102:e15–21.
32. Krishna S, Boren SA, Balas EA. Healthcare via cell phones: a systematic review. Telemed e-Health. 2009;15:231–40.

Information standards for recording alcohol use in electronic health records: findings from a national consultation

Shamil Haroon[1]*[id], Darren Wooldridge[2], Jan Hoogewerf[2], Krishnarajah Nirantharakumar[1], John Williams[2], Lina Martino[3] and Neeraj Bhala[4]

Abstract

Background: Alcohol misuse is an important cause of premature disability and death. While clinicians are recommended to ask patients about alcohol use and provide brief interventions and specialist referral, this is poorly implemented in routine practice. We undertook a national consultation to ascertain the appropriateness of proposed standards for recording information about alcohol use in electronic health records (EHRs) in the UK and to identify potential barriers and facilitators to their implementation in practice.

Methods: A wide range of stakeholders in the UK were consulted about the appropriateness of proposed information standards for recording alcohol use in EHRs via a multi-disciplinary stakeholder workshop and online survey. Responses to the survey were thematically analysed using the Consolidated Framework for Implementation Research.

Results: Thirty-one stakeholders participated in the workshop and 100 in the online survey. This included patients and carers, healthcare professionals, researchers, public health specialists, informaticians, and clinical information system suppliers. There was broad consensus that the Alcohol Use Disorders Identification Test (AUDIT) and AUDIT-Consumption (AUDIT-C) questionnaires were appropriate standards for recording alcohol use in EHRs but that the standards should also address interventions for alcohol misuse. Stakeholders reported a number of factors that might influence implementation of the standards, including having clear care pathways and an implementation guide, sharing information about alcohol use between health service providers, adequately resourcing the implementation process, integrating alcohol screening with existing clinical pathways, having good clinical information systems and IT infrastructure, providing financial incentives, having sufficient training for healthcare workers, and clinical leadership and engagement. Implementation of the standards would need to ensure patients are not stigmatised and that patient confidentiality is robustly maintained.

Conclusions: A wide range of stakeholders agreed that use of AUDIT-C and AUDIT are appropriate standards for recording alcohol use in EHRs in addition to recording interventions for alcohol misuse. The findings of this consultation will be used to develop an appropriate information model and implementation guide. Further research is needed to pilot the standards in primary and secondary care.

Keywords: Alcohol, Electronic health records, Information standards, Consolidated framework for implementation research, Consultation

* Correspondence: s.haroon@bham.ac.uk
[1]Institute of Applied Health Research, College of Medical and Dental
Sciences, University of Birmingham, Edgbaston, Birmingham B15 2TT, UK
Full list of author information is available at the end of the article

Background

Alcohol misuse remains a major cause of preventable disability and death and disproportionately affects those living in the most socioeconomically deprived areas [1]. In 2015 there were 8758 alcohol-related deaths in the UK and the rate of alcohol-related deaths has remained unchanged in recent years [2]. Health and care services have a role in identifying alcohol misuse among patients and providing brief interventions [3]. This has been shown to be effective at reducing alcohol misuse particularly in men seen in primary and secondary healthcare services [4, 5]. It may even reduce mortality among heavy alcohol users admitted to hospital [5]. However, recording information about alcohol use using validated measures in both primary and secondary care remains poor [6, 7].

The UK Academy of Medical Royal Colleges (AoMRC) standards for the clinical structure and content of patient records recommends recording information about alcohol use in the social context of the medical history [8]. However, it does not specify how this information should be recorded and there are currently no widely endorsed and validated standards pertaining to this. Consequently, researchers and clinicians at the University of Birmingham and Queen Elizabeth Hospital Birmingham, in partnership with the Royal College of Physicians Health Informatics Unit, embarked on a project to develop information standards for recording alcohol use in electronic health records (EHRs) in the UK. The objectives of the standards were as follows:

- Enable healthcare staff and clinical information systems to identify patients at risk of alcohol misuse, and provide preventative and therapeutic interventions.
- Is relevant to public health and healthcare organisations to inform commissioning and delivery of preventative services and clinical audit of health promotion practices.
- Enables epidemiological and clinical research on alcohol consumption among patients in primary and secondary care.
- Enables patient-relevant information to be shared across the health and care system to improve coordination and continuity of care.

To inform the proposed standards, an evidence review was conducted on alcohol screening in secondary care (unpublished but available upon request) [9]. This review included 97 articles, which evaluated a total of 38 screening tests. This identified that the Alcohol Use Disorders Identification Test (AUDIT) [10, 11] and AUDIT-Consumption questions (AUDIT-C, which consists of the first three questions of the full AUDIT questionnaire) [12] were the most widely validated screening tools for alcohol misuse, and had been evaluated in a total of 26 and 16 studies, respectively. They both demonstrated a high uptake (75%, 95% CI 64–85% based on a meta-analysis of 10 studies) in a range of clinical settings as well as high sensitivity (ranging from 72 to 100%) and specificity (71–100% for AUDIT and 72–77% for AUDIT-C) for alcohol misuse. We therefore proposed that all patients accessing healthcare have their alcohol use recorded in EHRs using AUDIT-C as standard and that those with a high score complete the full AUDIT questions at some point in their care. We consulted stakeholders nationally to ascertain the appropriateness of the proposed standards and to identify potential barriers and facilitators to their implementation in practice.

Methods

This was a qualitative analysis of responses to a national consultation on proposed information standards for recording alcohol use in EHRs. A consultation workshop was held at the Royal College of Physicians in London on 25th July 2016 to obtain the views of a wide range of stakeholders on the appropriateness of the proposed standards. Stakeholders were identified by the Royal College of Physicians Health Informatics Unit and the project team. They were invited from a range of relevant professional bodies (including medical royal colleges) and organisations representing patients and carers, clinicians, informaticians, public health specialists, and clinical information system suppliers. Attendees were provided background information on the proposed information standards and presented with the AUDIT and AUDIT-C questionnaires. They were asked to comment on their appropriateness as potential information standards for recording alcohol use in electronic health records and were asked five key questions (although participants were given the opportunity to comment beyond the scope of those questions):

1. How appropriate are the information standards?
2. What are the barriers to implementing the standards?
3. What are the facilitators to implementing the standards?
4. How might the standards be used to improve patient care?
5. Are there any patient safety issues with recording information in this way?

An online survey was launched on 17th January and closed on 05th March 2017 and disseminated to a wider range of stakeholders with the same questions and a number of additional questions that arose during the stakeholder workshop. A link to the consultation was also hosted on the Royal College of Physicians website. A full list of questions included in the online survey is provided in Additional file 1. All responses were anonymous, although basic information was captured about each respondent's profession. The survey was disseminated to stakeholders via a number of different communication channels including targeted emails, bulletins, newsletters, and social media.

Responses from the survey were extracted onto an Excel spreadsheet and thematically analysed by a single researcher (SH) using the Consolidated Framework for Implementation Research (CFIR) [13]. The raw data and the validity of the coding was then checked by a second investigator (LM). This was followed by a discussion to reach consensus on the coding scheme and the mapping of the codes to the CFIR. While there is a subjective element to coding and that some of the themes could also be placed elsewhere or overlap with other constructs, a consensus was reached on the most suitable coding scheme. The CFIR was used as a pragmatic framework for constructing a mind map to visually conceptualise and organise the emerging concepts and themes. The CFIR was specifically chosen because it brings together a number of important conceptual frameworks for implementation research and was recommended by an external collaborator with expertise in implementation science. The CFIR has five main domains, each having a number of underlying constructs: intervention characteristics, inner setting (context within the organisation through which the process of implementation will take place), outer setting (external context in which an organisation sits), characteristics of the individuals involved, and the process of implementation.

Results

Participants

Thirty-one stakeholders participated in the stakeholder consultation workshop and 100 participated in the online survey (Table 1). This included patients and carers, healthcare professionals, public health specialists, informaticians, researchers, and clinical information system suppliers. Their responses to the consultation are summarised below, thematically grouped by the CFIR domains and constructs (Table 2). Selected quotes and a mind map of the thematic analysis are also provided in Additional files 1 and 2.

Intervention

Relative advantage

A number of respondents highlighted the importance of the information standards being evidence based and demonstrating patient benefit. A number of advantages were reported of the proposed standards over the current, unstructured approach to recording information

about alcohol use, including improving the accuracy of estimating patients' alcohol use. AUDIT and AUDIT-C were viewed as objective measures that can standardise and improve the consistency in the way alcohol use is recorded by health services. Implementation of the proposed standards could normalise the process of taking an alcohol history and familiarise clinicians with the appropriate questions to ask about alcohol use. This could also improve communication between healthcare providers and patients about alcohol-related risk. It could provide clinicians, patients, researchers, and policy makers with a shared definition and understanding of alcohol misuse.

Participants reported that the information standards could be used to improve the identification of patients at risk of alcohol misuse and improve access to relevant interventions and services. They could facilitate the implementation of alcohol screening and brief interventions in health services, the provision of general health promotion about alcohol use, and help link alcohol support services with patients. They could also help identify patients who are at risk of alcohol withdrawal and aid

Table 1 Number of participants in the online survey by profession

Profession	N
Physician	51
General practitioner	7
Surgeon	5
Academic	4
Patient	4
Public health specialist	4
Midwife	3
Allied health professional	2
Data specialist	2
Healthcare manager	2
Homeopath	2
Nurse	2
System supplier	2
Alcohol trainer and consultant	1
Clinical informatician	1
Dental consultant	1
Dual Diagnosis Care Manager/Trainer	1
Healthcare commissioner	1
Paediatrician	1
Pharmacist	1
PhD student	1
Psychiatrist	1
Social enterprise founder	1
Total	100

Table 2 Summary of consultation findings

Domain	Construct	Description
Intervention	Relative advantage	Evidence based and validated
		Standardised and consistent
		Facilitate screening and brief interventions
		Diagnostic, prognostic, and social information
		Prescribing – drug interactions with alcohol
		Early recognition of alcohol withdrawal
		Temporal trends in alcohol use
		Audit, needs assessment, and research
	Adaptability – core components	Brief and simple
		User-friendly EHR interface
		Standard template
		Visual depiction of alcohol units
		Instant access to results and interpretation
		Frequency of recording is context dependent
		Lower AUDIT-C thresholds in pregnancy
		Age criteria
		Patient confidentiality
	Adaptability – adaptable periphery	Care pathways and support services
		Link with mental health services
		Wide range of health settings and health professionals potentially involved
		Self-completion of alcohol screening
		Direct patient access to EHRs and personal health records
		Inclusion in summary care records
		Electronic prompts for clinicians
	Other considerations	Costs and resources
		Piloting
Inner setting	Implementation climate	Integration with routine processes
		Clinical judgement
		Administrative burden
		Implementation of EHRs
		Integration of clinical information systems across health services
		IT infrastructure and digital connectivity
		Data governance
		Automation of care pathways
		Alignment with clinical coding standards and information models
		Organisational support and clear policy
		Clinical leadership
		Perceived importance among clinicians
		Financial incentives
		Key performance indicators
	Readiness for implementation	Training healthcare staff
		Implementation guide
		Access to EHRs
	Culture	Professional and cultural attitudes towards alcohol use

Table 2 Summary of consultation findings *(Continued)*

Domain	Construct	Description
		Perception of usual practice
		Normalise alcohol screening and brief interventions in practice
	Networks, communication, and structural factors	Communication of benefits and relevance to clinicians and patients
		Sensitive and non-judgemental communication
		Clear information on care pathways and best practice
		Integration of alcohol and mental health services
Outer setting	Patient needs and resources	Underreporting of alcohol use
		Stigma
		Poor understanding of alcohol units
		Confidentiality
		Consent for data sharing between healthcare providers
		Association with poor mental health
		Adverse implications for life insurance, driving, and employment
		Bias future clinical assessments
	External policies and incentives	Clinical guidelines
		Alcohol health campaigns
		Low risk drinking guidelines
		Financial incentives
		Key performance indicators
		Labelling of alcohol units lacking
	Cosmopolitanism and peer pressure	Communication and data sharing between health services
		Coordination and continuity of care
		Influence of peers in primary care

early prescription of alcohol withdrawal medication. The standards could potentially also improve access to mental health services and social care, and could be useful for identifying and managing cases of domestic violence, since alcohol misuse is an important risk factor.

Participants also commented that the standards could provide important diagnostic and social information and be useful for drug prescribing by highlighting potential drug-alcohol interactions. It may also have prognostic value by helping to estimate the risk of having or developing alcohol-related conditions. The quantitative nature of the proposed information standards (AUDIT-C or AUDIT score) would also enable access to temporal trends, which could help clinicians monitor alcohol use in their patients over time.

Implementation of the standards could improve the quality of data on alcohol use in EHRs. This would benefit epidemiological research and surveillance, allowing the derivation of more complete information on alcohol-related harms that could be accessed by patients, clinicians, public health specialists, and policymakers. The data could also be used for clinical audit, service evaluation, and quality improvement of alcohol support services.

Adaptability
Core components
Participants described a number of core features that the information standards should meet. This included the need for the standards to be brief and simple, with particular consideration to how alcohol units are communicated and understood. The wording of the screening questions should be simplified as far as possible, particularly when self-completion by patients is expected. Respondents highlighted the importance of the EHR interface being user-friendly, with the standards embedded in a standard template that includes a visual display of alcohol units as well as the date of last entry. Clinicians using the template should also have instant access to the results and their interpretation.

A number of comments were also made about the frequency of recording alcohol use. Several respondents emphasised that the frequency should be evidence-based and not so frequent that patients are aggravated and disproportionate opportunity costs are incurred, or so infrequent that the information is out-of-date. Some felt that information about alcohol use should be updated at fixed, regular intervals, while others felt that the frequency should be dynamic, based on clinical judgement (e.g. where risks of alcohol-related harm have been identified or major life events have been reported), on the basis of previous scores, with higher scores requiring more frequent recording than lower scores, and based on age, with younger patients requiring more frequent recording than older patients. Respondents also felt it would be beneficial for clinicians to ask about alcohol use when prescribing medications that interact with alcohol, and also when making mental health assessments.

The frequency of recording was also felt to be dependent on the health setting and context. For acute hospital admissions, a range of opinions were expressed from recording information about alcohol use in all acute episodes to only recording information for overtly alcohol-related admissions, or where patients are previously known to have problems with alcohol misuse. Similarly, some respondents felt that alcohol use should be asked at all outpatient visits while others felt that it would only need updating annually or based on clinical judgement. In primary care, respondents varied in how frequently they felt that information on alcohol use should be asked, ranging from every 1 to 10 years, and also at NHS health checks.

There was more consistency in views about recording information about alcohol use among women attending antenatal appointments, particularly during the first booking visit. Respondents felt thereafter that pregnant women could be asked about their alcohol use based on the clinical judgement of their midwife, at every antenatal visit, or specifically around the second or third trimester of pregnancy. Respondents also felt that AUDIT-C score thresholds should be lowered in pregnancy to align with the advice to be teetotal during pregnancy.

A number of comments also concerned the eligible population that the standards should apply to. Generally respondents felt that they would be appropriate for patients aged 16 years and older and potentially in those aged 10–16 years where alcohol misuse was being suspected, although this would require sensitive handling and would entail issues around obtaining parental consent. The standards were felt to be inappropriate for patients under the age of 10 years, during end-of-life care, and for patients with learning difficulties. Respondents also expressed the importance of ensuring patient confidentiality and where possible providing a private consultation setting when asking patients about their alcohol use.

Adaptable periphery

Some respondents emphasised the importance of having a whole systems approach to reducing alcohol-related harm, of which the information standards would form one component. The information standards were generally only considered to be useful in the presence of

appropriate care pathways and support services. This included the availability of alcohol liaison specialists and support workers, proactive signposting of patients to support services, provision of appropriate patient information, a clear process for management and referral, and for mental health assessment and treatment. Some respondents therefore felt that the information standards should incorporate some items related to recording the management of alcohol misuse.

A number of health settings were considered appropriate for the implementation of the standards including general practice and outpatient departments, with particular emphasis on making use of waiting rooms to gather relevant information prior to appointments. Other suggested settings included emergency care, medical and surgical assessment units, inpatient hospital wards, antenatal clinics, mental health services, pharmacies, sexual health clinics, dental practices, community nursing, addiction services, social care, health visiting, school nursing, paramedics, and paediatric services. Respondents generally felt that nurses, junior doctors, GPs, alcohol support workers, consultants, healthcare assistants, midwives, and even non-health professionals (e.g. social workers) had a responsibility for collecting information about their patient or client's alcohol use.

A number of respondents expressed the importance of patients being able to directly provide information about alcohol use, either by having access to their EHRs or personal health records, [14] or by paper-based questionnaires (including postal) or scratch cards that would later be entered onto their health records. Patient access to EHRs would require the development of appropriate online digital platforms (e.g. web portals or smartphone apps), and could include use of tablet computers or fixed computer terminals in waiting rooms. Digital platforms could be designed to help patients estimate their alcohol units and completion of the standards by patients could be encouraged through digital prompts. However this would require a degree of digital skills which not all patients would necessarily have and all modalities would require strict data protection and protect patient confidentiality.

Most respondents to the online survey agreed that the information standards should be incorporated into summary care records, provided that patient confidentiality was sufficiently protected. The summary care record is a copy of key information from the primary care record. It provides authorised care professionals with faster, secure access to essential information about patients when they need care. A smaller majority of respondents felt that the standards could be included in discharge summaries, although this was felt to be dependent on gaining patient consent, and when alcohol misuse was deemed to be relevant to the presenting problem, and was specifically identified during the clinical episode. Some respondents also felt that clinical information systems could be programmed to prompt healthcare providers to ask patients about alcohol use.

Other considerations concerning the intervention

Participants also commented on considering the costs of implementing the information standards, including the time taken for staff to ask about alcohol use, the resources needed to train staff on alcohol screening and brief interventions, and the cost of employing staff to provide alcohol support and associated administrative support. Respondents also highlighted the costs that would be associated with updating and adapting multiple clinical information systems with the information standards. Some also suggested that the standards could be piloted to ensure their feasibility in practice.

Inner setting

Implementation climate

A number of issues were raised about the implementation of the information standards in health settings. This principally concerned integration with routine processes, IT systems and infrastructure, and administrative burden. Respondents felt that the standards were more likely to be successfully implemented if completion was integrated with the admission pathway in secondary care, including nursing and medical clerking. In primary care, it was generally felt to be appropriate to include completion of the standards as part of GP registration. There was also felt to be an important role for clinical judgement in determining when it would be appropriate to ask about alcohol use and complete the screening questions. The additional administrative burden associated with capturing information about alcohol use and making referrals to alcohol support services would also have to be accounted for when planning the implementation of the standards.

IT systems and infrastructure were seen to be key factors that would determine the likely success of implementing the alcohol information standards in practice. This included the degree of implementation of EHRs, the integration of clinical information systems and shared EHRs across all elements of the health system (avoiding duplication of data entry), access to EHRs using mobile devices such as tablet computers, and ready patient access to EHRs and personal health records [14] to enable self-completion of information about alcohol use. Respondents also highlighted the importance of digital connectivity in health settings, as well as data security and governance (requiring patient consent for data sharing), standardisation of clinical coding, and the development of clinical information systems to automate referrals and signposting to support services. Variability in the current coding of alcohol use was seen as a barrier to understanding patient need. Some respondents also added that it was important to ensure the information standards were compatible with existing clinical coding standards and information models such as OpenEHR [15] and the national maternity and cancer information sets [16, 17].

A number of cultural and organisational factors that would influence implementation were also highlighted. This included the relative priority given by an organisation for delivering alcohol screening and brief interventions. Implementation of the standards would require organisational support, clinical leadership, and the provision of a clear policy for asking patients about their alcohol use using the recommended standards, as well as providing appropriate interventions. This would also depend on the perceived importance among clinicians of alcohol misuse in their patients and their role in preventing alcohol-related harm. Clinical champions potentially have an important role in fostering the clinical engagement needed for successful implementation in practice.

A number of organisational incentives and rewards were identified that might influence the implementation of the standards. Two key financial incentives include the Quality and Outcomes Framework (QOF) in primary care, [18] and Commissioning for Quality and Innovation (CQUIN) in secondary care [19]. Both are financial incentive schemes for achieving specific healthcare processes and outcomes in England. There are currently no QOF outcomes specifically related to recording alcohol use (except in the context of bipolar and psychotic disorders) or delivering brief interventions. However, the most recent CQUIN for England includes outcomes specific to alcohol screening and providing brief advice or referral in hospitals [19]. Some respondents suggested that implementation of the standards could also potentially be facilitated by healthcare organisations making them a mandatory requirement or by including related outcomes as part of their key performance indicators.

Readiness for implementation

A number of factors were reported by participants that could influence the readiness for implementation of the information standards in healthcare organisations. Respondents highlighted the importance of access to relevant information and knowledge, including healthcare staff having access to training on alcohol identification and brief advice. In order to implement the standards in practice, healthcare staff will need to have the necessary knowledge, skills, and confidence to ask patients about their alcohol use. An implementation guide was also viewed as important to provide operational clarity and should be targeted and adapted for both clinical information system suppliers and healthcare providers.

Respondents also commented on the importance of healthcare staff having the necessary level of digital literacy to use EHRs effectively in their practice and to have ready access to EHRs so that information about alcohol use can be recorded with relative ease.

Culture

Respondents felt that professional and cultural attitudes towards alcohol could influence the successful implementation of the data standards. Alcohol consumption and misuse among health professionals could plausibly reduce the likelihood of them asking their patients' about alcohol use. Similarly clinicians' perception of what constitutes usual practice, and viewing alcohol screening as beyond that, could act as a barrier to implementing the standards. Conversely, successful implementation of the standards in routine practice could help normalise alcohol screening and brief interventions in health and care services.

Networks, communication, and structural factors

Participants stressed the importance of clearly communicating the benefits of alcohol screening and brief interventions to both clinicians and patients. Patients would need to be explained why they were asked about alcohol use when presenting with unrelated (or seemingly unrelated) conditions, and that the information should be asked in a sensitive and non-judgemental way. Clinicians would also need to be informed of the available care pathways and guidance on best practice. A number of participants also expressed that implementation of the standards could be facilitated by better integration of alcohol and mental health services.

Outer setting

Patient needs and resources

Participants raised several patient-related factors that might influence the implementation of the information standards. A number highlighted the stigma associated with alcohol misuse and the importance of patient confidentiality. Patients may underreport their alcohol use for this reason but also because of a poor understanding of alcohol units. Conversely, implementation of the standards could help patients gain a better understanding of their level of alcohol use in relation to national guidelines [20]. The way information about alcohol use is ascertained will need to be acceptable to patients and culturally sensitive. Consent would need to be obtained for sharing this information with other healthcare providers. Participants also reported that healthcare providers would need to consider mental health when assessing patients for alcohol misuse since alcohol misuse frequently occurs in the context of poor mental health.

A number of potential adverse impacts were also identified from implementing the standards. Participants reported that information about alcohol misuse could have implications for life insurance, medical reports for the Driving and Vehicle Licence Authority (DVLA), prospects for employment, and interactions with the criminal justice system. If patients objected to having this information asked and recorded in their health records, this might negatively impact on their relationship with clinical services. Records of alcohol misuse could also potentially bias future clinical assessments towards diagnosing alcohol-related disorders.

External policies and incentives

A number of external policies and incentives that could influence the implementation of the alcohol information standards were highlighted. The National Institute for Health and Care Excellence (NICE) guidelines on prevention of alcohol-use disorders, [3] the NHS Digital Strategy, [21] and alcohol-related health campaigns, were all seen as potential facilitators. Similarly, implementation of the standards could help put the NICE guidelines on prevention of alcohol-use disorders into practice. Participants also felt that the standards should align with the UK Chief Medical Officers' low risk drinking guidelines [20]. Incorporation of outcomes on alcohol screening and brief interventions in key performance indicators for healthcare organisations could promote use of the standards, as could financial incentives such as the national CQUIN in England [19], as well as developing similar financial incentives for primary care. Beyond the context of health and care services, the lack of clear labelling of alcohol units on alcoholic beverages was seen as a barrier to implementation of the standards, since this impeded public understanding of alcohol intake and recommended low risk limits.

Cosmopolitanism and peer pressure

Implementation of the information standards could also be influenced by, or potentially facilitate communication and data sharing about alcohol use between primary care, secondary care, public health and other elements of the health service. This could potentially improve coordination and continuity of care for patients with alcohol misuse and facilitate an integrated approach to preventing further harms. Finally, awareness of local general practices actively implementing the standards and providing alcohol screening and brief interventions in primary care could potentially influence GPs to implement the standards in their own practices.

Discussion

Main findings

In this national consultation of 131 stakeholders, participants broadly agreed that recording the AUDIT-C and the full AUDIT questionnaire for patients with a high

AUDIT-C score, is an appropriate standard for recording information about alcohol use in EHRs. Participants also agreed that the standard should include some items about the management of patients identified as at-risk of alcohol misuse. Implementing this standard could improve the early identification of alcohol misuse, the delivery of brief interventions, and access to specialist services. They could also have a number of secondary uses for improving service quality, healthcare commissioning, and epidemiological research.

A number of factors were identified that are likely to influence the implementation of the standards in practice. In particular, the standards will need to be brief and simple and embedded within EHRs as a standard template with a visual illustration of alcohol units and will require clear care pathways for individuals identified with a high risk of alcohol misuse. The frequency of recording information about alcohol use will be context dependent and will vary by setting and prior risk. The standards are likely to be applicable in a wide range of health settings for patients aged 16 years and older and potentially in those aged 10 to 16 years where alcohol misuse is suspected.

The standards would work best if they were communicated effectively between primary and secondary care (through summary care records) as well as other relevant aspects of the health and care service to provide a more integrated approach to managing and preventing alcohol misuse. However, information sharing across the health service will require robust data governance and acquisition of patient consent. Implementation of the standards will require additional healthcare resources to cover training, support services, and development of clinical information systems.

Implementation of the standards could be facilitated by integrating them with existing clinical pathways, improving the accessibility of EHRs, and by providing training on alcohol screening and brief interventions, as well as a clear implementation guide. Organisational support and clinical engagement, implementation of relevant NICE guidelines, [3] and external financial incentives, would also encourage the implementation of the standards. The implementation strategy will also need to consider the stigma associated with alcohol misuse, the importance of ensuring patient confidentiality, under-reporting of alcohol use, and the cultural attitudes towards alcohol among both patients and health and care professionals.

Relationship to other studies

An analysis of free-text documentation of alcohol use in the social context module of EHRs in an academic hospital in the USA found that users had difficulty documenting alcohol use frequency, amount, and status within structured fields [22]. Free-text descriptions of frequency were commonly used, using variable terms and a significant proportion of those with suggestions of alcohol misuse did not have this documented in their past medical history or problem list. The authors highlighted the importance of improving clinical information systems, user training, decision support, and information standards to improve the documentation of alcohol use in EHRs. Participants in our consultation similarly reported that recording information about alcohol use in clinical records was currently highly variable and unstructured and that the development of standards could help improve the consistency of recording. Furthermore the quantitative nature of AUDIT-C and AUDIT should help clinicians record information about quantity and frequency of alcohol consumption using a more structured and validated approach.

A systematic review and meta-analysis of the clinical recognition and recording of alcohol disorders in primary care found that GPs were able to identify alcohol use disorders in 42% of cases, but recorded this correctly in only 27% of primary care records [23]. Secondary care clinicians were found to identify alcohol use disorders in 52% of cases and recorded this correctly in only 37% of medical records. The authors recommended considering the use of simple screening methods rather than relying solely on clinical judgement for identifying alcohol-related problems. This aligns with views expressed by stakeholders in our consultation that a more systematic approach is needed to identify alcohol misuse and fits with the proposed recommendations to use AUDIT-C and AUDIT as screening questions to incorporate within EHRs as the standard approach to asking patients about alcohol use.

Strengths and limitations

A large number of stakeholders from a wide range of relevant professions (including patients and carers) and organisations were consulted to inform the proposed standards for recording information about alcohol use in EHRs. The Consolidated Framework for Implementation Research was used to thematically analyse the responses, which provided a predefined and validated conceptual framework for organising the findings.

However, the findings of this consultation are prone to response bias since the stakeholders who accepted our invitation to participate are likely to have an interest in preventing and managing alcohol misuse and related disorders. The views expressed by the participants may therefore not necessarily reflect those of all patients, clinicians, and service providers. Furthermore, the majority of participants were physicians, which is likely due to the consultation being hosted by the Royal College of Physicians. The interpretation and analysis of the responses may also have been influenced by the authors who are all involved in a national project to develop information standards for recording alcohol use in EHRs. Finally, the proposed information standards were not evaluated by stakeholders against all the implementation considerations that arose from this consultation. This would be worth considering for future research. In addition, future work could assess the views of stakeholders on the relative utility of alternative screening tools for alcohol misuse.

Implications for policy, practice, and research

The findings of this consultation support use of AUDIT-C and AUDIT as information standards for recording alcohol use in EHRs. The findings will be used to develop an appropriate information model that can be used by system suppliers to implement the standards in clinical information systems and to develop an implementation guide for clinicians, service providers, and system suppliers. The proposed standards will need to be piloted in primary and secondary care to ensure that it can be feasibly implemented in real world practice and linked to appropriate care pathways. Further research will also be needed to evaluate how they can be best used to systematise the delivery of brief interventions and specialist referral for alcohol support in health and care services.

Conclusions

A wide range of stakeholders agree that use of AUDIT-C is a useful standard for recording information about alcohol use in EHRs among patients accessing health services and that AUDIT should be used for further risk assessment in those identified as at-risk of alcohol misuse. Further work is needed to incorporate the findings of this consultation into an information model and implementation guide and to pilot the proposed standards in primary and secondary healthcare settings.

Abbreviations

AoMRC: Academy of Medical Royal Colleges; AUDIT: Alcohol Use Disorders Identification Test; AUDIT-C: Alcohol Use Disorders Identification Test-Consumption; CFIR: Consolidated Framework for Implementation Research; CQUIN: Commissioning for Quality and Innovation; DVLA: Driving and Vehicle Licence Authority; EHR: electronic health record; IT: Information technology; NICE: National Institute for Health and Care Excellence; QOF: Quality and Outcomes Framework

Acknowledgements

We would like to thank all the stakeholders who participated in this consultation and the staff at the Royal College of Physicians Health Informatics Unit for hosting the stakeholder workshop and online survey. We would also like to thank Zarnie Khadjesari (Senior Postdoctoral Research Fellow Implementation Science, Kings College London) for advising us on the use of the Consolidated Framework for Implementation Research.

Funding

Funding to enable patient participation was provided by the NIHR Patient Involvement Fund.

Authors' contributions

SH, DW, JH, NB, KN, and JW jointly conceived the idea for this consultation. SH, DW, and JH drafted the survey, and DW and JH coordinated its dissemination. SH analysed the findings and wrote the manuscript with input from all co-authors. LM independently checked the analysis. All authors read and approved the manuscript.

Competing interests

The authors declare that they have no competing interest.

Author details

[1]Institute of Applied Health Research, College of Medical and Dental Sciences, University of Birmingham, Edgbaston, Birmingham B15 2TT, UK. [2]Health Informatics Unit, Royal College of Physicians, 11 St Andrews Place, Regent's Park, London NW1 4LE, UK. [3]Public Health Specialty Registrar, West Midlands, UK. [4]Queen Elizabeth Hospital Birmingham, Mindelsohn Way, Birmingham B15 2TH, UK.

References

1. Rehm J, Mathers C, Popova S, Thavorncharoensap M, Teerawattananon Y, Patra J. Global burden of disease and injury and economic cost attributable to alcohol use and alcohol-use disorders. Lancet. 2009;373:2223–33. Available from: http://www.ncbi.nlm.nih.gov/pubmed/19560604 Cited 24 Apr 2017
2. Campbell A. Alcohol-related deaths in the UK: registered in 2015 . Newport; 2015. Available from: https://www.ons.gov.uk/peoplepopulationandcommunity/healthandsocialcare/causesofdeath/bulletins/alcoholrelateddeathsintheunitedkingdom/registeredin2015
3. Alcohol-use disorders: prevention | Guidance and guidelines | NICE. NICE; Available from: https://www.nice.org.uk/guidance/ph24 Cited 24 Apr 2017.
4. Kaner EFS, Dickinson HO, Beyer FR, Campbell F, Schlesinger C, Heather N, et al. Effectiveness of brief alcohol interventions in primary care populations. Cochrane Database Syst Rev. 2007; Available from: https://doi.org/10.1002/14651858.CD004148.pub3 Cited 24 Apr 2017
5. McQueen J, Howe TE, Allan L, Mains D, Hardy V. Brief interventions for heavy alcohol users admitted to general hospital wards. Cochrane Database Syst Rev. 2011; Available from: https://doi.org/10.1002/14651858.CD005191.pub3 Cited 24 Apr 2017
6. Khadjesari Z, Marston L, Petersen I, Nazareth I, Walters K. Alcohol consumption screening of newly-registered patients in primary care: a cross-sectional analysis. Br J Gen Pract. 2013;63:e706–12. Available from: http://www.ncbi.nlm.nih.gov/pubmed/24152486 Cited 24 Apr 2017
7. Lee DJ, Knuckey S, Cook GA. Changes in Health Promot Pract in hospitals across England: the National Health Promotion in Hospital Audit 2009 and 2011. J Public Health. 2014;36:651–7. Available from: https://academic.oup.com/jpubhealth/article-lookup/doi/10.1093/pubmed/fdt120 Cited Apr 2017 24
8. Standards for the clinical structure and content of patient records [Internet]. London; 2015. Available from: https://www.rcplondon.ac.uk/projects/outputs/standards-clinical-structure-and-content-patient-records
9. Walsh S, Haroon S, Nirantharakumar K, Bhala N. Approaches to alcohol screening in secondary care: a review and meta-analysis. Lancet. 2017:390–S92. Available from: http://linkinghub.elsevier.com/retrieve/pii/S0140673617330271
10. Babor TF, Higgins-Biddle JC, Saunders JB, Monteiro MG. The Alcohol Use Disorders Identification Test Guidelines for Use in Primary Care. ; Available from: http://apps.who.int/iris/bitstream/10665/67205/1/WHO_MSD_MSB_01.6a.pdf Cited 24 Apr 2017.
11. Saunders JB, Aasland OG, Babor TF, De La Fuente JR, Grant M. Development of the Alcohol Use Disorders Identification Test (AUDIT): WHO Collaborative Project on Early Detection of Persons with Harmful Alcohol Consumption-II. AddictionBlackwell Publishing Ltd; 1993 ;88:791–804. Available from: https://doi.org/10.1111/j.1360-0443.1993.tb02093.x. Cited 8 Jun 2017

12. Bush K, Kivlahan DR, McDonell MB, Fihn SD, Bradley KA. For the ambulatory care quality improvement project (ACQUIP). The AUDIT alcohol consumption questions (AUDIT-C). Arch. Interal Med. 1998;158:1789–95.

13. Damschroder LJ, Aron DC, Keith RE, Kirsh SR, Alexander JA, Lowery JC, et al. Fostering implementation of health services research findings into practice: a consolidated framework for advancing implementation science. BioMed Central. 2009; Available from: https://implementationscience.biomedcentral.com/articles/10.1186/1748-5908-4-50. Cited 24 Apr 2017.

14. Wyatt J, Sathanandam S, Rastall P, Hoogewerf J, Wooldridge D. Personal health record (PHR) - Landsc Rev. London; 2016. Available from: https://www.rcplondon.ac.uk/projects/outputs/personal-health-record-phr-landscape-review.

15. openEHR [Internet]. [cited 2017 Apr 24]. Available from: http://www.openehr.org/

16. Maternity Services Secondary Uses Data Set. NHS Digital; [cited 2017 Jul Available from21].http://content.digital.nhs.uk/maternityandchildren/maternity.

17. Cancer Outcomes and Services Dataset (COSD). Public Heal. Engl. 2017 [cited 2017 Jul 21]. Available from: http://www.ncin.org.uk/collecting_and_using_data/data_collection/cosd

18. NHS Digital, 1 Trevelyan Square, Boar Lane, Leeds, LS1 6AE UK. Quality and Outcomes Framework [Internet]. NHS Digital, 1 Trevelyan Square, Boar Lane, Leeds, LS1 6AE, United Kingdom; Available from: https://digital.nhs.uk/data-and-information/data-collections-and-data-sets/data-collections/quality-and-outcomes-framework-qof. Cited Apr 25 2017.

19. NHS England » 2017/19 CQUIN . Available from: https://www.england.nhs.uk/nhs-standard-contract/cquin/cquin-17-19/

20. UK Chief Medical Officers' Low Risk Drinking Guidelines . 2016. Available from: https://www.gov.uk/government/uploads/system/uploads/attachment_data/file/545937/UK_CMOs__report.pdf

21. Our Strategy - NHS Digital. 2015 . Available from: https://digital.nhs.uk/article/249/Our-Strategy

22. Chen E, Garcia-Webb M. An analysis of free-text alcohol use documentation in the electronic health record: early findings and implications. Appl Clin Inform. 2014;5:402–15. Available from: http://www.ncbi.nlm.nih.gov/pubmed/25024757 Cited 24 Apr 2017

23. Mitchell AJ, Meader N, Bird V, Rizzo M. Clinical recognition and recording of alcohol disorders by clinicians in primary and secondary care: meta-analysis. Br J Psychiatry. 2012;201 Available from: http://bjp.rcpsych.org/content/201/2/93.full Cited 24 Apr 2017

5

Time series model for forecasting the number of new admission inpatients

Lingling Zhou, Ping Zhao, Dongdong Wu, Cheng Cheng and Hao Huang*(iD)

Abstract

Background: Hospital crowding is a rising problem, effective predicting and detecting managment can helpful to reduce crowding. Our team has successfully proposed a hybrid model combining both the autoregressive integrated moving average (ARIMA) and the nonlinear autoregressive neural network (NARNN) models in the schistosomiasis and hand, foot, and mouth disease forecasting study. In this paper, our aim is to explore the application of the hybrid ARIMA-NARNN model to track the trends of the new admission inpatients, which provides a methodological basis for reducing crowding.

Methods: We used the single seasonal ARIMA (SARIMA), NARNN and the hybrid SARIMA-NARNN model to fit and forecast the monthly and daily number of new admission inpatients. The root mean square error (RMSE), mean absolute error (MAE) and mean absolute percentage error (MAPE) were used to compare the forecasting performance among the three models. The modeling time range of monthly data included was from January 2010 to June 2016, July to October 2016 as the corresponding testing data set. The daily modeling data set was from January 4 to September 4, 2016, while the testing time range included was from September 5 to October 2, 2016.

Results: For the monthly data, the modeling RMSE and the testing RMSE, MAE and MAPE of SARIMA-NARNN model were less than those obtained from the single SARIMA or NARNN model, but the MAE and MAPE of modeling performance of SARIMA-NARNN model did not improve. For the daily data, all RMSE, MAE and MAPE of NARNN model were the lowest both in modeling stage and testing stage.

Conclusions: Hybrid model does not necessarily outperform its constituents' performances. It is worth attempting to explore the reliable model to forecast the number of new admission inpatients from different data.

Keywords: New admission inpatients, Time series forecasting, SARIMA model, NARNN model, Hybrid model

Background

With an increasing global population and economy, the demand for healthcare continues to rise. Hospital crowding has become a major problem faced by large hospitals. Hospital adverse events increase with crowding, and have further effects on patient satisfaction, quality of nursing, treatment, wait time, and length of stay [1–4]. A vast literature about overcrowding focus on the outpatient wards [1, 5] and emergence departments [4, 6]. Overcrowding appearing in the inpatient wards should also be paid attention to. When no inpatient beds are available to

admit new inpatients, overcrowding would occur. Often, inpatient beds may be scarce as a result of too many patients with non-urgent medical conditions seeking healthcare.

The prediction of admissions is one piece of larger equation in the using hospital census, patient acuity, disease burden, allocation of resources and general management to improve hospital performance and improve patient outcomes. Much of research on hospital management focuses on the emergence of demand predicting [7–10], forecasting of outpatient visits [11, 12], inpatients discharge [13], and patient volume [14]. However, little published research is available regarding predicting the number of new admission inpatients. Monitoring and forecasting for new admission inpatients

* Correspondence: m13608388426@163.com
Department of Information, Research Institute of Field Surgery, Daping Hospital of Army Medical University, 10 Changjiang Access Road, Chongqing 400042, China

are important processes in making feasibility decisions for hospital resource management, reducing crowding, and improving the quality of medical care delivered.

Time series forecasting approaches have been adopted in other research fields, such as infectious disease [15–18], power and energy [19], finance and economy [20, 21], traffic [22], environment [23], and hydrology [24]. Among these approaches, for problems involving linear time series forecasting, the autoregressive integrated moving average (ARIMA) model is linear in that predictions of the future values are constrained to be linear functions of past observations. However, the prediction accuracy of ARIMA model is restricted due to its inability to capture the nonlinear relationships of time series in the real world. For nonlinear problems, the artificial neural network (ANN) has enhanced forecasting accuracy due to its intrinsic properties that can approximate any sort of arbitrary nonlinear function [25]. More recently, hybrid forecasting models that combine the ARIMA and ANN models to handle linear and nonlinear relationships that exist in time series data have been extensively applied in many fields with high predictive performance [16, 17, 19, 21, 26–28] . These previous studies remind us that the number of new admission inpatients as time series could also be predicted by hybrid models.

Our team has successfully applied the hybrid model with ARIMA and the nonlinear autoregressive neural network (NARNN) to the field of infectious diseases, for example forecasting the prevalence of schistosomiasis in humans in Qianjiang City and Yangxin City, China [17, 28], and the incident cases of hand, foot, and mouth disease in Shenzhen, China [29]. Wu [16] also verified the feasibility of a hybrid ARIMA-NARNN model in forecasting the incidence of hemorrhagic fever with renal syndrome in Jiangsu Province, China. These literatures indicate combining both the ARIMA and NARNN models could improve the forecasting performance due to incorporate both the linear and nonlinear patterns found in the real world.

In this paper, we will explore whether the ARIMA-NARNN hybrid model is reliable for forecasting the number of new admission inpatients to a large hospital. Our aim is to forecast the monthly and daily new admission inpatients using time series models. This will enable hospitals to provide more efficient and better quality care to their patients.

Methods

Data sources
Our hospital, as a member of the first batch of public tertiary hospitals in Chongqing, China, is a large-scale comprehensive medical institution involves in medical care, education and scientific research. By now our hospital opens with 2628 inpatient beds, and there are almost 2,000,000 outpatients, 100,000 emergency admissions and 100,000 discharges during a year. Like most other tertiary hospitals in China, we are faced with the growing challenge of overcrowding. Between 2010 and 2015, the amount of outpatient-emergency patients, new admissions and surgeries increased by 96.75, 37.59, 37.13%, respectively. Although the largest increase was observed in the number of outpatient-emergency patients, allocation of hospital resourcesis also greatly effected by admitted patients. Therefore, we chose to focus on new admissions in this study.

To analyze the "day of the week" effect and the "month of the year" effect of new admission inpatients, we included data from two different time series: monthly data from January 2010 to October 2016 (82 months) and daily data from January 4 to October 2, 2016 (273 days). The data was obtained from the Hospital Information System (Additional file 1). The study was approved by the ethics committee of Daping Hospital of Third Military Medical University.

Methods

The SARIMA model construction
Taking into account the characteristics of seasonal fluctuation of new admission inpatients, the seasonal ARIMA (SARIMA) model was constructed. The SARIMA $(p, d, q)(P, D, Q)s$ model is developed from the ARIMA model [15]. There are seven main parameters in the SARIMA model: the order of autoregressive (p) and seasonal autoregressive (P), the order of regular difference (d) and seasonal difference (D), and the order of moving average (q) and seasonal moving average (Q), and finally, the length of seasonal period(s). Stationarity is a necessary condition in building a SARIMA model and differencing is often used to stabilize the time series data. The main methods to check the stationarity of time series include the sequence trend diagram, autocorrelation function (ACF), partial autocorrelation function (PACF), augmented dickey-fuller (ADF) unit root test, phillips and perron (PP) test, nonparametric test and so on. In this study, the ACF, PACF plots, and ADF test were used to identify the stationarity of time series and the possible order of autoregression and moving average. The most suitable model was selected according to the akaike information criterion (AIC), schwarz bayesian criterion (SBC) and the Ljung-Box Q-test. Both monthly and daily seasonal periodicities were taken into account in this analysis. The two time series are nonstationary. Regular difference and seasonal difference are used to stabilize them. The new stationary series after difference are as the target sequence of the SARIMA model.

Before the modeling process, the time series were split into two sets each: one (modeling data set) was used to develop the models and the other (testing data set) to test the model. The modeling monthly set included data from January 2010 to June 2016 (1/2010–6/2016), while data from July to October 2016 (7/2016–10/2016) was used as the corresponding testing data set. The modeling daily data set was from January 4 to September 4, 2016 (1/4/2016–9/4/2016), while the testing data was collected within 1 week from September 5 to September 11, 2016(9/5/2016–9/11/2016) and four-weeks from September 5 to October 2, 2016 (9/5/2016–10/2/2016). The SARIMA model was developed with SAS Software version 9.4.

The NARNN model construction
The NARNN model is capable of predicting a simple time series given past values of the same time series, $y_t = f(y_{t-1}, y_{t-2}, \cdots, y_{t-d})$. NARNN incorporates a default two-layer FFBP with a sigmoid transfer function in the hidden layer, a linear transfer function in the output layer. The output of the NARNN, $y(t)$, is fed back to the input of the network (through delays). The configuration is showed in Fig. 1. The NARNN model was performed with the Neural Network Toolbox in MATLAB version 7.11(R2010b). The following steps describe how to build the NARNN model.

Step 1: Inputted the target series to generate a command-line script.
Step 2: Used the default data division function type to divide the data randomly to three parts: the training subset (training the network), the validation subset (stopping training before over-fitting) and the testing subset (testing the network generalization). Set the ratios for training (80%), validation (10%), and testing (10%).
Step 3: Adjusted the arguments feedback delays and hidden units by trial and error. Set the hidden units (10~ 18) and feedback delays (4~ 10) depending on our experience with the amount of data. In total of 63 architectures were tested to obtain the optimal model according to the error autocorrelation plot, the time series response plot, the MSE and the correlation coefficient (R).

Step 4: According to the feedback delays, we inputted the targets of the closed loop network for multi-step-ahead prediction.

The hybrid SARIMA-NARNN model construction
The hybrid SARIMA-NARNN model was developed in two stages. In the SARIMA model stage, the main goal was to extract the linear relationships between the original data. The SARIMA model was then used to generate the residuals. In the NARNN model stage, the chief aim was to model the nonlinear relationships that exist in the residuals. The eventual combined forecasting values of the time series were the sum of predictions from SARIMA model and adjusted residuals from NARNN model: $\hat{y}_t = \hat{L}_t + \hat{N}_T$, where $\hat{y}_t$ was the predicted value by the SARIMA-NARNN model at time t, $\hat{L}_t$ denoted the predicted value by the SARIMA model at time t, and $\hat{N}_t$ denoted the residuals predicted by the NARNN model.

Performance statistic index
The modeling errors and testing errors were used to compare the fitness and prediction performance of the SARIMA, NARNN and SARIMA-NARNN models. The three indices: root mean square error (RMSE), mean absolute error (MAE) and mean absolute percentage error (MAPE), were selected for evaluation of the errors. The formulas for calculation are defined as follows:

$$RMSE = \sqrt{\frac{1}{n}\sum_{t=1}^{n}\left(y_t - \hat{y}_t\right)^2} \tag{1}$$

$$MAE = \frac{1}{n}\sum_{t=1}^{n}\left|y_t - \hat{y}_t\right| \tag{2}$$

$$MAPE = \frac{1}{n}\sum_{t=1}^{n}\frac{\left|y_t - y_t^{\wedge}\right|}{y_t} \tag{3}$$

Results
SARIMA model analysis
The monthly time series achieved stationary state after regular difference of 1 order, followed by seasonal difference of 1 order and length of seasonal period of 12.

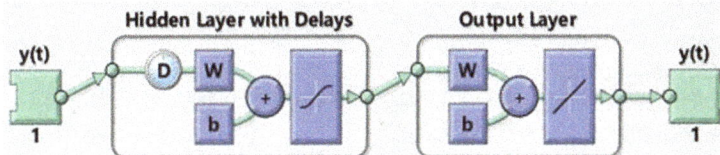

Fig. 1 The configuration of the NARNN. The NARNN consists of one output layer with 1 unit and one hidden layer with n units and D delays

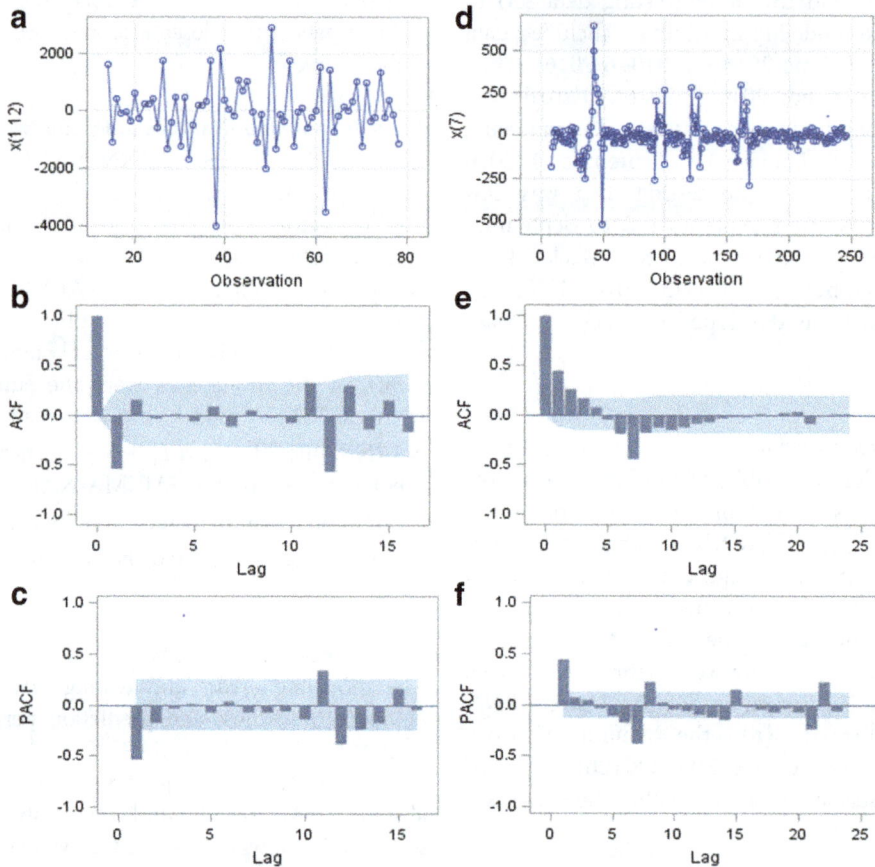

Fig. 2 Trend and Correlation Analysis for different time series. **a**, **b** and **c** show the trend of new admission inpatients per month from January 2010 to June 2016, ACF and PACF plots of monthly original time series (MOS) respectively after one order of regular difference and one order of seasonal difference with the length of seasonal period 12. **d**, **e** and **f** show the trend of new admission inpatients per day from January 4 to September 4, 2016, ACF and PACF plots of daily original time series (DOS) respectively after one order of seasonal difference with the length of seasonal period 7

The daily time series achieved stationary state after seasonal difference of 1order and length of seasonal period of 7 without regular difference. Fig. 2 a and d show the stationary monthly original time series (MOS) and daily original time series (DOS) after difference. The ACF and PACF plots of MOS and DOS after difference are displayed in Fig. 2 b, c, e, and f. Most of the correlations were at around zero within a 95% confidence interval, suggesting that the time series achieved stationarity. Results of ADF test of MOS and DOS after difference was considered are shown in Table 1. All the P-values were less than 0.05 supporting the absence of unit root. This provided further confirmation that the difference in the series was stationary.

Results of the parameter estimation are shown in Table 2. All of the estimated parameter values were statistically significant ($P < 0.05$). These results showed that using the model SARIMA$(1,1,0)(0,1,1)_{12}$ with the smallest AIC (1049.72) and SBC (1054.07) for forecasting the monthly new admission inpatients and the model

SARIMA$(2,0,1)(0,1,1)_7$ (AIC = 1049.72, SBC = 1054.07) for daily predicting were appropriate.

The autocorrelation of residuals is presented in Table 3. All the P-values were more than 0.05, showing that the residuals were all white noises, which indicated the information was extracted sufficiently.

Table 1 Augmented dickey-fuller unit root (ADF) test of two time series

Type	Lag	Monthly		Daily	
		t	P	t	P
Zero Mean	0	−14.60	< 0.0001	−9.56	<.0001
	1	−8.15	< 0.0001	−7.55	<.0001
Single Mean	0	−14.48	0.0001	−9.54	<.0001
	1	−8.09	0.0001	−7.54	<.0001
Trend	0	−14.37	< 0.0001	−9.52	<.0001
	1	−8.02	< 0.0001	−7.52	<.0001

Note: Monthly = monthly time series from January 2010 to June 2016
Daily = daily time series from January 4 to September 4,2016

Table 2 Parameter estimations of two time series from SARIMA model

Time series	Parameter	Estimate	Standard error	t	P	Lag
Monthly	MA1,1	0.90	0.08	11.54	<.0001	12
	AR1,1	−0.50	0.11	−4.52	<.0001	1
Daily	MA1,1	−0.45	0.06	−7.05	<.0001	1
	MA2,1	0.81	0.04	21.32	<.0001	7
	AR1,1	0.23	0.07	3.34	0.0010	2

Table 4 Optimum network parameters of different target series

Time series	Target series	Hidden units	Delays	RMSE			R
				training	validation	testing	
Monthly	OS	11	8	53.74	309.8	280.89	0.92
	RS	16	6	113.58	187.02	221.44	0.82
Daily	OS	13	10	30.07	36.01	46.48	0.96
	RS	14	7	33.91	51.35	41.90	0.87

Note: OS = original series, RS = residual series

All predicted values are available in the Additional file 2. We then computed the monthly residual series (MRS) and daily residual series (DRS), which were subsequently applied as the target series of the NARNN model.

NARNN model analysis

The optimal NARNN models we applied to forecast the MOS, MRS, DOS and DRS are shown in Table 4: target series MOS with hidden units 11 and delays 8, MRS with hidden units 16 and delays 6, DOS with hidden units 13 and delays 10, and DRS with hidden units 14 and delays 7. All MSE of the training, validation, and testing subsets were relatively small, and all the R values were greater than 0.8.

The error autocorrelation function plot of different target series are displayed in Fig. 3. The correlation coefficients for all the models, except for the one at zero lag, fell within the 95% confidence limits, demonstrating that the models were applicable. The time series response plots are displayed in Fig. 4, showing that the outputs were distributed evenly on both sides of the response curve and the errors were small in the training, testing, and validation subsets, indicating that the model reliably reflected the data. We observed that the predicted residuals from July to October 2016 were – 240.47, 35.31, – 132.87 and 189.98, respectively. In addition, the predicted residuals, from September 5 to October 2, 2016 were 3.86, 3.65, 7.93, 6.17, 5.50, 5.46, 10.44, 10.65, 11.41, 14.96, 14.14, 17.08, 18.08, 21.26, 23.60, 24.68, 29.83, 29.77, 35.42, 37.97, 41.36, 48.66, 47.95, 60.84, 58.58, 71.15, 79.63 and 71.89 respectively. The predicted monthly and daily new admission inpatients by NARNN model are presented in the Additional file 2.

Table 3 White noise check of residuals of two time series from SARIMA model

Lag	Monthly		Daily	
	X^2	P	X^2	P
6	4.35	0.36	3.06	0.38
12	7.20	0.71	6.45	0.69
18	11.04	0.81	9.80	0.83
24	13.52	0.92	13.14	0.90

SARIMA-NARNN model analysis

The monthly and daily values predicted by the SARIMA-NARNN model are shown in the Additional file 2. The point-to-point comparison between original observations and predicted values from the SARIMA, NARNN and SARIMA-NARNN models are shown in Fig. 5 and Fig. 6. The curve of the original observations and predicted series from the SARIMA-NARNN model was closer than those from the SARIMA and NARNN models (Fig. 5 a, b and c), indicating that the hybrid model was well fitted to the data of monthly new admission inpatients. However, among the three models, the predicted curve from the NARNN model was the closest to the original curve (Fig. 6 a, b and c), indicating that the NARNN model was appropriate for forecasting the daily new admission inpatients.

Comparing analysis

The differences in modeling errors and testing errors between the original observations and predicted values of monthly and daily new admission inpatients are presented in Table 5.

For the monthly data, the modeling RMSE and the testing RMSE, MAE and MAPE of the SARIMA-NARNN model were less than those obtained from the single SARIMA or NARNN model, but the MAE and MAPE were more than those obtained from NARNN model.

For the daily data, we calculated the testing errors of one-week and four-weeks. The NARNN model was the best with the lowest RMSE, MAE and MAPE in modeling stage and testing stage, indicating that the NARNN model was well fitted to the data of daily new admission inpatients.

Discussion

To our knowledge, this study was the first to develop and apply the time series models in admission patients research, with the specific purpose of forecasting the number of new admission inpatients trends and guiding management strategies. We sought to construct a single SARIMA model, a single NARNN model, and a hybrid SARIMA-NARNN model based on the monthly and daily data of an entire hospital. The NARNN model and

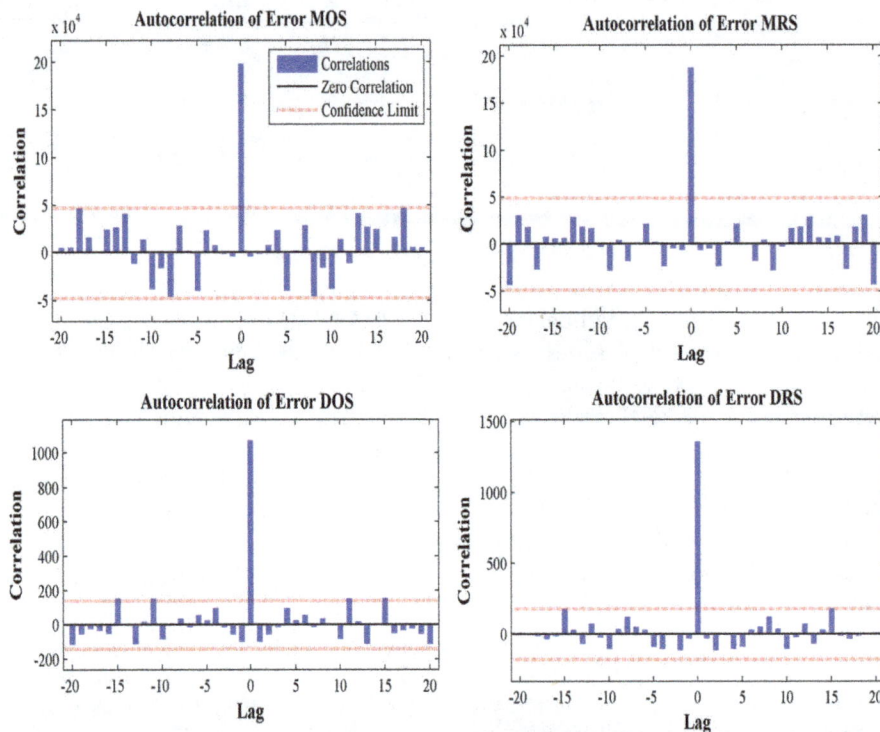

Fig. 3 Error autocorrelation plots of different time series from NARNN model. The error autocorrelation was one of the evaluation indices in the modeling process. The red dotted line indicate 95% confidence intervals. MOS = monthly original time series, MRS = monthly residual series, DOS = daily original time series, DRS = daily residual series

SARIMA-NARNN model were appropriate to forecast the number of new admission inpatients. But the results of forecasting performance were compared by using the RMSE, MAE, MAPE showing that the hybrid model does not necessarily achieved better prediction accuracy than either of the models used separately.

As shown in Fig. 5, the original new admission inpatients fluctuated every year based on the monthly data. However, an upward trend was observed overall. The result of the SARIMA model analysis incorporated a 12-step seasonal differencing operation. The monthly time series analysis supports a "month of the year" effect. The lowest numbers were observed in January or February each year, presumably due to the Spring Festival holiday. The numbers reached the maximum in March 2010, 2012, 2015 and 2016, and greater numbers in March compared to other months were also observed in other years, a phenomenon that could potentially be attributed to long holiday and seasonal replacement. Based on these findings, we suggest that hospital management should strategize and assign medical resources accordingly. The modeling RMSE, MAE, MAPE of the SARIMA-NARNN model decreased by 42.89, 47.85, 48.86% and the corresponding testing error decreased by 11.35, 20.25, 19.99%, respectively as compared to using the SARIMA model alone. When compared to the

NARNN model, the modeling RMSE of the SARIMA-NARNN model decreased by 3.12%, and the testing RMSE, MAE, MAPE decreased by 57.35, 52.66, 52.11%, respectively. Interestingly, the modeling MAE and MAPE of the SARIMA-NARNN model increased by 28.47 and 27.26%, respectively. As mentioned in the article [30, 31], the RMSE is not always a superior parameter over the MAE, a combination of metrics is often required to accurately evaluate model performance. However, all testing errors of the SARIMA-NARNN model were the lowest among the three models and overall, the predicted curves of the hybrid model was close to the original curves (Fig. 5 a, b and c). Therefore, we concluded that the hybrid model was the most appropriate for forecasting the monthly new admission inpatients.

As shown in Fig. 6a, b and c, our analysis of daily data indicates an obvious "day of the week" effect. Maximum values were usually observed on Mondays, while the minimum values tended to fall on Saturdays or Sundays every week. Some fluctuations were found under the influence of various festals. For examples, the lowest number was observed during the 7th to the 13th of February likely due to the Spring Festival holiday and the one-week maximum was observed on Tuesday (3th of May) probably because this was the first day after the

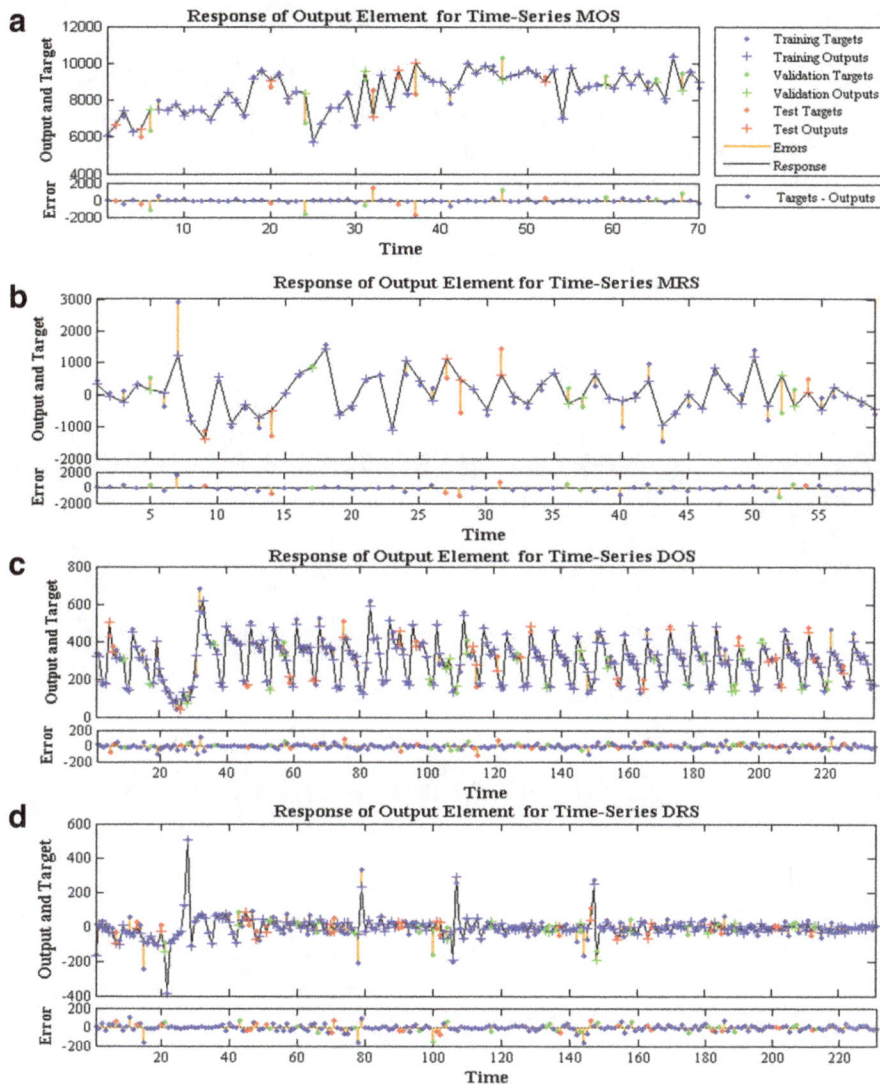

Fig. 4 The time-series response plots of different time series from NARNN model. **a**, **b**, **c** and **d** show the inputs, targets, and errors versus time and also give which time points were selected for training, testing, and validation

May Day holiday. In addition, the maximum value was also found on Sunday (18th of September) potentially due to the Mid Autumn Festival holidays from Thursday to Saturday prior. Forecasting performance could be greatly influenced by these fluctuations. If the time series predictions were within the range of these holidays, extra cautions should be paid on interpreting prediction results. As compared to using the SARIMA model alone, the modeling RMSE, MAE, and MAPE of the NARNN model decreased by 55.28, 44.01, and 49.01% and the corresponding one-week and four-weeks testing errors dropped by 34.20, 30.65, 30.05 and 0.15%, 3.66, and 4.45%, respectively. When compared to the SARIMA-NARNN model, the modeling RMSE, MAE, MAPE of the NARNN model decreased by 10.54, 8.22 and 9.23%, respectively,

while the corresponding one-week and four-weeks testing errors reduced by 31.50, 24.74, 33.33 and 11.56%, 22.37, 31.72%, respectively. We, therefore, concluded that the NARNN model was suitable for forecasting the daily new admission inpatients.

According to the development trend of new admission inpatients, we can make some following suggestions for the hospital managers. Try to avoid the medical staff leave at the peak of admission; Carry out the repair work for the inpatient beds on Saturday or Sunday; Provide vacant beds by clinical departments with fewer admission inpatients to other departments with more admission inpatients. Set up some waiting beds for turnover in the whole hospital; Make an "emergence plan about overcrowding"- once overcrowding occur the "overcrowding

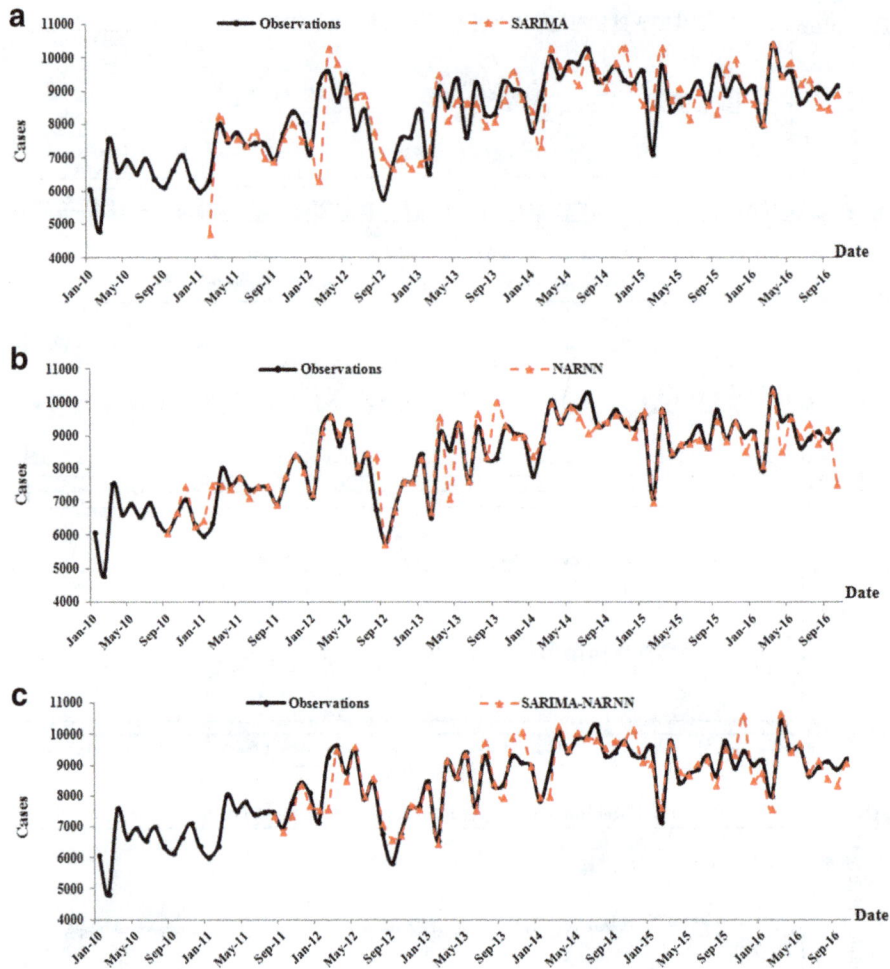

Fig. 5 The change trend of the monthly number of new admission inpatients from three models. **a**, **b** and **c** show the observations and predicted values from the SARIMA model , NARNN model and SARIMA-NARNN model respectively

beds" are opened. When the forecasting results indicate that the new admission inpatients are increasing, the plan is in a state of vigilance.

Although the ARIMA model is one of the most mature time series forecasting methods, our study [17, 28] and other studies [32] have indicated that its forecasting performance for predicting real world cases is slightly lower than other models. Therefore, we do not recommend using the ARIMA model exclusively. The NARNN model is capable of successfully simulating some time series due to its dynamic property, high fault tolerance performance, and ability to capture nonlinear information [25, 33]. In practical data analysis, the NARNN model should be construct. In addition, our results were consistent with previous publication, which reported the comparative study of autoregressive neural network hybrids, showing that hybrid models are not always better and the model construction process should remain an important step despite the popularity of hybrid models [34]. The four-weeks testing errors were much greater than those of one-week, showing that the prediction accuracy was obviously reduced with the increase of forecasting time. It is the inherent disadvantages of the time series forecasting model-the forecasting ability to extrapolate is limited, the longer the forecasting time, the lower the prediction accuracy. Further studies are needed to develop synthetic approaches combining various types of models to improve the ability of forecasting the new admission inpatients from different data.

From a clinical perspective, our research shows that it is benefit to monitor the change trend of admission inpatients by adding time series model to the hospital information system. When the predicted new admission inpatients are increasing, hospital managers can open more preparation beds or let doctors reduce the admissions. From a methodology perspective, our research shows that the time series model can be applied to study the development trend of admission inpatients. NARNN model was implemented based on the neural network time series tool of MATLAB which provided a graphical

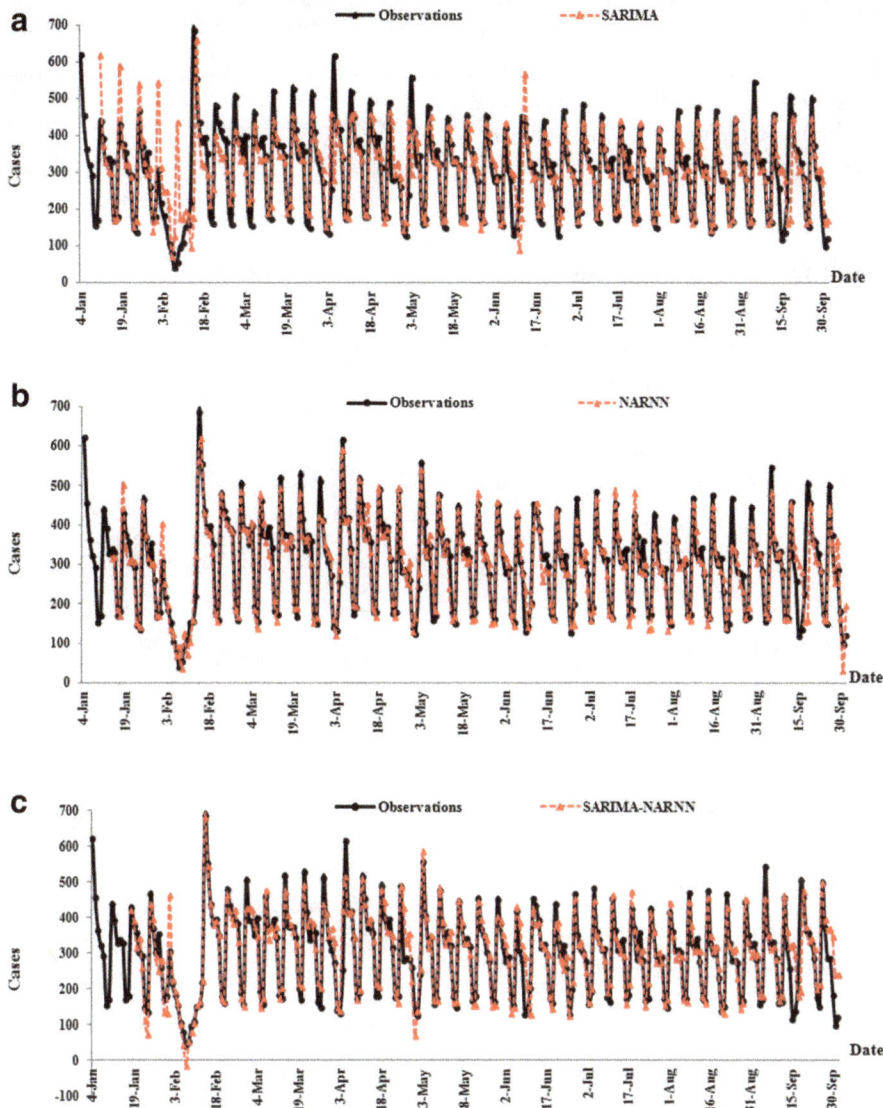

Fig. 6 The change trend of the daily number of new admission inpatients from three models. **a**, **b** and **c** show the observations and predicted values from the SARIMA model , NARNN model and SARIMA-NARNN model respectively

Table 5 Prediction performance results of three models

Time series	Model	Modeling error			Testing error		
		RMSE	MAE	MAPE*	RMSE	MAE	MAPE*
Monthly	SARIMA	759.67	573.75	6.81	426.45	410.97	4.56
	NARNN	448.04	232.92	2.73	886.39	692.29	7.61
	SARIMA-NARNN	433.82	299.22	3.48	378.03	327.75	3.64
Daily	SARIMA	73.73	42.01	18.50	37.29 [a]	20.36 [a]	4.91 [a]
					87.01 [b]	51.11 [b]	24.22 [b]
	NARNN	32.97	23.49	9.42	24.54 [a]	14.12 [a]	3.44 [a]
					86.88 [b]	49.24 [b]	23.14 [b]
	SARIMA-NARNN	36.86	25.59	10.37	35.82 [a]	18.76 [a]	5.15 [a]
					98.24 [b]	63.43 [b]	33.90 [b]

*MAPE values should be multiplied by 10^{-2}. [a]the testing error in one-week, [b]the testing error in four-weeks

environment to make the design process of model easy. Although many researches have indicated hybrid models could improve the forecasting performance, our results do not support this point. Understanding how and which models could be implemented in which data requires hospital managers prudent choice.

Conclusions

In summary, the SARIMA-NARNN model for forecasting did not always provide better estimates than the single NARNN model. Our results show that combined models do not necessarily outperform the individual constituents. Therefore, it is worth attempting to explore different reliable models with high degree of accuracy for forecasting the number of new admission inpatients using different data.

Abbreviations
ARIMA: Autoregressive Integrated Moving Average; MAE: Mean Absolute Error; NARNN: Nonlinear Autoregressive Neural Network; RMSE: Root Mean Square Error; SARIMA: Seasonal Autoregressive Integrated Moving Average; MAPE: Mean Absolute Percentage Error; ANN: Artificial Neural Network; ACF: Autocorrelation Function; PACF: Partial Autocorrelation Function; ADF: Augmented Dickey-Fuller; PP: Phillips and Perron; AIC: Akaike Information Criterion; SBC: Schwarz Bayesian Criterion; MOS: Monthly Original Time Series; DOS: Daily Original Time Series; MRS: Monthly Residual Series; DRS: Daily Residual Series

Acknowledgments
The authors would like to thank all of staffs from Information Department, Inpatient department and Medical-record department, for their collecting and providing data.

Authors' contributions
HH and LLZ conceived the study. LLZ and PZ wrote and edited the manuscript. LLZ and DD Wu participated in data collection and analysis. LLZ, HH and CC participated in interpretation of results. All authors read and approved the final manuscript.

Competing interests
The authors declare that they have no competing interests.

References
1. Bahadori M, Teymourzadeh E, Ravangard R, Raadabadi M. Factors affecting the overcrowding in outpatient healthcare. J Educ Health Promot. 2017; 6(1):21.
2. Guttmann A, Schull MJ, Vermeulen MJ, Stukel TA. Association between waiting times and short term mortality and hospital admission after departure from emergency department: population based cohort study from Ontario, Canada. BMJ (Clinical research ed). 2011;d2983:342.
3. Schull M, Vermeulen M, Guttmann A, Stukel T. Better performance on length-of-stay benchmarks associated with reduced risk following emergency department discharge: an observational cohort study. Cjem. 2015;17(3):253-62.
4. Phillips JL, Jackson BE, Fagan EL, Arze SE, Major B, Zenarosa NR, Wang H: Overcrowding and its association with patient outcomes in a median-low volume emergency department. J Clin Med Res 2017, 9(11):911-916.
5. Bao Y, Fan G, Zou D, Wang T, Xue D. Patient experience with outpatient encounters at public hospitals in shanghai: examining different aspects of physician services and implications of overcrowding. PLoS One. 2017;12(2): e0171684.
6. MH Y, Rezaei F, Haghshenas A, Tavakoli N. Overcrowding in emergency departments: a review of strategies to decrease future challenges. J Res Med Sci. 2017;22(1):23.
7. Mai Q, Aboagye-Sarfo P, Sanfilippo FM, Preen DB, Fatovich DM. Predicting the number of emergency department presentations in Western Australia: a population-based time series analysis. Emerg Med Australas. 2015;27(1): 16-21.
8. Aboagye-Sarfo P, Mai Q, Sanfilippo FM, Preen DB, Stewart LM, Fatovich DM. A comparison of multivariate and univariate time series approaches to modelling and forecasting emergency department demand in Western Australia. J Biomed Inform. 2015;57:62-73.
9. Rosychuk RJ, Youngson E, Rowe BH. Presentations to emergency departments for COPD: a time series analysis. Can Respir J. 2016;2016: 1382434.
10. Xu M, Wong TC, Chin KS. Modeling daily patient arrivals at emergency department and quantifying the relative importance of contributing variables using artificial neural network. Decis Support Syst. 2013;54(3): 1488-98.
11. Cheng C-H, Wang J-W, Li C-H. Forecasting the number of outpatient visits using a new fuzzy time series based on weighted-transitional matrix. Expert Syst Appl. 2008;34(4):2568-75.
12. Hadavandi E, Shavandi H, Ghanbari A, Abbasian-Naghneh S. Developing a hybrid artificial intelligence model for outpatient visits forecasting in hospitals. Appl Soft Comput. 2012;12(2):700-11.
13. Zhu T, Luo L, Zhang X, Shi Y, Shen W. Time series approaches for forecasting the number of hospital daily discharged inpatients. IEEE J Biomed Health Informs. 2015:2168-94.
14. Abdel-Aal RE, Mangoud AM. Modeling and forecasting monthly patient volume at a primary health care clinic using univariate time-series analysis. Comput Meth Prog Bio. 1998;56(3):235-47.
15. Song X, Xiao J, Deng J, Kang Q, Zhang Y, Xu J. Time series analysis of influenza incidence in Chinese provinces from 2004 to 2011. Medicine. 2016;95(26):e3929.
16. Wu W, Guo J, An S, Guan P, Ren Y, Xia L, Zhou B. Comparison of two hybrid models for forecasting the incidence of hemorrhagic fever with renal syndrome in Jiangsu Province, China. PLoS One. 2015;10(8):e0135492.
17. Zhou L, Xia J, Yu L, Wang Y, Shi Y, Cai S, Nie S. Using a hybrid model to forecast the prevalence of Schistosomiasis in humans. Inter J Env Res Pub Heal. 2016;13(4):355.
18. Siriyasatien P, Phumee A, Ongruk P, Jampachaisri K, Kesorn K. Analysis of significant factors for dengue fever incidence prediction. BMC Bioinformatics. 2016;17(1):166.
19. Liu H, H-q T, Li Y-f. Comparison of two new ARIMA-ANN and ARIMA-Kalman hybrid methods for wind speed prediction. Appl Energy. 2012;98:415-24.
20. Qiu M, Song Y. Predicting the direction of stock market index movement using an optimized artificial neural network model. PLoS One. 2016;11(5): e0155133.
21. Omar H, Hoang VH, Liu DR. A hybrid neural network model for sales forecasting based on ARIMA and search popularity of article titles. Comput Intell Neurosci. 2016;2016:9656453.
22. Zhang X, Pang Y, Cui M, Stallones L, Xiang H. Forecasting mortality of road traffic injuries in China using seasonal autoregressive integrated moving average model. Ann Epidemiol. 2015;25(2):101-6.
23. Song Y, Wang Y, Liu F, Zhang Y. Development of a hybrid model to predict construction and demolition waste: China as a case study. Waste Manag. 2017;59:350-61.
24. Araujo P, Astray G, Ferrerio-Lage JA, Mejuto JC, Rodriguez-Suarez JA, Soto B. Multilayer perceptron neural network for flow prediction. J Environ Monit. 2011;13(1):35-41.
25. Cross SS, Harrison RF, Kennedy RL. Introduction to neural networks. Lancet. 1995;346:1075-9.
26. Yolcu U, Egrioglu E, Aladag CH. A new linear and nonlinear artificial neural network model for time series forecasting. Decis Support Syst. 2013;54: 1340-7.

27. Khashei M, Bijari M. A new class of hybrid models for time series forecasting. Expert Syst Appl. 2012;39(4):4344–57.

28. Zhou L, Yu L, Wang Y, Lu Z, Tian L, Tan L, Shi Y, Nie S, Liu L. A hybrid model for predicting the prevalence of schistosomiasis in humans of Qianjiang City, China. PLoS One. 2014;9(8):e104875.

29. Yu L, Zhou L, Tan L, Jiang H, Wang Y, Wei S, Nie S. Application of a new hybrid model with seasonal auto-regressive integrated moving average (ARIMA) and nonlinear auto-regressive neural network (NARNN) in forecasting incidence cases of HFMD in Shenzhen, China. PLoS One. 2014; 9(6):e98241.

30. Willmott CJ, Matsuura K. Advantages of the mean absolute error (MAE) over the root mean square error (RMSE) in assessing average model performance. Clim Res. 2005;30(1):79.

31. Chai T, Draxler RR. Root mean square error (RMSE) or mean absolute error (MAE)? – arguments against avoiding RMSE in the literature. Geosci Model Dev. 2014;7(3):1247–50.

32. Purwanto EC, Logeswaran R. An enhanced hybrid method for time series prediction using linear and neural network models. Appl Intell. 2012;37(4): 511–9.

33. Kaastra I, Boyd M. Designing a neural network for forecasting financial and economic time series. Neurocomputing. 1996;10(3):215–36.

34. Taskaya-Temizel T, Casey MC. A comparative study of autoregressive neural network hybrids. Neural Netw. 2005;18(5–6):781–9.

6

Developing a tablet computer-based application ('App') to measure self-reported alcohol consumption in Indigenous Australians

KS Kylie Lee[1,2*], Scott Wilson[3,1], Jimmy Perry[3], Robin Room[2], Sarah Callinan[2], Robert Assan[4], Noel Hayman[5,6,7], Tanya Chikritzhs[8], Dennis Gray[8], Edward Wilkes[8], Peter Jack[9] and Katherine M. Conigrave[9,1]

Abstract

Background: The challenges of assessing alcohol consumption can be greater in Indigenous communities where there may be culturally distinct approaches to communication, sharing of drinking containers and episodic patterns of drinking. This paper discusses the processes used to develop a tablet computer-based application ('App') to collect a detailed assessment of drinking patterns in Indigenous Australians. The key features of the resulting App are described.

Methods: An iterative consultation process was used (instead of one-off focus groups), with Indigenous cultural experts and clinical experts. Regular (weekly or more) advice was sought over a 12-month period from Indigenous community leaders and from a range of Indigenous and non-Indigenous health professionals and researchers.

Results: The underpinning principles, selected survey items, and key technical features of the App are described. Features include culturally appropriate questioning style and gender-specific voice and images; community-recognised events used as reference points to 'anchor' time periods; 'translation' to colloquial English and (for audio) to traditional language; interactive visual approaches to estimate quantity of drinking; images of specific brands of alcohol, rather than abstract description of alcohol type (e.g. 'spirits'); images of make-shift drinking containers; option to estimate consumption based on the individual's share of what the group drank.

Conclusions: With any survey platform, helping participants to accurately reflect on and report their drinking presents a challenge. The availability of interactive, tablet-based technologies enables potential bridging of differences in culture and lifestyle and enhanced reporting.

Keywords: Aboriginal, Indigenous, Alcohol, Measurement, Survey

Background

Data on the context in which people drink, what they drink, how much and how often, inform efforts to prevent and treat unhealthy alcohol use. While Aboriginal and Torres Strait Islander (Indigenous) Australians face up to eight times increased risk of harms from alcohol

* Correspondence: kylie.lee@sydney.edu.au
[1]University of Sydney, Discipline of Addiction Medicine, Indigenous Health and Substance Use, NHMRC Centre of Research Excellence in Indigenous Health and Alcohol, King George V Building, 83-117 Missenden Road, Camperdown, NSW 2050, Australia
[2]Centre for Alcohol Policy Research, La Trobe University, 215 Franklin Street, Melbourne, VIC 3000, Australia
Full list of author information is available at the end of the article

[1], there is a lack of good data on alcohol consumption itself [2, 3]. Some experts say that one national survey (published in 2008) underestimates consumption by more than 700% for females and 200% for males [4]. The national survey that is described as having the most suitable methods, and therefore most accurate data is more than two decades old and is specific to urban settings [2]. On a local level, communities and health services do not have a good way to monitor patterns of drinking and how well they are going with prevention or treatment efforts [5, 6].

Estimating how much alcohol an individual consumes is challenging in any population [7] and many approaches have been studied [2, 3, 8, 9]. None are perfect. Many methods require the drinker to convert their consumption into standard drinks or units. This requires awareness of the size of a standard drink (in Australia, equivalent to 10 g of ethanol), and then, awareness of the volume and strength, or standard drink content, of the beverage the person has consumed. The person then needs the mathematical skills to convert their consumption to standard drinks. Discomfort with reading or with numbers can be a significant [10, 11], which is more common in disadvantaged population subgroups. Estimating drinking by self-report is made more difficult if alcohol is shared, which can be common in the developing world and among indigenous peoples [11]. Episodic drinking patterns (e.g. due to geography, social or financial reasons or local alcohol restrictions) are also more common among Indigenous Australians, and make it difficult to answer questions on 'usual' drinking.

There is a need for a survey tool to collect comparable, standardised data on alcohol use, but which is flexible enough in terms of design and administration to be employed in, and responsive to, varying Indigenous contexts [3]. Alcohol tracker applications installed on a smartphone have been used to allow an individual to prospectively record their alcohol use [12]. However, this requires sustained participant engagement, and the availability of smartphones and internet, and so may not be feasible for large scale household surveys in indigenous or disadvantaged populations. Accordingly, a household survey tool which relies on retrospective reporting of drinking is likely to typically required. Compared to pen and paper surveys, or computer surveys which are purely text based, audio computer-assisted self-interviewing using tablet-computer technology or a similar platform may increase respondents' engagement with survey items and increase their confidence in the anonymity and confidentiality of survey answers [13, 14]. Visual and audio opportunities offered by tablet-technologies may help counteract the need for individuals to be comfortable with numbers and the written word (in English; as is required with existing national alcohol paper and pen surveys). This paper discusses the processes used to develop a tablet computer-based application ('App') to collect a detailed assessment of drinking patterns in Indigenous Australians as a survey tool. The key features of the resulting App are described.

Methods
Overview
Study methods were designed by investigators in consultation with the Aboriginal Drug and Alcohol Council of South Australia (ADAC); the Aboriginal Drug and Alcohol Network New South Wales (ADAN), representing Aboriginal alcohol and other drug workers in New South Wales (NSW); and the Aboriginal Health Council

of South Australia (AHCSA), the peak body for Aboriginal community controlled health services in South Australia (SA). Half the authors of this paper are themselves Aboriginal. Ethical approval was obtained from three ethics committees, including the the Aboriginal Health Council of South Australia (ACHSA) and Metro South Health Human Research Ethics Committee (Queensland).

The App was developed as part of a 5-year Australian National Health and Medical Research Council (NHMRC) project grant. That larger study aims to develop, test and re-test a tablet computer-based survey for Indigenous Australians (aged 16 years or older) to report on their drinking.

Steps taken to consult with experts during App development
An iterative process was used during App development (instead of formal focus groups) with weekly or more frequent advice sought over a 12-month period from clinicians and other health professionals. This included from Indigenous alcohol and other drug, health, mental health, or health promotion workers; addiction medicine physicians; a nurse; a psychiatrist; Indigenous community leaders; and researchers of various expertise (including: epidemiology, sociology, survey design, psychometrics). Advice was also iteratively sought from other individuals from a range of backgrounds (see Table 1), by a smaller group of researchers (Lee, Conigrave, Wilson, Perry) and then relayed back to the App developers once consensus was reached. In particular, the Aboriginal Drug and Alcohol Council SA

Table 1 Grid showing skill area of individuals ($n = 44$) who advised on the development or testing of a tablet-based survey 'App' to help Indigenous Australians describe their drinking patterns

Skill area[a]	Indigenous (n)	Non-Indigenous (n)
Drug and alcohol (clinical)	7	4
Drug and alcohol (non-clinical)	11	–
Drug and alcohol (policy)	3	2
Mental health	1	1
Health promotion	2	1
Medicine	1	4
Psychology	–	2
Justice	2	–
Research (alcohol and other drugs)	5	11
Research (alcohol surveys, epidemiology, biostatistics, sociology, anthropology)	–	6
Proof reading	–	4
Community member	3	–
Total	**35**	**35**

[a]Some individuals have multiple skill areas, so total numbers in this table are greater than the number of individuals (n = 44) who advised on development of the App

(ADAC; Wilson and Perry) played a lead advisory role in App development and in its deployment for validation.

The main steps taken to develop the App are described below:

- Review of the design of key selected national and international alcohol surveys using peer-reviewed and grey literature to compile a broad list of potential survey items
- Review of relevant websites and Apps to compile a list of potential technical features
- An external company ("We are the Nest/Frost Collective") awarded the tender to develop and build the App
- Survey items drafted and comment sought from investigators and other colleagues
- Two-day consultation workshop for 25 participants from around Australia (Indigenous, *n* = 16; and non-Indigenous, *n* = 9; see Fig. 1)
- Survey items finalised using feedback from the workshop, from investigators and relevant colleagues. Questions selected on demographics, alcohol consumption (see Table 2), dependence, harms to self or others, treatment access and collecting feedback about the experience of using the App

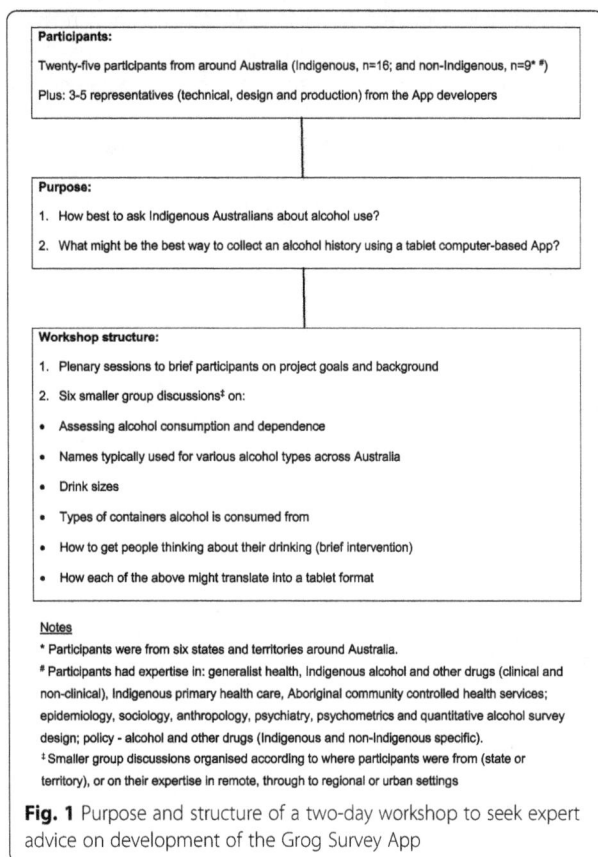

Participants:

Twenty-five participants from around Australia (Indigenous, n=16; and non-Indigenous, n=9* #)

Plus: 3-5 representatives (technical, design and production) from the App developers

Purpose:

1. How best to ask Indigenous Australians about alcohol use?

2. What might be the best way to collect an alcohol history using a tablet computer-based App?

Workshop structure:

1. Plenary sessions to brief participants on project goals and background

2. Six smaller group discussions‡ on:

- Assessing alcohol consumption and dependence
- Names typically used for various alcohol types across Australia
- Drink sizes
- Types of containers alcohol is consumed from
- How to get people thinking about their drinking (brief intervention)
- How each of the above might translate into a tablet format

Notes

* Participants were from six states and territories around Australia.

Participants had expertise in: generalist health, Indigenous alcohol and other drugs (clinical and non-clinical), Indigenous primary health care, Aboriginal community controlled health services; epidemiology, sociology, anthropology, psychiatry, psychometrics and quantitative alcohol survey design; policy - alcohol and other drugs (Indigenous and non-Indigenous specific).

‡ Smaller group discussions organised according to where participants were from (state or territory), or on their expertise in remote, through to regional or urban settings

Fig. 1 Purpose and structure of a two-day workshop to seek expert advice on development of the Grog Survey App

- Development of the App and user testing: Workshop participants, investigators and colleagues tested the App, with comments reviewed by two authors (Lee and Conigrave) then submitted to the developers

Results

Here results of consultations are summarized and the general principles and key features underpinning the survey items and their delivery in the App are described.

General principles

Consultation suggested that the App would need to:

1) Be suitable for an Indigenous Australians aged from 16 to old-age, including those who are unfamiliar with computers or tablets;
2) Be suitable for individuals in urban through to isolated or traditional areas;
3) Help individuals to be comfortable telling their drinking story (e.g. how often or how much);
4) Reassure participants of confidentiality;
5) Work offline, then data from each iPad can be 'pushed' to a secured computer server at the University of Sydney when WIFI is available;
6) Provide a de-identified summary of completed surveys periodically (sex, age, community, drinking status), with remote access to data for principal investigators; and
7) Be comparable with (some items of) existing national and international alcohol surveys or screening tools.

Suitability of existing approaches to measure alcohol consumption

Examples of national and international alcohol surveys were reviewed, and potential items that might be adapted for use on the App were discussed with Indigenous and non-Indigenous experts. International tools included: Alcohol Use Disorders Identification Test (AUDIT) [15]; Composite International Diagnostic Interview Version 7.1 (CIDI) [16]; Alcohol, Smoking and Substance Involvement Screening Test Version 3.0 (ASSIST) [17]; 2007 Gender Alcohol and Culture: An International Study Survey Version 6.1 (GENACIS) [18]; and the International Alcohol Control Policy Evaluation Study (IACS) [19]. Australian tools included: the 2008 National Aboriginal and Torres Strait Islander Social Survey (NATSISS) [20]; the 2013 National Drug Strategy Household Survey [21]; the Indigenous Risk Impact Screen (IRIS) [22]; the Harms From Others' Drinking Study [23]; and a community survey on alcohol consumption in Indigenous populations in remote Western Australia [24].

Table 2 Comparisons between a selection of consumption items on the Australian National Drug Strategy Household Survey, AUDIT and the Grog[a] Survey App

Existing survey item	Response categories	Wording changes	Response categories	Technical solutions	Survey delivery solutions
Have you had an alcoholic drink of any kind in the last 12 months?[b] [NDSHS]	Yes, No	Have you had any grog[a] at all in the last 12 months? (Since the [Easter holidays] last year)[c]	Yes, No	The App dynamically calculates which reference point to use (for 'in the last 12-months e.g. Easter holidays versus New Year) and inserts this into the survey question (text on screen and in audio)	Headphones supplied for privacy and anonymity; research assistant sitting a little away if assistance needed
In the last 12 months, how often did you have an alcoholic drink of any kind?[b] [NDSHS]	• Every day • 5 to 6 days a week • 3 to 4 days a week • 1 to 2 days a week • 2 to 3 days a month • About 1 day a month • Less often • No longer drink	Some people drink grog most days while others drink 'once in a blue moon'[d]. How often do you drink grog at all?[e]	• 'Once in a blue moon'[d] • Sometimes • A few times a week • Most days or every day	—	—
How often do you have a drink containing alcohol? [AUDIT Q1]	• Never • Monthly or less • 2-4 times a month • 2-3 times week • 4 or more times a week				
How often do you have six or more standard drinks on one occasion? [AUDIT Q3]	• Never • Less than monthly • Monthly • Weekly • Daily or almost daily	Thinking of the last 12-months [since Easter last year], how often would you drink [this much grog or more] in 1 day (24 h)?[e]	• Never • 'Once in a blue moon'[d] (less than once a month) • Sometimes (1-3 times a month) • A few times a week (1-3 times a week) • Most days or every day	Interactive Dynamically shows image equivalent of 5 standard drinks (50 g) of the alcohol type most often consumed based on the last 4 drinking occasions.	—

[a]Slang for 'alcohol'

[b]From the 2013 Australian National Drug Strategy Household Survey

[c]Example of reference points used to anchor answers reflecting on 'in the last 12-months' time period

[d]Slang for 'rarely'

[e]Example of using a conversational way to ask about drinking, often with a gentle introduction to the question

Two other internationally validated approaches to assessing alcohol use were considered, as they appeared to have particular relevance to Indigenous Australian contexts. The 'Timeline follow back' approach [25] encourages the individual to recall where they were and who they were with, to help elucidate a detailed history of drinking. The interviewer works backwards, day-by-day for the past month or up to a year. This recounting of real life context and linking of drinking to events and people was considered relevant and approachable in an Indigenous context. However, substantial time is needed to use this approach in its entirety. Another approach, the "Finnish" method, only enquires into the last four drinking occasions [26] and so is less time consuming. Again, the Finnish method asks the person to think over the events or context that were associated with drinking, and does not assume regularity of drinking pattern. However, it is possible that the past four drinking occasions may not be typical of the rest of the year: for example, a person might have 4 days of heavy drinking associated with a trip to the city, while the rest of the year was spent in a 'dry' (alcohol-restricted) area.

Item selection was then guided by Indigenous and non-Indigenous colleagues' advice, for example that:

1) It should take no more than 20 min to complete the survey App (due to competing demands on participants);
2) The app should make it easier for individuals to describe their drinking without requiring skills in numeracy or literacy; and
3) Survey items should cater to a range of drinker types (e.g. including those who drink episodically).

For quantifying alcohol consumption: 10 items are enquired into. This consisted of:

1) Any alcohol consumption in the last year;
2) Frequency of consumption in the last year (The Alcohol Use Disorders Identification Test [AUDIT] Q1-modified);
3-6) The frequency and timing of the last four occasions of drinking and what was consumed, using the 'Finnish method' [25], combined with elements of 'time line follow back' [24] to help participants remember where they were and who they were with in each drinking occasion;
7) Reasons why participants sometimes might drink more;
8) Quantity and types of alcohol consumed in a heavy drinking occasion (24-h period);
9) Length of the longest period of no drinking in the last year; and.

10) Frequency of consuming five or more standard drinks (24 h period) in the last year? (AUDIT Q3-modified) with visual cues to quantify.

We were advised that AUDIT-Q2 was problematic as it asks into 'usual' consumption, and in some traditional regions, the concept of 'usual' does not exist. The app also collected other data on alcohol use behaviours that are the not the focus of this paper (on: alcohol dependence, harms to self or others and treatment access).

Presenting questions in a conversational way

Indigenous colleagues and other clinicians stressed the importance of asking questions in a conversational manner. This was based on clinical and research experience, and on the work of one author (Assan and colleagues) on training clinicians in the use of the Indigenous Risk Impact Screen (IRIS; a screening tool for alcohol, drug and mental health issues developed by and for Indigenous Australians [22]). Accordingly, sensitive survey items were introduced with a short scenario (where appropriate), to assist the individual to reflect on their own life experience (see Table 2).

To ensure privacy, each participant would be presented with an iPad and headphones and be supported by an Indigenous research assistant to open the survey. The individuals would then work through the questions, with a research assistant sitting a little distance away in case problems or questions arose.

Reference points used to 'anchor' time periods

Time is not universally understood as a linear concept in Australia [10, 11]. In traditional communities time of year may be marked more by the seasons or a tree flowering, or times when shops are shut rather than by a calendar. So reference points were used to help individuals to anchor their answers in time. Based on a small group discussion focused on this issue at the workshop, reference points that are widely recognised across Indigenous Australia were agreed upon. As a result, the 'last 12-months' is divided into quarters with the help of four key time points: a) Christmas or New Year (December/January); b) Easter (April); c) National Aboriginal and Islander Day of Celebration (NAIDOC) week (July); and d) Australian Football League (AFL) or National Rugby League (NRL) grand finals (September/October; see Table 2). There was consensus that individuals who do not celebrate Christmas or Easter, or who do not follow sport, would know when in a calendar year these events occur.

The survey app calculates which reference point (for 'in the last 12-months') to use depending on the date when the App is being completed. This then enables an individual to focus on what they were doing, for example, at 'Easter last year', rather than trying to remember what they were doing '12-months ago'. A visual timeline was used to allow respondents to select dates moving back in time, of their four recent drinking occasions. The reference points are converted to dates 'behind' the App for data analysis.

Response categories for questions on frequency of drinking

Indigenous colleagues and other clinicians advised that response categories typically used in alcohol surveys posed difficulties, as they are reliant on individuals counting days, weeks or months [10]. Instead, modified response categories were used that included colloquial English that would be commonly understood by the target population (e.g. 'once in a blue moon (less than once a month)' instead of 'less than monthly'; see Table 2).

Asking about pattern and quantity of drinking on the iPad App

The last four occasions approach [26] was adapted for a user-friendly and visual approach. This combined elements of 'Timeline follow back' [25], and was seen by our advisers as compatible with a conversational or story telling approach.

On the iPad screen, a retrospective "grog diary" appears as a strip. The participant selects when (in the last 12-months) each of their last four drinking occasions occurred. The time periods displayed on the first screen are: "Yesterday, 2 days ago [.... up to], 1 week ago etc". The user moves backwards in time to select the day. The App uses the timing of drinking and the quantity selected (see below) to calculate average quantity consumed.

In addition, to better describe drinking which may stop and start according to geographic location or circumstance, participants are asked about their longest gap without alcohol in the last 12-months (indicating the actual length of time using the same retrospective grog diary and nominating reasons for this dry period).

Each individual is also asked about a 'heavy' drinking occasion: "In the last 12 months, when you drank a lot of grog, would you ever drink more than [this–]?". An image depicting the largest amount of alcohol that the person reported consuming in the last four drinking occasions is then shown. If the person responds that they sometimes drink more than that amount, they can select items of alcohol to describe their level of consumption at that higher level of drinking. The individual then reports how *often* they drink a lot for them (see 'Response categories for questions on frequency of drinking' above).

Identifying the type of alcohol a person drinks

Some drinkers are not familiar with the names for some categories of alcohol type, for example, 'fortified wines', but rather they identify type of alcohol by its brand or container. To address this issue, a simplified classification of

alcohol types was agreed on: beer, wine, port or sherry, spirits or other. Pictures of common local brands in each alcohol type would be displayed. The 'other' category included cocktails, methylated spirits and drinks not listed elsewhere.

A listing of common alcohol brands and drinking containers was created for each alcohol type in each surveyed state. With the help of colleagues from those states, this guide was refined to reflect popular alcohol brands but also sufficient choice in each alcohol type. State-based drinking preferences were reflected. For example, "XXXX" was a beer choice made available for Queensland individuals, but instead, "West End" appeared in SA. It was not possible to present every choice, so research assistants were instructed to encourage participants who cannot find their choice to select an alcohol type of similar strength to their preferred brand, or to choose the "other" category.

Beer posed particular challenges as Indigenous colleagues and other clinicians reported confusion around terms such as 'regular strength' versus 'mid strength' or 'low alcohol' [21]. The term 'low carb' was sometimes incorrectly understood to mean 'low alcohol'. To reduce confusion, pictures of several actual beer brands were used. Brand recognition is typically strong. For example, workshop participants advised that in more isolated settings, some types of alcohol are known by the colour of the packaging. So, if hand drawn images were to be used, extra care would need to be taken to ensure comprehension of brand names in different geographical settings.

Drink containers

Indigenous colleagues stressed the importance of offering a broad range of containers from which alcohol might be consumed. For example, many individuals do not drink wine from a wine glass, especially in remote communities. Instead they may use a container sold for other purposes, ranging from a pannikin (metal mug; 355 mL), slurpee/slushy cup (490 mL), empty water bottle (600 mL), through to a large soft drink bottle (1.25 L; see Fig. 2).

Working out individual consumption based on a share of what the whole group drank

Indigenous and non-Indigenous clinicians reported that when collecting an alcohol history, some clients spontaneously report what the whole group had to drink, rather than on what they alone consumed. The clinician then assists the individual to estimate their share. So, when asked about the last drinking occasion, the App enables the participant to choose to describe what they consumed as an individual or to describe what the group drank (see Fig. 3).

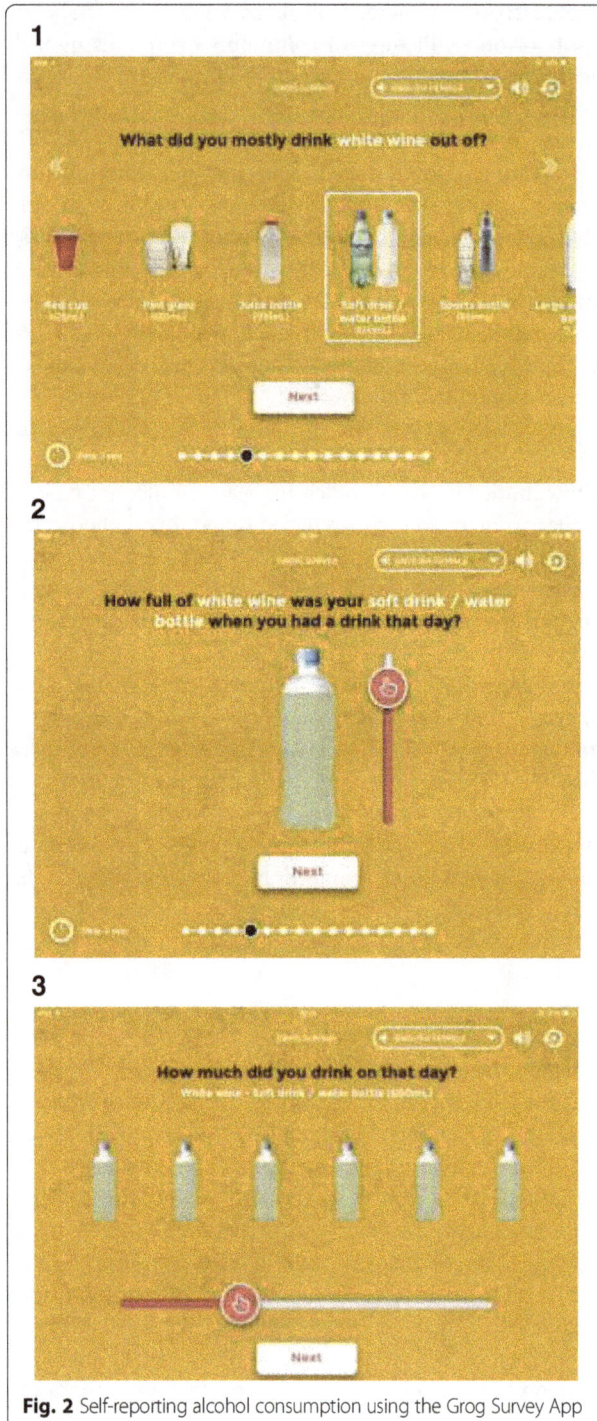

Fig. 2 Self-reporting alcohol consumption using the Grog Survey App

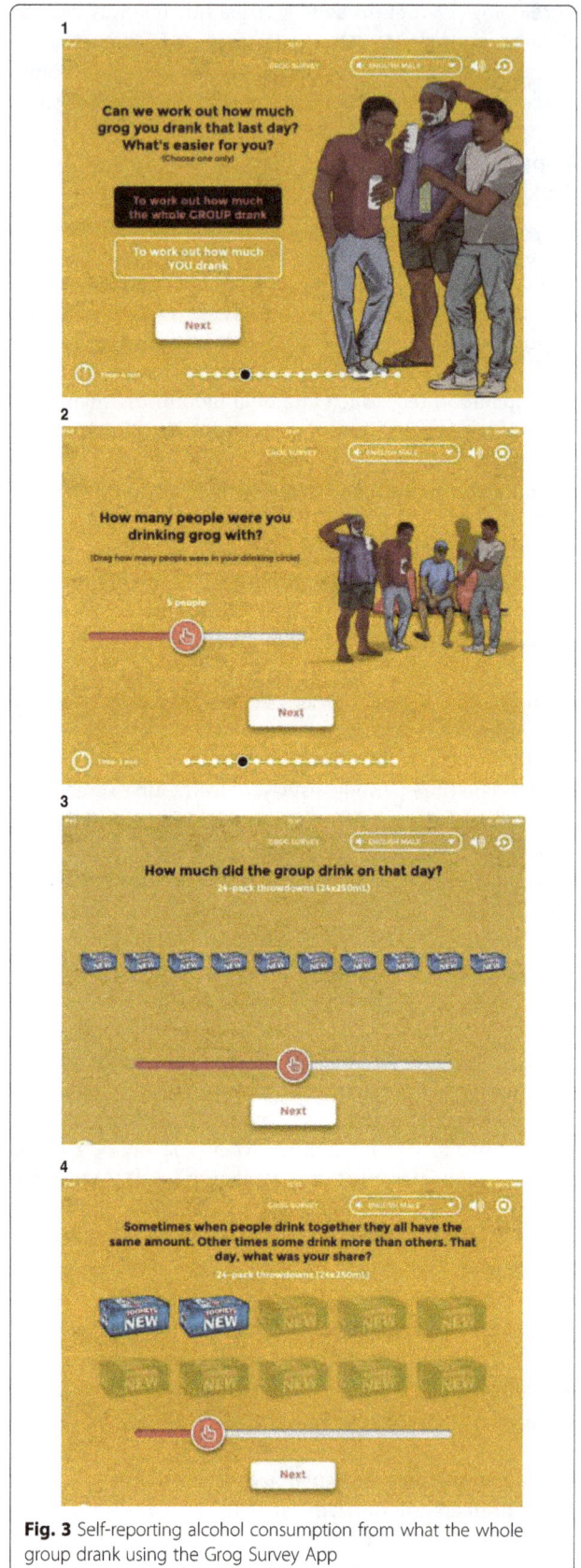

Fig. 3 Self-reporting alcohol consumption from what the whole group drank using the Grog Survey App

After selecting when in the last 12-months the last drinking occasion took place (on the retrospective grog diary), an individual is asked: "How many people were you drinking with?". A 'slider' (from left to right) enables the individual to select: "Just you" through to a group of "10+ people". The accompanying image changes as the slider is moved to show the number of people in the drinking group. The individual then chooses 1) To work out how much the whole group drank or 2) To work out how much they themselves drank.

Then, for example, if an individual selects that the last time they drank, the group consumed ten cases or slabs (24-cans) of full strength beer. The App then asks: "Sometimes when people drink together they all have the same amount. Other times some drink more than others. That day, what was your share?" In the screen-shot below (Fig. 3), an individual reported a total of five people in their drinking group. So, the next screen defaults to showing an image of two out of ten cases as that individual's share (i.e. the App assumes an equal share of beer on this occasion). The individual can then slide a meter to adjust their individual portion. Invisible to the user, each container is divided into 10 to calculate standard drinks. For example, of the ten cases of full strength beer consumed by the group, the individual consumed two cases (see Fig. 3). Estimated at 4.8% alcohol/volume at 0.789 g/mL, this equates to 45.5 standard drinks consumed by that individual on that occasion.

Modifying AUDIT Q3

This item was modified to be in keeping with Australian drinking guidelines (i.e. to ask about consuming *five* drinks or more on an occasion) [7]. Also, instead of relying on participants to convert what they drink into 'standard drinks', the App dynamically produces an image of 50 g or more of ethanol based on the type of alcohol that each individual consumed the most of (i.e. the maximum grams of alcohol) from their last four drinking occasions (see Table 2).

Image and audio options

When a survey is started, each participant identifies their gender. The images, audio and lifestyle references are then matched with that gender. For example, female participants predominantly see women and girls in the images on screen and the audio is spoken by a woman. Original artwork featured on the app was commissioned from an artist employed by the Aboriginal Drug and Alcohol Council SA.

Two language options are offered in the Stage 1 version of the App – English or Pitjantjatjara, a language of Indigenous Australians used in a region of South Australia, Northern Territory and Western Australia. To begin with, two experienced Indigenous alcohol and other drug professionals recorded the English female and then the English male audio. During recording, there was further refinement of the wording of survey items, for example, to check that phrasing was comfortable. Suggestions made by these clinicians during the recording process were checked at the time with three researchers (Lee, Conigrave and Perry).

The Pitjantjatjara language program at the University of South Australia facilitated translation of survey items from English to Pitjantjatjara (including 'back translation' of key items). Audio was provided by two Pitjantjatjara language speakers/interpreters (a male and a female). This team and a researcher (Perry) met face-to-face to workshop the translation of survey items. Where there was differing opinion, clarification was sought on intended meaning from a researcher (Perry or Conigrave), until consensus was reached. Efforts were made to ensure suitability of survey items for Pitjantjatjara speakers from adolescence to old age. Further workshopping of survey items occurred in the recording studio. To ensure consistency, one researcher (Perry, who speaks some Pitjantjatjara) was present for one of the English and both of the Pitjantjatjara (male and female) recordings. Suggestions made during the recording process were checked at the time by two researchers (Lee and Perry).

Discussion

This study describes for the first time the process taken to develop a tablet-based survey 'App' to help Indigenous Australians to describe and measure their drinking. The approach described is consistent with earlier interactive touch screen-based platforms that screen for alcohol use (and other risk factors) in Indigenous Australians [27, 28]. However, it extends this work in several ways. While previous studies have focused on screening [27, 28] or health promotion [28], this study sets out to create an alternative way to measure self-reported alcohol consumption in a detailed manner that is similar to approaches used in a household survey. This potentially will provide a gold standard against which shorter screening tools can be validated. Validation of the survey App itself, comparing it with a clinical assessment and also test-retest, is currently being conducted as well as an assessment of its acceptability. These will be reported separately.

Worldwide there are challenges in recording an accurate assessment of drinking [9]. This challenge is greater if alcohol is shared, for example, as is described in Africa and in Indigenous Australia [29–31]. Reliance on individuals to convert their consumption to standard drinks (or units) is fraught. Even in higher socio-economic status populations, comfort with mathematics varies. In lower socio-economic status groups, or in subpopulations with lower literacy in the mainstream language or numeracy, the challenge is greater. This situation is likely to occur increasingly in multicultural societies and with rising numbers of displaced persons.

With any survey platform, getting participants to accurately reflect on their drinking presents a challenge [32]. A survey-based App can harness available technologies to dynamically customize the survey experience for each participant. For example, a conversational style of questions in plain English text can be augmented by audio in the local language with pictures customized to gender and community setting, to help create a relaxed friendly and responsive 'interview' environment [33].

Mathematical formulae embedded in the programming back-end can convert the library of images showing actual alcohol products and range of containers in the front-end into standard drinks (or grams of alcohol). This can help the individual to recall what they were drinking without the need to use mental arithmetic to convert drinks consumed into "standard" drinks.

In busy Indigenous primary care settings, some Indigenous health professionals have been reticent to conduct alcohol screening because they may be required to screen their own family members or friends [34]. Also, individuals may be reticent to take part in alcohol screening (or surveys) because of past experience of racism and discrimination [35]. The App enables participants to 'anonymously' tell their alcohol story without needing to make personal disclosures to a research assistant or health professional. Even if the research assistant knows the individual, individuals are informed during recruitment and explanation of the study that data cannot be accessed or linked to an individual once entered into the App.

This appealing format of the App is also likely to result in higher response rates. In field-testing to date, research assistants report being inundated by community members wanting to try out the App having heard about it via 'word of mouth' (personal communication with J Perry, S Wilson, N Hayman; qualitative feedback from staff will be reported in a later paper).

Limitations

In this work, an iterative process of advice seeking was used to develop the App instead of formal focus groups or semi-structured interviews. However, such an approach allowed us to work from the 'ground up', collaborating with the broadest range of colleagues and to reflect varied viewpoints [6, 36].

The number of survey items that could be included was limited, as it was recommended that the duration of the App survey should be no more than 20 min. This suited the target population who are often time-poor and where there can be many distractions (such as the needs of children or relatives). It also suited the Indigenous primary care services and other drug and alcohol facilities where recruitment occurred, where time pressure is reported as a significant barrier to alcohol screening [34, 37].

Validation of the App

Between August 2016 to May 2017, a pilot version of the survey is being administered to Aboriginal or Torres Strait Islander respondents in three rural and remote sites in South Australia and one urban site in Queensland. The Queensland site was likely to recruit Aboriginal or Torres Strait Islander respondents, given its proximity to the Torres Strait and Papua New Guinea. The Aboriginal field research assistants who administered the survey in Queensland are known to the community and are aware of particular issues in relation to alcohol and other drug use in individuals from a Torres Strait background [10]. The responses to the app will be compared with a clinical assessment conducted by an Indigenous health professional, and with a repeat administration of the survey App (2-7 days later). Analysis will examine the internal and external validity of the app, test-re-test reliability, acceptability and feasibility. The App converts the amount and strength of alcohol consumed into the equivalent number of Australian standard drinks (each 10 g ethanol). The consumption on each of the last four drinking sessions, and the number of days between sessions are used to estimate the average number of standard drinks per drinking day, the number of drinking days per year and total volume consumed for the year in grams of ethanol (and then in Australian standard drinks). In addition, consumption on the heaviest drinking session is calculated. Efforts will then be made to further shorten the duration of the App survey.

Future applications

Household surveys: The App could be a cost-effective way to collect and store confidential survey data, even on a national level. It can operate 'off line' so is suitable for isolated settings where there may be little or no internet access. There would be an initial outlay to conduct comprehensive translations and back translations [38] and audio recordings in different languages. However, such recordings are cheaper than having translators present during each administration of the survey. Also, audio recording ensures standardization of instructions across all surveys.

Research in general populations: The technology used to create the survey App could have broader benefits beyond this field of research. Instead of needing to store confidential paper surveys while out in the field, data are simply synchronized daily from each tablet-computer to a secure central point (e.g. university or government server). This can be performed using wireless internet tethered to a smart phone or other wireless modem. Study leaders can also access data remotely during data collection. This allows for monitoring of study progress in 'real' time (e.g. to check quotas of data collected, better support research assistants in the field).

Computer screening in clinic waiting rooms: The App could be modified to improve the way alcohol screening and assessment is conducted with clients. For example, clients could be handed a tablet (and headphones) in the waiting room and asked to complete a survey. Completed surveys could then be shared with the treating health professional with the client's consent. This could help the health professional to become aware of possible unhealthy drinking [39] including any risk of alcohol withdrawal. Further work is needed to better understand the effectiveness of brief intervention among Indigenous populations [40]. However, more accurate assessment of drinking will improve both screening and outcome measurement.

The guidance into ways of asking an alcohol history, obtained from consultation for this app, is very relevant to clinicians. This includes making it easier for patients to relate to time points marking the last 12-months. Also, clinicians can avoid making patients do mental arithmetic, in either self-reporting their drinking or when the clinician is conveying drinking guidelines.

Health promotion role: National drinking guidelines are often expressed in standard drinks or units, which can be hard for the individual to relate to their own drinking. The Grog Survey App could help a person to first quantify their drinking, and then to compare this against current drinking guidelines.

Conclusion

Estimating alcohol consumption is challenging in any setting [41]. It is made more so when alcohol is shared or there may be only intermittent access to alcohol. This requires a 'shake up' of existing ways of asking about alcohol consumption in surveys or clinical practice. Interactive tablet-based technologies potentially enable some of these challenges to be overcome. The detailed and iterative advice provided by a range of content experts helped to create a survey App that was respectful of a range of viewpoints (cultural, clinical, health promotion, policy, research etc). The approach taken to develop the App and its key features are likely to be useful for a wide range of marginalized populations. They are also relevant to assessing drinking in the developing world, where drinking is often in unstandardized containers. Among vulnerable groups the need for an accurate estimation of alcohol consumption is particularly important to inform prevention and treatment efforts.

Acknowledgements
This work was supported by the National Health and Medical Research Council (NHMRC) through a Project Grant (#1087192), the Centre of Research Excellence in Indigenous Health and Alcohol (#1117198) and a Practitioner Fellowship for K Conigrave (#1117582). Chikritzhs, Gray and Wilkes are supported by funding from the Australian Government under the Substance Misuse Prevention and Service Improvement Grants Fund. We would also like to acknowledge the help of: the communities and services who took part and who remain anonymous; and of Mustafa Al-Ansari, Alexandra Carr, Teagan Weatherall, Monika Dzidowska and John Redmond from the University of Sydney; and of Mira Branezac from NSW Health's Drug and Alcohol Health Services Library.

Funding
This work was supported by the Australian National Health and Medical Research Council (NHMRC; Project Grant ID#1087192 and a Practitioner Fellowship for K Conigrave).

Authors' contributions
KL: literature review, drafted paper, designed tables and figures, synthesised co-authors' comments. SW: initiated idea for grant application that this study is funded by, reviewed drafts of paper, key to process of developing and implementing the iPad application. JP: reviewed drafts of paper, key to process of developing and implementing the iPad application, reviewed draft of paper. RR: key to reviewing alcohol survey items featured in the iPad application, reviewed draft of paper. SC: key to reviewing alcohol survey items featured in the iPad application, reviewed draft of paper. RA: key input to ensure alcohol survey items fit with Aboriginal health professional best practice, reviewed draft of paper. NH: key to reviewing alcohol survey items featured in the iPad application, and ensuring that alcohol survey items fit with Aboriginal health professional best practice, reviewed draft of paper. TC: key to reviewing alcohol survey items featured in the iPad application, reviewed draft of paper. DG: key to reviewing alcohol survey items featured in the iPad application, and ensuring that alcohol survey items fit with Aboriginal health professional best practice, reviewed draft of paper. EW: key to reviewing alcohol survey items featured in the iPad application, and ensuring that alcohol survey items fit with Aboriginal health professional best practice, reviewed draft of paper. PJ: key input to ensure alcohol survey items fit with Aboriginal health professional best practice, reviewed draft of paper. KC: key to reviewing alcohol survey items featured in the iPad application, and ensuring that alcohol survey items fit with best clinical practice, reviewed several drafts of paper including tables and figures. All authors have read and approved the manuscript.

Competing interests
The authors declare that they have no competing interests.

Author details
[1]University of Sydney, Discipline of Addiction Medicine, Indigenous Health and Substance Use, NHMRC Centre of Research Excellence in Indigenous Health and Alcohol, King George V Building, 83-117 Missenden Road, Camperdown, NSW 2050, Australia. [2]Centre for Alcohol Policy Research, La Trobe University, 215 Franklin Street, Melbourne, VIC 3000, Australia. [3]Aboriginal Drug and Alcohol Council (ADAC) South Australia, 155 Holbrooks Road Underdale, Adelaide, South Australia 5032, Australia. [4]Alcohol, Tobacco and other Drugs Service, Queensland Health, 190 Palmerston Vincent, Townsville, QLD 4814, Australia. [5]Southern Queensland Centre of Excellence in Aboriginal and Torres Strait Islander Primary Health Care, 37 Wirraway Parade, Inala, QLD 4077, Australia. [6]School of Medicine, University of Queensland, Herston Road, Brisbane, QLD 4006, Australia. [7]School of Medicine, Griffith University, Gold Coast Campus, Gold Coast, Brisbane, QLD 4222, Australia. [8]National Drug Research Institute, Curtin University, 10 Selby St, Shenton Park, WA 6008, Australia. [9]Drug Health Services, Royal Prince Alfred Hospital, Sydney Local Health District, KGV Building, Missenden Road, Camperdown, NSW 2050, Australia.

References
1. Australian Institute of Health and Welfare. Substance use among aboriginal and Torres Strait islander people. Canberra: AIHW; 2011.
2. Chikritzhs T, Brady M. Fact or fiction? A critique of the National Aboriginal and Torres Strait islander social survey 2002. Drug and Alcohol Review. 2006;25(3):277–87.
3. Lee K, et al. Better methods to collect self-reported alcohol and other drug use data from aboriginal and Torres Strait islander Australians. Drug and Alcohol Review. 2014;33:466–72.
4. Chikritzhs T, Liang W. In: Hunter B, Biddle N, editors. Does the 2008 NATSISS underestimate the prevalence of high risk Indigenous drinking?, in Survey analysis for indigenous policy in Australia: Social science perspectives. Canberra: ANU E Press; 2012. p. 49–64.

5.   Gray D, et al. Managing alcohol-related problems among indigenous Australians: what the literature tells us. Aust N Z J Public Health. 2010; 34(S1):S34–5.

6.   Ministerial Council on Drug Strategy. National Drug Strategy Aboriginal and Torres Strait islander peoples complementary action plan 2003-2009 (background paper). Canberra: Commonwealth of Australia; 2006.

7.   Haber P, et al. Guidelines for the treatment of alcohol problems. Canberra: Australian Government Department of Health and Ageing; 2009.

8.   Chikritzhs T, Brady M. Postscript to 'fact or fiction: a critique of the National Aboriginal and Torres Strait islander social survey 2002' (letter). Drug and Alcohol Review. 2007;26:221–2.

9.   Dawson D, Room R. Towards agreement on ways to measure and report drinking patterns and alcohol-related problems in adult general population surveys: the SkarpoÈ conference overview. J Subst Abus Treat. 2000;12:1–21.

10. Conigrave K, Lee K, Freeburn B. In: Haber P, Day C, Farrell M, editors. Aboriginal and Torres Strait Islander Australians, in Addiction medicine: principles and practice, vol. 464. Melbourne: IP Communications; 2015.

11. Lee K, et al. Handbook for aboriginal alcohol and drug work. Sydney: University of Sydney; 2012. p. 446.

12. Zhang MW, Fang P, Ho RC. Global outreach and user preferences of a smartphone application developed for drinkers. Technol Health Care. 2016; 24(4):495–501.

13. Islam M, et al. The reliability of sensitive information provided by injecting drug users in a clinical setting: clinician administered versus audio computer-assisted selfinterviewing (ACASI). AIDS Care. 2012;24(12):1496–503.

14. Ward, J., et al., Findings from the GOANNA study. HIV Australia (online), 2013. 11.

15. Saunders J, et al. Development of the alcohol use disorders identification test (AUDIT): WHO collaborative project on early detection of persons with harmful alcohol consumption–II. Addiction. 1993;88:791–804.

16. Cottler LB, Robins LN, Helzer JE. The reliability of the CIDI-SAM: a comprehensive substance abuse interview. Br J Addict. 1989;84(7):801–14.

17. Humeniuk R, Ali R. Validation of the alcohol, smoking and substance involvement screening test (ASSIST) and pilot brief intervention: a technical report of phase II findings of the WHO ASSIST project. Geneva: World Health Organization (WHO); 2006.

18. Wilsnack RW, et al. Gender and alcohol consumption: patterns from the multinational GENACIS project. Addiction. 2009;104(9):1487–500.

19. Casswell S, et al. The international alcohol control (IAC) study-evaluating the impact of alcohol policies. Alcohol Clin Exp Res. 2012;36(8):1462–7.

20. Australian Bureau of Statistics. 2008 National Aboriginal and Torres Strait islander social survey. Cat. 4714.0. Canberra: Australian Bureau of Statistics; 2009.

21. Australian Institute of Health and Welfare. 2013 National Drug Strategy Household Survey Questionnaire. Canberra: AIHW; 2013.

22. Schlesinger CM, et al. The development and validation of the indigenous risk impact screen (IRIS): a 13-item screening instrument for alcohol and drug and mental health risk. Drug and Alcohol Review. 2007;26:109–17.

23. Laslett A-M, et al. Surveying the range and magnitude of alcohol's harm to others in Australia. Addiction. 2011;106(9):1603–11.

24. Hunter E, Hall W, Spargo R. The distribution and correlates of alcohol consumption in a remote Aboriginal population. Sydney: National Drug and Alcohol Research Centre; 1991.

25. Sobell L, Sobell M. In: Litten R, Allen J, editors. Timeline Follow Back: A technique for assessing self-reported alcohol consumption, in Measuring Alcohol Consumption: Psychosocial and Biochemical Methods. Totowa: Humana Press; 1992. p. 41–72.

26. Alanko T. In: Smart R, et al., editors. An overview of techniques and problems in measurement of alcohol consumption, in Research advances in alcohol and drug problems (Volume 8). New York: Plenum Press; 1984. p. 209–26.

27. Noble N, et al. Does a retrospective seven-day alcohol diary reflect usual alcohol intake for a predominantly disadvantaged Australian aboriginal population? Subst Use Misuse. 2015;50(3):308–19.

28. Hunter E, et al. Bridging the triple divide: performance and innovative multimedia in the service of Behavioural health change in remote indigenous settings. Australasian Psychiatry. 2007;15:S44.

29. Oishi T, Hayashi K. From ritual dance to disco: change in habitual use of tobacco and alcohol among the Baka hunter-gathers of south eastern Cameroon. African Study Monographs. 2014;47:143–63.

30. May P, et al. Epidemiology of fetal alcohol syndrome in a south African Community in the Western Cape Province. Am J Public Health. 2000; 90(12):1905–12.

31. Room R, et al. Alcohol and developing societies: a public health approach. Geneva: Finnish Foundation for Alcohol Studies World Health Organization; 2002. p. 86–94.

32. Casswell S, Huckle T, Pledger M. Survey data need not underestimate alcohol consumption. Alcoholism. 2002;26:1561–7.

33. Moyo V, et al. Traditional beer consumption and the iron status of spouse pairs from a rural Community in Zimbabwe. Blood Journal. 1997;89(6):2159–66.

34. Brady M, et al. The feasibility and acceptability of introducing brief intervention for alcohol misuse in an urban aboriginal medical service. Drug and Alcohol Review. 2002;21:375–80.

35. Deloitte Access Economics. An economic analysis for aboriginal and Torres Strait islander offenders: prison vs residential treatment. Canberra: Deloitte Access Economics; 2012.

36. Wild R, Anderson P. Ampe Akelyernemane Meke Mekarle: little children are sacred, report of the northern territory Board of Inquiry into the protection of aboriginal children from sexual abuse. Darwin: Northern Territory Government; 2007. p. 320.

37. Clifford A, Shakeshaft A. Evidence-based alcohol screening and brief intervention in aboriginal community controlled health services: experiences of health-care providers. Drug and Alcohol Review. 2011;30:55–62.

38. World Health Organisation. Management of substance abuse: process of translation and adaptation of instruments. 2017; Available from: http://www.who.int/substance_abuse/research_tools/translation/en/. [cited 2017 16 April].

39. Bonevski B, et al. Randomized controlled trial of a computer strategy to increase general practitioner preventive care. Prev Med. 1999;29(6 Pt 1):478–86.

40. Leske S, et al. Systematic review of interventions for indigenous adults with mental and substance use disorders in Australia, Canada, New Zealand and the United States. Aust N Z J Psychiatry. 2016;50(11):1040–54.

41. Gmel G, Rehm J. Measuring alcohol consumption. Contemporary Drug Problems. 2004;31:467–540.

Development and validation of a model for the adoption of structured and standardised data recording among healthcare professionals

Erik Joukes[1]* , Ronald Cornet[1], Martine C. de Bruijne[2], Nicolette F. de Keizer[1] and Ameen Abu-Hanna[1]

Abstract

Background: Healthcare professionals provide care to patients and during that process, record large quantities of data in patient records. Data in an Electronic Health Record should ideally be recorded once and be reusable within the care process as well as for secondary purposes. A common approach to realise this is to let healthcare providers record data in a standardised and structured way at the point of care. Currently, it is not clear to what extent this structured and standardised recording has been adopted by healthcare professionals and what barriers to their adoption exist. Therefore, we developed and validated a multivariable model to capture the concepts underlying the adoption of structured and standardised recording among healthcare professionals.

Methods: Based on separate models from the literature we developed a new theoretical model describing the underlying concepts of the adoption of structured and standardised recording. Using a questionnaire built upon this model we gathered data to perform a summative validation of our model. Validation was done through partial least squares structural equation modelling (PLS-SEM). The quality of both levels defined in PLS-SEM analysis, i.e., the measurement model and the structural model, were assessed on performance measures defined in literature.

Results: The theoretical model we developed consists of 29 concepts related to information systems as well as organisational factors and personal beliefs. Based on these concepts, 59 statements with a 5 point Likert-scale (fully disagree to fully agree) were specified in the questionnaire. We received 3584 responses. The validation shows our model is supported to a large extent by the questionnaire data. Intention to record in a structured and standardised way emerged as a significant factor of reported behaviour ($\beta = 0.305$, $p < 0.001$). This intention is influenced most by attitude ($\beta = 0.512$, $p < 0.001$).

Conclusions: This model can be used to measure the perceived level of adoption of structured and standardised recording among healthcare professionals and further improve knowledge on the barriers and facilitators of this adoption.

Keywords: Electronic health records, Adoption, Intention, Structured, Standardised, Recording, Structural equation modelling

* Correspondence: e.joukes@amc.uva.nl
[1]Department of Medical Informatics, Amsterdam Public Health research institute, Academic Medical Center, University of Amsterdam, P.O. Box 22700, 1100 DE Amsterdam, The Netherlands
Full list of author information is available at the end of the article

Background

Healthcare professionals provide care to patients and record large quantities of data in patient records during that process. These data are used in daily care practice as records of the history of a patient, parts of the thought process of the physician, and the planned course of treatment. These data are used to make informed decisions about diagnosis and treatment. These data are increasingly recorded digitally in electronic health records (EHRs). These systems, and their underlying databases, enable storage and easy retrieval of data. By storing the data in an electronic form, the possibilities of data reuse increase. The data can be reused for other purposes such as decision support, generation of discharge letters, scientific research, management information, quality assurance through auditing registries, and reimbursement. However, for data to be fully reusable they have to be stored structured and standardised. A common approach to realise this is to let healthcare providers record data in a standardised and structured way at the point of care.

The main focus of our study is recording at the point of care of structured and standardised data that are reusable within the care process as well as for secondary purposes. This means that healthcare professionals must record data in an Electronic Health Record once, in a standardised and structured way by using structured forms and coding systems. This specific method of recording differs from the way of working that numerous physicians have been used to for decades, using free text for precisely recording the patient status, combined with sometimes multiple ways of coding for research. This means that structured and standardised data recording is not automatically and fully adopted by healthcare professionals. In addition, the actual data recording might take more time than current working procedures. The efficiency effect of reusing data is not always clear to the physicians, and they have concerns about a higher recording burden [1]. An additional barrier may be that physicians who record the data are not always the ones benefitting from the profits of structured and standardised data recording. For example, physicians might require more time to record in a structured manner, while administrative staff benefits using the data for financial reimbursement or management purposes.

Currently, it is not clear to what extent structured and standardised data recording has been adopted by healthcare professionals. For the management of hospitals the largest impediments for this adoption are unclear. Therefore, in this study, we aim to develop a multivariable model to capture the interrelating concepts underlying the adoption of structured and standardised data recording among healthcare professionals. The model includes concepts related to information systems as well as organisational factors and personal beliefs and can be used to identify those concepts relevant to the adoption of structured and standardised recording and barriers that currently limit the adoption. The results of our model should further our understanding of the underlying theory pertaining to structured and standardised data recording. Additionally, this might help hospital management and national coordinating organizations to improve the adoption by working on identified barriers, thereby using the limited available resources of these organizations to solve the most limiting factors holding back the adoption.

To evaluate the validity of our theoretical model we performed a summative evaluation. The results of this evaluation indicate to what extent the model is supported by the collected data obtained by questionnaires. Additionally, this evaluation can give leads to where future research can update and improve our theoretical model.

Methods

Our method consists of four steps. First, we developed the model based on other validated models from the literature. A number of models have described the usage intention or acceptance of a specific system by the users, or the system's success [2–5]. Our main outcome is, however, not the intention to use a system but the intention to record data in a certain way (i.e. structured and standardised). Therefore, we need to develop and validate a new model that can be used to measure those healthcare professionals' intentions. Second, based on this model we created a questionnaire. Third, we used our questionnaire to collect data from healthcare professionals. Finally, we use partial least squares structural equation modelling to empirically validate our model using data we collected in the third step. Further details on all four steps are described below.

Development of the theoretical model

The outcome of our model will be the (self-reported) adoption of structured and standardised data recording. We performed an exploratory literature search to identify models that describe the acceptance of electronic healthcare systems and human-computer interactions. From those models we selected two models [6, 7] that were relevant to our goal. The model of Wixom and Todd [7] describes an integrated model combining user satisfaction and technology acceptance. The model of Hsieh [6] targets the acceptance of electronic medical records exchange. Since these two models are both based on the Technology Acceptance Model (TAM), we were able to link them on matching concepts (perceived usefulness, perceived ease of use, attitude, and intention). Both models have been validated with structural equation modelling [6, 7]. Based on other literature [8] we added specific concepts that the models were lacking, addressing the goal of our model.

Questionnaire development and data collection

For each theoretical concept in our model, we specified at least one concrete question that covers the concept. Together with demographic questions this set of questions were presented in an online questionnaire. This questionnaire was sent to healthcare professionals from seven out of the eight Dutch university hospitals. All professions working with patient data or the EHR were included (e.g. physicians, nurses, researchers). In five hospitals, all personnel working with patient data were included, in two hospitals a random selection of 1000 people were included. Data were collected between May and November 2015. The first question of the questionnaire was whether the respondent was an active or passive user of the questionnaire. Passive users only read data from the EHR, whereas active users also record data in the system. The active users received the full questionnaire, the passive users only a selection of relevant questions. Only the active user respondents were included in the current analysis.

Model validation

To validate our model we performed structural equation modelling (SEM) using the partial least squares (PLS) method [9]. SEM is a group of multivariate techniques combining aspects of factor analysis and regression where relationships among observed variables (the questions in the questionnaire) and latent variables (the concepts in the model), as well as among latent variables are analysed [9]. The PLS variant of SEM is especially suitable for models with a high number of latent and observed variables. Additionally, PLS does not require the data to be normally distributed. The technique is used both within [6, 10] and outside [7] of the healthcare domain.

In SEM the distinction is made between the measurement model and the structural model (see Fig. 1a and b). The structural model was obtained from the development

of the theoretical model. This structural model (Fig. 1a) shows the latent variables and their interrelations as we have defined them a priori. These latent variables are the concepts of our theoretical model which are not measured directly by the questions in the questionnaire.

Each question in our questionnaire, called an observed variable, reflects an aspect of one of the latent variables in the model. In the measurement model (Fig. 1b) the observed variables are linked to the latent variables. This model indicates which observed variables are related to which latent variables. For example, the questions 'format1' (corresponding to the statement "The format of the patient record is clear") and 'format2' ("Because of clear formatting, data in the patient record can easily be recognised") are observed variables referring to format of the data. These are linked to 'format', the corresponding latent variable, in the measurement model. The latent variable 'format' is linked to the other latent variable 'information satisfaction' through the structural model. All the latent variables in our model are reflective (rather than formative), indicating the assumption that the latent variable is responsible for the variability in the observed variables.

We will separately validate the measurement model and the structural model. Validating the measurement model will show whether we actually measure what we want to measure within each concept. For this validation we determined the performance measures as described by Hair et al. [9] and listed in Table 1. The criteria for the validation of the measurement model are not applicable to single-item concepts [9]. Therefore we can only calculate the measures for latent variables that had more than one observed variable.

The validation of the structural model based on the data that we collected will show whether our a priori defined model is valid. In this step, we evaluated: the coefficients of determination (R^2) and the size and relevance of the path coefficients.

We used the statistical environment R (version 3.3.1) [11] with the plspm package version 0.4.7 [12]. To adjust for the missing values in our dataset we used stochastic multiple imputation methods from the mice package to

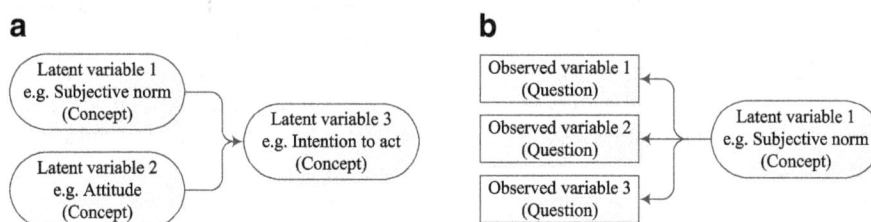

Fig. 1 a Structural model - showing the relation between three latent variables (concepts from our theoretical model). **b** Measurement model - showing the relation between three observed variables (questions from our questionnaire) and one latent variable (concept from the theoretical model).

Table 1 Used performance measures and targets to validate the measurement model from Hair et al. [9]

Type of validation	Measure	Target
internal consistency / composite reliability	Dillon Goldstein's rho (alternatives are Cronbach's alpha and eigenvalues)	> 0.60 are acceptable in exploratory research
indicator reliability	outer loadings	> 0.708
convergent validity	Average Variance Extracted (AVE)	> 0.5
discriminant validity	A) outer loadings	A) the outer loading of an observed variable on its concept is higher than its cross loadings with other concepts
	B) Fornell-Larcker criterion	B) the square root of the AVE of a concept should be higher than its correlations with all other concepts

create five datasets without missing values. All analyses were performed on one dataset. To determine the effect of this imputation we performed a sensitivity analysis by repeating all analyses on the four additional imputed datasets. We compared the results of the different analyses.

Different types of healthcare providers have different ways of interacting with patient data and EHRs. This means that the performance of the model might be different if we use data of a subgroup based on a specific type of healthcare provider. Therefore in addition to using the full dataset we repeated the model validation using two subsets of the data: data of either medical specialists or nurses, as these are the largest groups of healthcare providers that actively use the EHR. We compared the performance measures for these two subgroups with those of the overall model and evaluated the performance of the two additional models based on the same targets as listed in Table 1. The latter indicates whether the final conclusion concerning the performance of our model would be different when it is based on a subgroup of healthcare providers.

The study design was submitted to the ethics committee of the VU University Medical Center Amsterdam, and was exempt from review (reference 2015.185).

Results
Development of the theoretical model
Figure 2 shows the proposed theoretical model based on the literature. All other hypothesised relations, based on the underlying validated models [6, 7], are depicted therein. For example; system satisfaction influences perceived ease of use and information satisfaction. Table 2 provides the origin and a description of all concepts.

The main outcome of our theoretical model is the self-reported behaviour of care professionals, i.e. whether they report to have adopted structured and standardised data recording. Behaviour is influenced by the professional's intention to act. This intention is based on attitude, subjective norm, perceived behavioural control, institutional trust, and perceived risk. All concepts on the

right-hand side of the model, are related to working processes and human attitudes. The concepts influencing attitude describe the professional's knowledge of structured and standardised data recording and whether they think this way of working is usable, useful, and aligned with their own working processes. The items in the lower right quadrant describe the environmental factors such as the promotion of structured and standardised data recording by supervisors and colleagues, the level of control the professional has, and the perceived risks that the work processes might pose. Improvements in this part of the model need to come from changing the way people perceive their working environment, their work processes, and structured and standardised data recording.

The concepts in the model on the left-hand side of the diagram are all related to the documentation system in place in the organization, in most cases an EHR. These are the concepts that can be influenced by changing aspects of the EHR itself. The items information reliability (from [8]), completeness, accuracy, format, and currency, all indicate separate facets of information quality. They all describe a specific aspect of the stored data or information in an EHR that influences whether the users of the system trust the data (reliability, accuracy, currency) and whether they can actually understand and work with the data (completeness, format). All these items influence whether the user is satisfied with the information that is presented (information satisfaction). The concepts system reliability, flexibility, integration, accessibility, and timeliness represent aspects of system satisfaction. They influence the opinion of the EHR users on the quality of the system.

Finally, we removed two concepts from the Wixom and Todd model (information quality and system quality). For these two items, the questions in our questionnaire were too similar to those that belong to the items information satisfaction and system satisfaction.

Questionnaire development and data collection
The questionnaire included 59 questions based on all 29 concepts of our model, supplemented with 17 questions

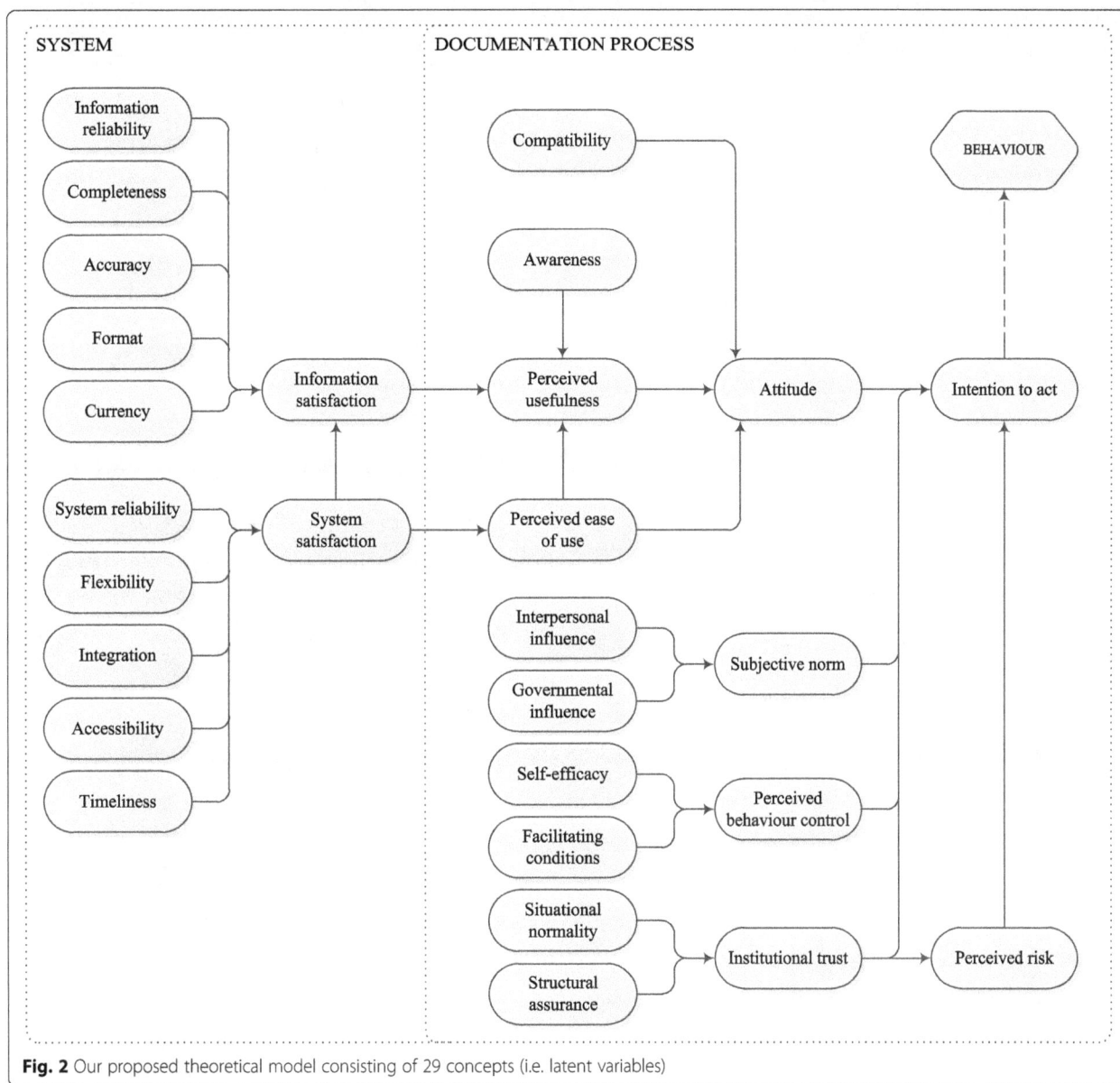

Fig. 2 Our proposed theoretical model consisting of 29 concepts (i.e. latent variables)

on demographic data. Additional file 1 shows an English translation of the original Dutch version of the 59 questions based on the model. We received responses to our questionnaire from 5011 participants of which only the 3584 active users were included in the analyses described in this paper. The demographics of our respondents are summarised in Table 3. The number of missing values was between 6 and 57% (IQR 22–33%) per variable. For more detailed information on missing data see Additional file 2: Table S1.

Model validation
The measurement model
The results of the validation of the measurement model are listed in Tables 4 and 5, and Additional file 2.

First, we evaluated the composite reliability by calculating the Dillon Goldstein's rho. All relevant latent variables had a Dillon Goldstein's rho of more than 0.7, apart from attitude which had a score of 0.62. Hence, all these scores were above the limit of 0.6 suggested for indicating composite reliability. Evaluation of the Cronbach's alpha and eigenvalues showed qualitatively similar results.

To estimate the indicator reliability, we calculated the loadings of the observed variables on the latent variables. In six of the 12 blocks of latent variables all loadings were > 0.708 (accuracy, format, integration, intention to act, perceived ease of use, and structural assurance). Although the other six blocks (attitude, awareness, behaviour, information reliability, perceived risk, and

Table 2 All concepts in our model, including origin and explanation of each concept

Model concepts	Wixom and Todd [7]	Hsieh [6]	This study	Explanation
Information reliability			X	Whether the information in the EHR is reliable
Completeness	X			Whether the information in the EHR is complete
Accuracy	X			Whether the information in the EHR is accurate
Format	X			Whether the information in the EHR is in an understandable format
Currency	X			Whether the information in the EHR is up to date
System reliability	X			Whether the user can trust that the EHR works
Flexibility	X			Whether the user can use the EHR flexibly in different situations
Integration	X			Whether the user needs to open multiple computer programs to gather all information on patients
Accessibility	X			Whether the user can access the patient data in every place in the organization
Timeliness	X			Whether the system responds to user input in a timely manner
System satisfaction	X			The overall opinion of the user on the quality of the EHR
Compatibility		X		Whether the EHR supports the work processes of the user
Awareness			X	Whether the user knows why it is important that their data are recorded correctly
Perceived ease of use	X	X		The overall opinion of the user on the usability of the EHR
Information satisfaction	X			Whether the user is satisfied with the information that the EHR provides
Perceived usefulness	X	X		Whether the EHR aids in the user's daily work
Attitude	X	X		What the user thinks of structured and standardised recording
Interpersonal influence		X		Whether the supervisor promotes correct recording
Governmental influence		X		Whether the government (i.e. the inspectorate) promotes correct recording
Subjective norm		X		Whether the user records correctly because colleagues expect this
Self-efficacy		X		Whether the user is capable of correct recording
Facilitating conditions		X		Whether there is enough time to record data correctly
Perceived behavioural control		X		Whether it is within the user's control to record data correctly
Situational normality		X		Whether it is normal in the organisation to record correctly
Structural assurance		X		Whether the organisation ensures that data are stored safely and cannot be lost
Institutional trust		X		Whether the user trusts that the organisation stores the records safely
Perceived risk		X		Whether the reuse of data can harm the patients' privacy and or safety
Intention to act	X	X		Whether the user wants to record data structured and standardised and wants to reuse data
Behaviour			X	A number of facets that indicate whether the user is already recording structured and standardised data

perceived usefulness) had at least one observed variable that is > 0.708, one or more loadings in these blocks were < 0.708, see Table 5. These loadings varied from − 0.034 to 0.703. Especially behaviour had a number of very low loadings.

The convergent validity is based on the Average Variance Extracted (AVE) of the concepts. In Table 6 these AVEs are reported. Of the 12 concepts that have multiple indicators, seven had an AVE of > 0.5. The other five concepts (information reliability, awareness,

Table 3 Demographics of the included respondents

	n (%)
Total respondents	3584 (100)
Gender	
Male	889 (25)
Female	2413 (67)
Age	
< 30	461 (13)
30–39	879 (25)
40–49	743 (21)
50–59	868 (24)
> =60	270 (8)
Function	
Analytical staff	57 (2)
Clinical (co-)care provider	336 (9)
Medical support staff	223 (6)
Management	90 (3)
Medical specialists	856 (24)
Administrative staff	247 (7)
Nurses	1358 (38)
Scientific research	251 (7)
Other	265 (7)

perceived usefulness, attitude, and behaviour) had AVEs ranging from 0.250 (behaviour) to 0.481 (awareness).

Discriminant validity is based on the cross loadings of all indicators and concepts that are depicted in Additional file 2: Table S2. It shows that five of the 59 indicators had a cross loading that is higher than

Table 4 Composite reliability measures of latent variables with more than one observed variable

	number of observed variables	Dillon-Goldstein's rho
Attitude	4	0.620
Information reliability	4	0.711
Awareness	3	0.730
Perceived usefulness	5	0.766
Integration	2	0.782
Structural assurance	2	0.802
Behaviour	11	0.804
Accuracy	2	0.825
Perceived risk	2	0.831
Intention to act	2	0.831
Perceived ease of use	3	0.866
Format	2	0.925

Latent variables not mentioned in this table have only one observed variable and therefore no scores on these measures

Table 5 All observed variables, their latent variable, and their loadings

Observed variable	Latent variable	loading
InformationReliability1	information reliability	**0.719**
InformationReliability2	information reliability	0.461
InformationReliability3	information reliability	0.540
InformationReliability4	information reliability	0.703
Accuracy1	accuracy	**0.850**
Accuracy2	accuracy	**0.825**
Format1	format	**0.930**
Format2	format	**0.926**
Integration1	integration	**0.750**
Integration2	integration	**0.847**
Awareness1	awareness	**0.746**
Awareness2	awareness	0.534
Awareness3	awareness	**0.775**
PerceivedEaseOfUse1	perceived ease of use	**0.804**
PerceivedEaseOfUse2	perceived ease of use	**0.865**
PerceivedEaseOfUse3	perceived ease of use	**0.808**
PerceivedUsefulness1	perceived usefulness	0.576
PerceivedUsefulness2	perceived usefulness	**0.800**
PerceivedUsefulness3	perceived usefulness	**0.774**
PerceivedUsefulness4	perceived usefulness	**0.817**
PerceivedUsefulness5	perceived usefulness	0.090
Attitude1	attitude	0.297
Attitude2	attitude	**0.737**
Attitude3	attitude	0.554
Attitude4	attitude	0.689
StructuralAssurance1	structural assurance	**0.737**
StructuralAssurance2	structural assurance	**0.886**
PerceivedRisk1	perceived risk	**0.943**
PerceivedRisk2	perceived risk	0.701
IntentionToAct1	intention to act	**0.750**
IntentionToAct2	intention to act	**0.917**
Behaviour1	behaviour	−0.034
Behaviour2	behaviour	**0.721**
Behaviour3	behaviour	0.689
Behaviour4	behaviour	**0.731**
Behaviour5	behaviour	0.446
Behaviour6	behaviour	0.340
Behaviour7	behaviour	0.240
Behaviour8	behaviour	0.206
Behaviour9	behaviour	0.536
Behaviour10	behaviour	0.623
Behaviour11	behaviour	0.356

Loadings in bold cells satisfy the prescribed threshold (> 0.708). Each observed variable is a question in our questionnaire, the actual questions are available in Additional file 1

Table 6 Latent variables, mean, sd, and Average Variance Extracted (AVE)

Latent variable	mean	sd	AVE
information reliability	3.74	0.63	0.379
completeness	3.54	1.02	1
accuracy	3.44	0.74	0.701
format	3.12	0.97	0.861
currency	3.52	0.90	1
system reliability	3.47	0.90	1
flexibility	3.23	0.97	1
integration	3.00	0.91	0.640
accessibility	3.67	1.07	1
timeliness	3.15	1.05	1
system satisfaction	2.96	1.03	1
compatibility	3.66	0.87	1
awareness	3.60	0.60	0.481
perceived ease of use	2.99	0.91	0.683
information satisfaction	3.27	0.88	1
perceived usefulness	2.93	0.97	0.449
attitude	3.90	0.51	0.353
interpersonal influence	3.43	0.94	1
governmental influence	3.21	0.89	1
subjective norm	3.62	0.88	1
self-efficacy	3.78	0.84	1
facilitating conditions	2.79	1.02	1
perceived behavioural control	3.63	0.88	1
situational normality	3.50	0.91	1
structural assurance	3.49	0.73	0.664
institutional trust	3.97	0.71	1
perceived risk	2.84	0.75	0.690
intention to act	4.04	0.59	0.701
behaviour	3.42	0.56	0.250

the loading on its own concept. Three were situated in the behaviour block, one in awareness, and one in perceived usefulness. The difference between the loadings and cross loadings ranged from 0.325 to 0.035. Additionally, the square root of the AVE and the inter-concept correlations are shown in Additional file 2: Table S3. It shows that the square roots of all AVEs were higher than the inter-concept correlations (Fornell-Larcker criterion).

The structural model
To validate our structural model, we evaluated the coefficients of determination (R^2) and the size and relevance of the path coefficients. Figure 3 shows the resulting structural model with all the path coefficients and the

coefficients of determination. All but three path coefficients were significant at $p < 0.001$. Only accessibility ($p = 0.0531$), perceived ease of use ($p = 0.0012$), and perceived behavioural control ($p = 0.0202$) had higher p-values. The coefficients of determination (R^2) ranged from 0.013 (perceived risk) to 0.448 (information satisfaction).

To evaluate the impact of missing values in our dataset we repeated all tests on four additional imputed datasets. The results showed similar outcomes for all used validation measures (available from authors).

To investigate whether the performance of the model would be different based on only the data from medical specialists or nurses we did two additional validations using the data of only these subgroups. The results and distribution of performance measures of these two validations were comparable to the original measures (see Additional file 2 for the results). More importantly, when we apply the same target values for these additional validations as described in Table 1, the performance of the additional models is the same as that of our general model using all available data.

Discussion
In this study, we constructed and validated a theoretical model representing underlying concepts that influence the adoption of structured and standardised data recording by healthcare professionals. The model includes concepts related to information systems as well as organisational factors and personal beliefs. The results of the model validation give credence to the model's concepts and interrelationships. Additional validation of two models based on subsets of the respondents (either medical specialists or nurses) show comparable performance of these models.

First we validated the measurement model showing whether our questions (from the questionnaire) reliably measure the concepts (from our theoretical model). We found the measurement model had satisfactory composite reliability for exploratory models (i.e. models developing theory). The measurement model does satisfy the Fornell-Larcker criterion, which is a measure of discriminant validity. For six of our 12 relevant variables (i.e. blocks) the loadings of our observed variables are satisfactory for all items. For the other six variables, the loadings of one or more items were less than the required threshold, especially behaviour scores low in this respect. However, for all variables, at least one item scored above the threshold. The loadings indicate that a number of observed variables (i.e. questions from the questionnaire) could be removed from the model to improve both the efficiency of the questionnaire and the accuracy of the model. This could also improve the Average Variance Extracted (AVE) of the latent variables that are too low at this moment. The cross-loadings indicate a similar pattern

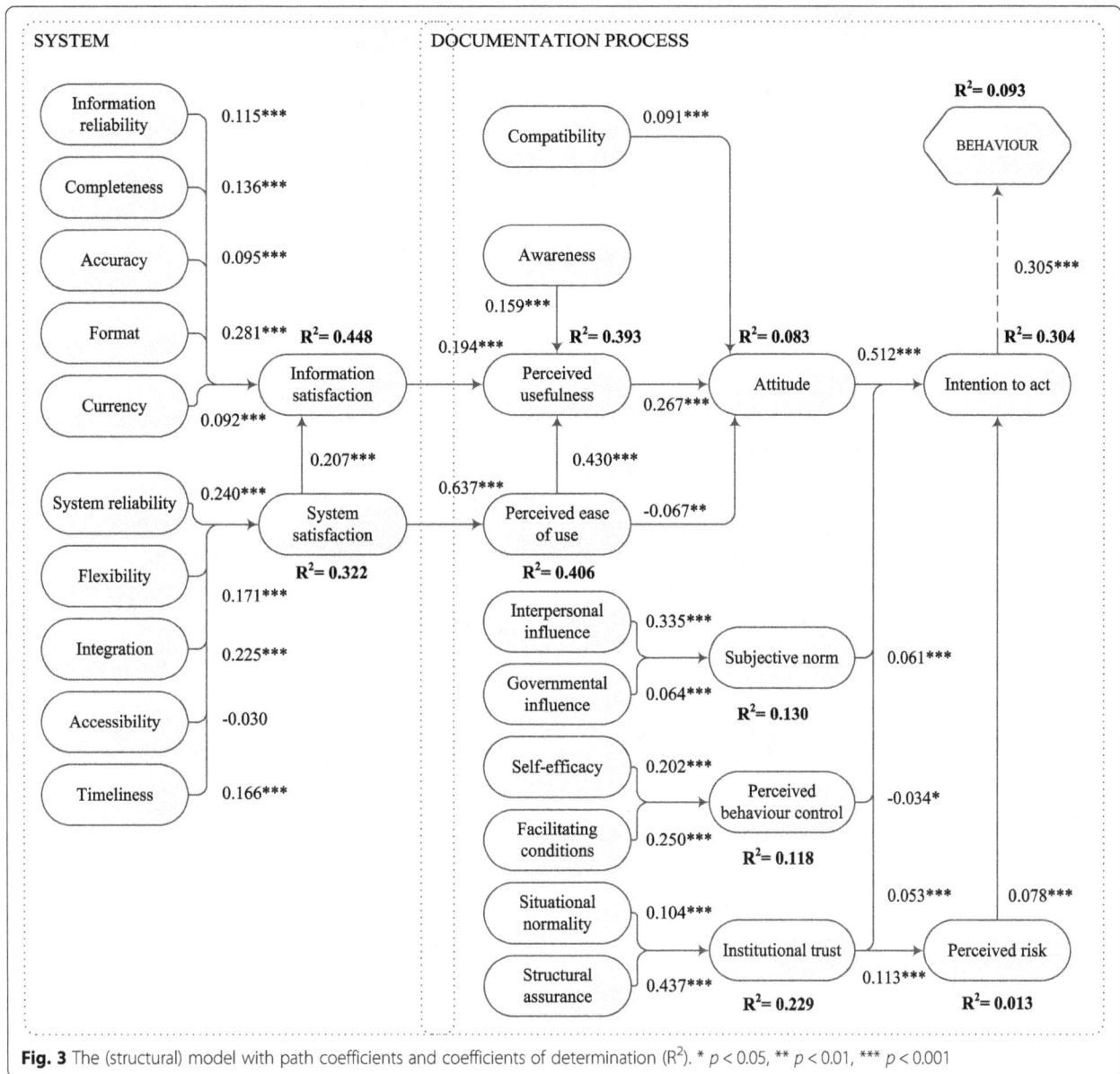

Fig. 3 The (structural) model with path coefficients and coefficients of determination (R^2). * $p < 0.05$, ** $p < 0.01$, *** $p < 0.001$

that a small number of observed variables could be removed, most notably within the latent variable behaviour. In this study we performed a summative evaluation to validate our theoretical model. Future research should investigate the effect of model adaptations on the performance of the model.

Second, we validated the structural model, showing whether the variables of our theoretical model and their interrelations are valid. The validation shows that the R^2 of the concepts are higher in the left part of the model. This is the part with concepts that have been developed and validated in multiple other studies (e.g. information and system satisfaction [13]). The lower scores are most prominent for attitude (0.083), behaviour (0.093), and perceived risk (0.013). These three concepts need further

research to find the missing explaining underlying variables. The strongest indicator for intention to act is attitude. This means that it is important that the attitude of the healthcare professionals is positive with respect to structured and standardised data recording.

The only coefficient that was not significant at all was that of accessibility (to system satisfaction). The questionnaire was used in a high resource setting (the Netherlands) where the EHR and power are available 24/7. Therefore, although accessibility is not significant in our setting, it might become more significant in lower-resource settings. All other path coefficients were significant ($p < 0.05$ for perceived behavioural control and perceived ease of use) to very significant ($p < 0.001$).

A main strength of our study is that we based our model on existing and validated models. In particular, the underlying Technology Acceptance Model (TAM), commonly used outside [14] and within healthcare [15]. As Holden and Karsh state TAM "predicts a substantial portion of the use or acceptance of health IT" [15] however they also mention that the theory might benefit from additions and modifications [15]. Or, as concluded by Legris et al., it is has to be integrated into a broader model [14] as we did in this study. Another major strength is the large number of respondents to our questionnaire. This created a large sample size for our validation with structural equation modelling using the partial least squares method. By including healthcare professionals from seven out of eight different university hospitals we gathered data independent of the centre-specific context, such as the used documentation processes or EHRs.

A limitation of our study is the large proportion of missing data in our dataset. However, we used four additional imputed datasets in the analyses to evaluate the effect of imputing the missing data on the results of the validation. These analyses showed very similar results to the ones presented in this paper, thus justifying the robustness of the findings. Another limitation is that we cannot precisely calculate the response rate of our questionnaire since we do not definitively know who has received the email with the invitation to participate in our study.

If we compare our results with those from the two underlying models to our model [6, 7] we find that our model has lower coefficients of determination than the original models. The different focus, standardised and structured recording at the point of care, instead of system acceptance, and the different population (work field and country) could probably have attributed to this difference. Perceived risk is the lowest scoring concept and information satisfaction the highest matching concept in both our own model and the original source models.

Our questionnaire is based on self-reported outcomes and intentions. Further research will have to measure the exact compliance of healthcare professionals to structured and standardised data recording. When self-reported outcomes can be compared to the actual uptake of structured and standardised data recording we can evaluate whether the respondents are capable of a good assessment of their own compliance.

Conclusions

First and foremost, our model helps to further understand the barriers and facilitators for healthcare professionals to adopt structured and standardised data recording. Additionally, our model and accompanying questionnaire can be used by hospitals to measure their own adoption and progress over time. When measuring in multiple centres, the results can be used to benchmark the scores and to identify best practice hospitals. Based on what best performing centres do differently, other hospitals can consider to adopt promising practices to improve their own adoption. Repeating the measurement at some other time in the future may indicate whether the changes have had effect on the adoption.

Additional files

Additional file 1: English translation of used questionnaire (PDF 111 kb)

Additional file 2: Three additional tables showing 1) The percentage of missing data from each question in the questionnaire, 2) the cross loadings of the model, and 3) the Fornell-Larcker criterion. Also contains the performance measures of the two validations based on subgroups of our respondents (either medical specialists or nurses). (XLSX 125 kb)

Abbreviations
AVE: Average Variance Extracted; EHR: Electronic Health Records; PLS: Partial Least Squares; SEM: Structural Equation Modelling; TAM: Technology Acceptance Model

Acknowledgements
The authors gratefully acknowledge the healthcare professionals that took the time to respond to our questionnaire.

Funding
This research was funded by the Netherlands Federation of University hospitals through the Citrienfonds. The funding body was not involved in the design of the study, the collection, analysis, and interpretation of the data, or the writing of the manuscript.

Authors' contributions
Study conception and design: EJ, RC, MdB, NdK. Acquisition of data: EJ, MdB. Analysis and interpretation of data: EJ, AAH. Drafting of manuscript: EJ, AAH. Critical revision: MdB, NdK, RC, AAH. All authors read and approved the final manuscript.

Competing interests
The authors declare that they have no competing interests, even though physicians from their own hospitals were included in the questionnaire.

Author details
[1]Department of Medical Informatics, Amsterdam Public Health research institute, Academic Medical Center, University of Amsterdam, P.O. Box 22700, 1100 DE Amsterdam, The Netherlands. [2]Department of Public and Occupational Health, Amsterdam Public Health research institute, VU University Medical Center, Van der Boechorststraat 7, 1081 BT Amsterdam, The Netherlands.

References
1.   Joukes E, De Keizer N, Abu-Hanna A, De Bruijne M, Cornet R. End-User Experiences and Expectations regarding data registration and reuse before the implementation of a (new) electronic health record: a case study in two university hospitals. In: Studies in Health Technology and Informatics; 2015. p. 997.
2.   Aggelidis VP, Chatzoglou PD. Using a modified technology acceptance model in hospitals. Int J Med Inform. 2009;78:115–26. https://doi.org/10.1016/j.ijmedinf.2008.06.006.

3. Garcia-Smith D, Effken JA. Development and initial evaluation of the clinical information systems success model (CISSM). Int J Med Inf. 2013;82:539–52. https://doi.org/10.1016/j.ijmedinf.2013.01.011.

4. Melas CD, Zampetakis LA, Dimopoulou A, Moustakis V. Modeling the acceptance of clinical information systems among hospital medical staff: an extended TAM model. J Biomed Inf. 2011;44:553–64. https://doi.org/10.1016/j.jbi.2011.01.009.

5. Ketikidis P, Dimitrovski T, Lazuras L, Bath PA. Acceptance of health information technology in health professionals: an application of the revised technology acceptance model. Heal Informat J. 2012;18:124–34. https://doi.org/10.1177/1460458211435425.

6. Hsieh PJ. Physicians' acceptance of electronic medical records exchange: an extension of the decomposed TPB model with institutional trust and perceived risk. Int J Med Inf. 2014; https://doi.org/10.1016/j.ijmedinf.2014.08.008.

7. Wixom BH, Todd PA. A theoretical integration of user satisfaction and technology acceptance. Inf Syst Res. 2005;16:85–102.

8. Winter A, Haux R, Ammenwerth E, Brigl B, Hellrung N, Jahn F. Health Inf Syst. 2nd ed. London: Springer-Verlag London; 2011. https://doi.org/10.1007/978-1-84996-441-8.

9. Hair JFJ, Hult GTM, Ringle C, Sarstedt M. A primer on partial least squares structural equation modeling (PLS-SEM). Thousand Oaks: Sage Publications Inc.; 2014.

10. Tavares J, Oliveira T. Electronic health record portal adoption: a cross country analysis. BMC Med Inform Decis Mak. 2017;17:97. https://doi.org/10.1186/s12911-017-0482-9.

11. R Core Team. R: a language and environment for statistical computing. 2017 https://www.r-project.org/.

12. Sanchez G, Trinchera L, Russolillo G. plspm: Tools for Partial least squares path modeling (PLS-PM). 2017. https://cran.r-project.org/package=plspm.

13. Aggelidis VP, Chatzoglou PD. Hospital information systems: measuring end user computing satisfaction (EUCS). J Biomed Inform. 2012;45:566–79. https://doi.org/10.1016/j.jbi.2012.02.009.

14. Legris P, Ingham J, Collerette P. Why do people use information technology? A critical review of the technology acceptance model. Inf Manag. 2003;40:191–204. https://doi.org/10.1016/s0378-7206(01)00143-4.

15. Holden RJ, B-TT K. The technology acceptance model: its past and its future in health care. J Biomed Inform. 2010;43:159–72. https://doi.org/10.1016/j.jbi.2009.07.002.

8

Evidence-based usability design principles for medication alerting systems

Romaric Marcilly[1]* (iD), Elske Ammenwerth[2], Erin Roehrer[3], Julie Niès[4] and Marie-Catherine Beuscart-Zéphir[1]

Abstract

Background: Usability flaws in medication alerting systems may have a negative impact on clinical use and patient safety. In order to prevent the release of alerting systems that contain such flaws, it is necessary to provide designers and evaluators with evidence-based usability design principles. The objective of the present study was to develop a comprehensive, structured list of evidence-based usability design principles for medication alerting systems.

Methods: Nine sets of design principles for medication alerting systems were analyzed, summarized, and structured. We then matched the summarized principles with a list of usability flaws in order to determine the level of underlying evidence.

Results: Fifty-eight principles were summarized from the literature and two additional principles were defined, so that each flaw was matched with a principle. We organized the 60 summarized usability design principles into 6 meta-principles, 38 principles, and 16 sub-principles. Only 15 principles were not matched with a usability flaw. The 6 meta-principles respectively covered the improvement of the signal-to-noise ratio, the support for collaborative working, the fit with a clinician's workflow, the data display, the transparency of the alerting system, and the actionable tools to be provided within an alert.

Conclusions: It is possible to develop an evidence-based, structured, comprehensive list of usability design principles that are specific to medication alerting systems and are illustrated by the corresponding usability flaws. This list represents an improvement over the current literature. Each principle is now associated with the best available evidence of its violation. This knowledge may help to improve the usability of medication alerting systems and, ultimately, decrease the harmful consequences of the systems' usability flaws.

Keywords: Human engineering, Usability, Alerting system, Decision support, Design

Background

Medication alerting systems "provide real-time notification of errors, potential hazards or omissions" related to the prescription of medications, and thus help clinicians to make informed decisions (*nota bene*: in the present report, a "clinician" is defined as any healthcare professional who interacts with the patient; the term therefore encompasses physicians, nurses and pharmacists) [1]. These promising technologies can change prescribers' behavior by helping them avoid errors [2] and, ultimately, can improve the quality of the medication management process [3]. Nonetheless, the design and the implementation of these tools may introduce negative, unforeseen side effects: poor integration into the clinical workflow [4], acceptance issues, and decreased safety and quality of care, for example [5]. Some of these issues are related to the usability of the alerting systems [6]; they are caused by defects in the design of the system, i.e. usability flaws. For instance, alerts may be poorly integrated into the workflow and may appear too late in the decision-making process – rendering the alerting system useless [7, 8]. In other cases, the content of the alert is either incomplete or not visible enough to adequately support a clinician's decision making – leading to incorrect clinical decisions [9]. This lack of information also increases the clinician's cognitive load [10]. Alerts may be poorly written or explained - causing

* Correspondence: romaric.marcilly@univ-lille.fr
[1]Univ. Lille, INSERM, CHU Lille, CIC-IT / Evalab 1403 - Centre d'Investigation clinique, EA 2694, F-59000 Lille, France, Maison Régionale de la Recherche Clinique, 6 rue du professeur Laguesse, 59000 Lille France
Full list of author information is available at the end of the article

misunderstandings or at least creating difficulties in understanding them. These cognitive issues may also lead to incorrect clinical decisions [11–13]. In summary, these and other usability flaws in the alerting system may have severe consequences, such as rejection of the alerting system, and incorrect clinical decisions. Therefore, the usability of an alerting system warrants special scrutiny, with a view to avoiding usability-induced use errors at least.

To prevent the usability of alerting systems from introducing errors, usability activities (e.g. design specifications and prototype evaluation) must be undertaken during the technology development process [14]. The implementation of those activities requires a sound knowledge of good usability design principles (also known as usability heuristics and usability criteria). Violation of those principles may generate usability flaws in the technology. With a view to helping companies to avoid the release of medication alerting systems that contain unintentional violations of these principles, it is necessary to provide designers and evaluators with easy access to relevant, illustrated usability design principles and to convince them of the value of applying these principles to design decisions. In summary, designers and evaluators of medication alerting systems need to access evidence-based usability design principles, i.e. usability design principles that have proven their value in practice [15]. As far as we know, the present study is the first to have provided evidence-based usability design principles for medication alerting systems.

Putting together a body of evidence relies on the accumulation of results that demonstrate the positive value of applying design principles. Unfortunately, publications in the field of usability evaluation tend to report only negative results, i.e. instances of usability flaws. This reporting bias prevents the collection of evidence to show that applying principles is beneficial. Hence, although it is not yet possible to demonstrate the positive value of applying usability design principles, it is still possible to demonstrate the negative consequences of violating them.

In previous research, we started to develop a usability knowledge framework (Fig. 1; [16]). We have used this framework to gather evidence-based usability design principles for medication alerting systems. In a first step, we performed a systematic review of the literature to identify the usability flaws in medication alerting systems used in hospital and/or primary care (active or passive alerts, and use as a standalone system or integrated into a larger information system) [17]. In a second step, we searched for the consequences of these flaws on users (usage problems; e.g. alert fatigue and missed information) and on the work system (negative outcomes; e.g. a decrease in effectiveness, and patient safety issues), and linked them to their cause [6].

The third step involves identifying, summarizing, and organizing published design principles so as to avoid "reinventing" principles as far as possible. The fourth step (in line with previous work by Nielsen [18]) seeks to match usability flaws to the usability design principles that could fix them and thus obtain empirical illustrations of the principles' violation. The present study tackled the third and fourth steps. The results will help to establishing evidence in support of these principles.

The present study had two objectives. Firstly, it sought to identify and organize literature reports of usability design principles for medication alerting systems in hospital or primary care settings into a comprehensive, structured list of design principles. Secondly, the study sought to match this list with the set of usability flaws identified in the systematic review [17], in order to assess the fit between known usability flaws and known existing design principles and thus illustrate violations of these principles.

Methods

A two-step methodology was applied.

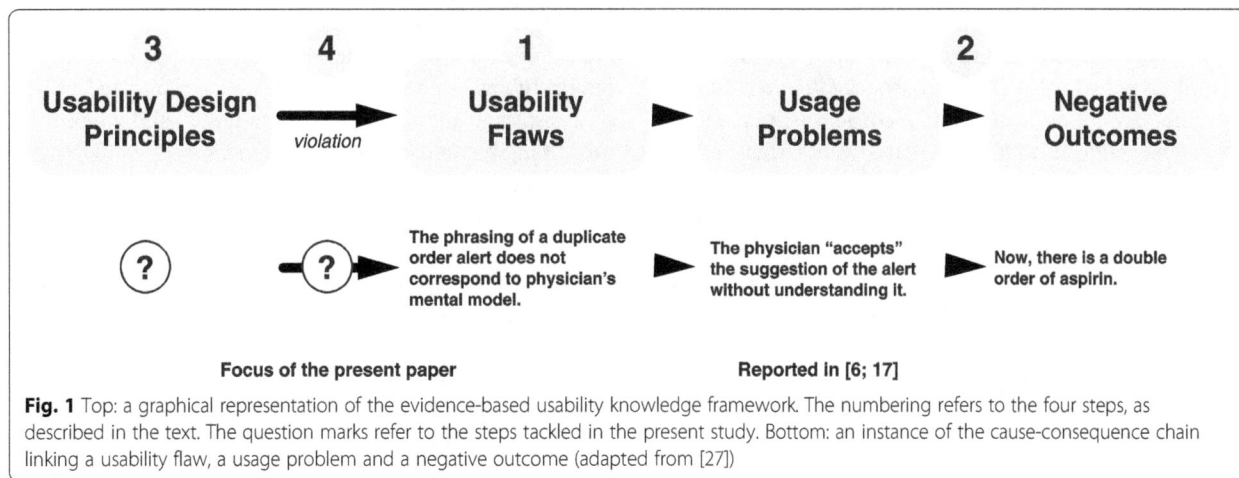

Fig. 1 Top: a graphical representation of the evidence-based usability knowledge framework. The numbering refers to the four steps, as described in the text. The question marks refer to the steps tackled in the present study. Bottom: an instance of the cause-consequence chain linking a usability flaw, a usage problem and a negative outcome (adapted from [27])

Gathering and structuring usability design principles

We searched peer-reviewed journals and conference papers for published consensus sets of usability design principles for medication alerting systems (i.e. principles that experts in the field had agreed on). The "grey" literature was excluded because the quality of the information may vary. Hence, we searched PubMed, Scopus, and Ergonomics Abstracts databases for articles addressing both "medication alerting systems" and "usability" topics. With this goal in mind, we used the screening and eligibility assessment steps from our previous systematic review [17] to identify papers purposefully providing at least one usability design principle dedicated to medication alerting systems. We excluded system-specific papers providing recommendations on improving usability because these principles are not applicable to a broad range of systems. This task was updated on March 30th 2016. The literature search was intended to provide an overview of published sets of usability design principles for medication alerting systems, rather than being systematic and reproducible. The database search was completed by examining the investigators' personal libraries and by screening the references of the selected publications. Two investigators (MCBZ and RM) decided on the final list of publications by consensus.

Once relevant publications had been identified, one investigator (RM) extracted all items referring to usability design principles from each publication. Next, the investigator grouped together principles with similar purposes and organized them hierarchically. A second investigator (MCBZ) independently crosschecked the hierarchical organization of the principles. Disagreements were solved by discussion until a consensus was reached. Lastly, the two investigators summarized the principles that had been grouped together.

Matching usability design principles to known usability flaws

One investigator (RM) checked the list of usability flaws published in the on-line appendices of Marcilly et al. [17] against the structured list of usability design principles. A second investigator (MCBZ) crosschecked the results. Disagreements were discussed until a consensus was reached. The items referring to usability flaws were either descriptions of the technology's defects observed during field studies or usability tests, answers to interviews/questionnaires, or users' positive or negative comments about the characteristics of the technology collected during their interaction with the system. A usability flaw was matched to a given usability design principle if it was an instance of a violation of the said principle. Reciprocally, a usability design principle matched a usability flaw if the application of the principle stopped the flaw from occurring. If a flaw did not match any of the usability design principles, then

we considered the possible extension (broadening) of an existing principle to other contexts so that it covered a wider range of flaws. If no principles could be extended to cover the flaw, we defined a new principle.

The matching process was intended to be as unequivocal as possible, i.e. one flaw matched one principle. However, if a given usability flaw violated several principles (e.g. at different levels of granularity), we matched that flaw to the most significantly violated principles (based on our experience). It should be noted that a given principle could be matched with several instances of the same flaw.

Figure 2 illustrates the matching process. Both investigators performed the descriptive analysis of the matches.

Results

Gathering and structuring usability design principles

We identified 9 publications on design principles dedicated to medication alerting systems (Table 1).

Figure 3 describes the sets of publications analyzed. One publication (Zachariah et al. [22]) was included in both sets; although this publication was an extension of another set of design principles described by Phansalkar et al. [20], it contained a few usability design principles not found in the original publication [20]. The publication also gave a list of usability flaws detected using heuristics. Despite the potential for self-matching bias, this publication was included because our objective was to obtain the most comprehensive possible list of design principles. Moreover, it was found that virtually all first authors of the set of usability design principles were co-authors of one or more studies included in the review of usability flaws (e.g.[1, 4, 20, 23]).

A total of 345 items referring to usability design principles were extracted from the 9 publications (see Additional file 1: Appendix 1) and then organized. The level of agreement between the two investigators regarding the organization of the items was very high, with full agreement for 92.6% of the combinations, discussion needed for 6%, and disagreement for 1.3%. After a consensus meeting, the items were summarized into 58 principles. No significant inconsistencies between principles from different publications were noticed. The summarized principles displayed different granularity levels, and some were more tangible and precise than others; they could therefore be organized hierarchically into 6 meta-principles, 36 principles, and 16 sub-principles (Fig. 4, Table 2).

Overall, the 9 publications contributed to different extents to the set of summarized principles: the contributions ranged from 12% [22] to 69% [24] (see Additional file 2: Appendix 2).

The level of support for each of the summarized principles (in terms of number of publications in which they were found) varied: one summarized principle was supported by all 9 papers (#49 "Include actionable tools

Usability Design Principles

Meta-principle E: (#44) Make the system transparent for the user. The system must not be a black-box and its coverage must be accessible to its user [19]. Inform users when necessary data are missing (e.g. severity of the unsafe event) [24].

Make accessible:

#48 The events that are checked by the alerting system [20] ...

... and the type and format of data (e.g. free-text, origin of the data (other hospital data), name of the drugs vs. ATC codes).

Corresponding Usability Flaws

The decision support is invisible to users [42]: capabilities and limitations of the system along with types of data that are checked are not shown to the users [10; 27; 42]

Corresponding Usability Flaws

The system does not explain which interactions are actually checked [10], ...

... which patient's data are analyzed [31], whether orders in free text are checked [10] and whether checking is based on drugs' names or on ATC codes [13]

Fig. 2 Illustration of the matching process, using meta-principle E (#44) and one of its sub-principles (#48). The usability design principles found in the literature were summarized and organized hierarchically (left). The usability flaws identified in the systematic review were collated by topic (right). Next, the correspondence between a given type of flaw and a given summarized principle was established based on the principle's ability (if applied) to fix the usability flaw. This correspondence is represented by a double arrow. When a usability flaw could not be fixed by any of the design principles in the literature, we either extended an existing principle or created a new one (single arrow). The illustration presents an extension of principle #48 (in italics)

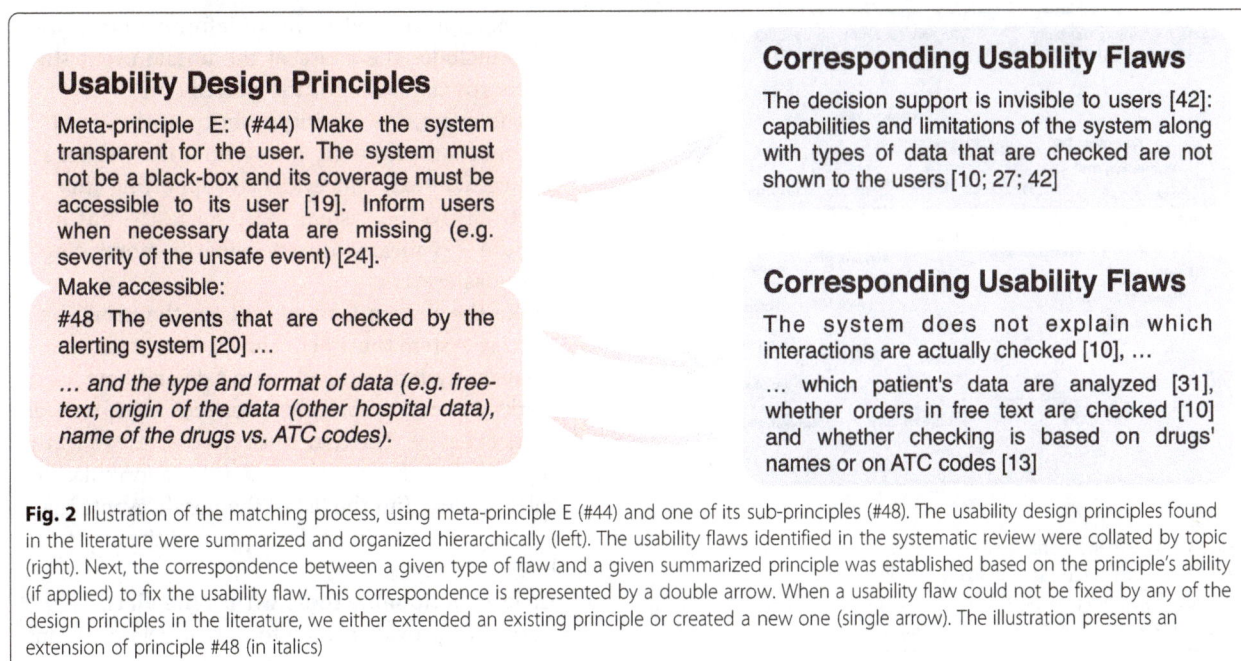

within the alert"), "Suggest, do not impose" (#42) was supported by 8 publications, and 6 principles were found in 1 publication. When considering the overall meta-principles and their components (i.e. related principles and sub-principles), the level of support ranged from 5 publications for meta-principle E ("Make the system transparent for the user") to 9 publications for meta-principle D ("Display relevant data within the alert") and meta-principle F ("Include actionable tools within the alert").

Matching usability design principles with known usability flaws

The two investigators agreed well on the matching between usability flaws and usability design principles, with full agreement for 54.6% of matches, partial agreement for 31% (agreement on the main corresponding principle but a need to match the flaw with a second principle), discussion needed for 13.4%, and disagreement for 1%. Of the 58 principles, 34 directly matched at least one instance of a usability flaw, nine were broadened to cover a flaw, and 15 were not matched at all (see Additional file 3: Appendix 3). Two new principles were defined so that all flaws matched a principle (#46, provide "a description of the characteristics of the tools included in the alert" to users, and #57, include a "send the alert into the clinical note template" function in the alert).

After the addition of the 2 new principles, the final set comprised 60 summarized usability design principles: 6 meta-principles, 38 principles, and 16 sub-principles. The 6 meta-principles were as follows:

Table 1 Main characteristics of the publications on usability design principles

	First author	Year	Focus	Method used to provide the principles
[2]	Bates DW	2003	Design, implementation, monitoring	Lessons learned
[19]	Kuperman GJ	2007	Design, implementation	Expert consensus
[4]	Sittig DF	2008	Design, implementation, research	Lessons learned / expert consensus
[20]	Phansalkar S	2010	Usability	Targeted review
[21]	Pelayo S	2011	Usability	Targeted review & analysis of cognitive and collaborative tasks
[22]	Zachariah M	2011	Development of a usability evaluation instrument	Phansalkar et al.s' review and feedback from a preliminary evaluation
[1]	Horsky J	2012	Usability	Targeted review
[23]	Horsky J	2013	Usability	Targeted review
[24]	Payne T	2015	Usability	Expert consensus

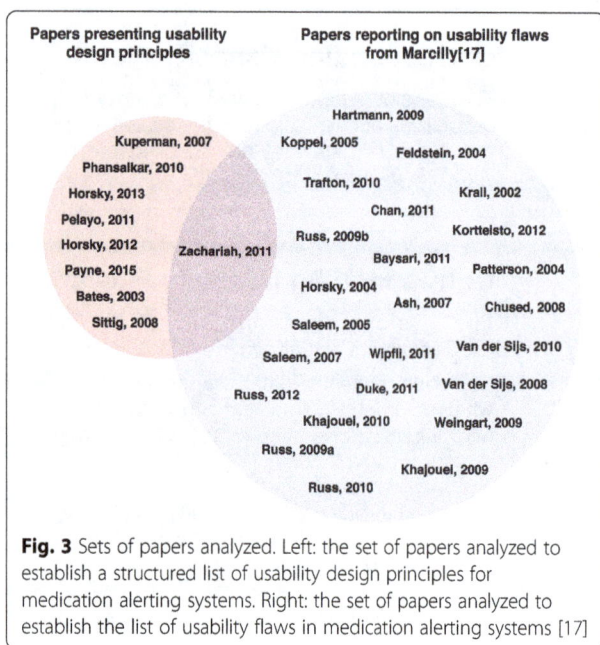

Fig. 3 Sets of papers analyzed. Left: the set of papers analyzed to establish a structured list of usability design principles for medication alerting systems. Right: the set of papers analyzed to establish the list of usability flaws in medication alerting systems [17]

A. **Improve the system's signal-to-noise ratio**, in order to decrease the frequency of over-alerting. In addition to the drugs ordered, the alert strategy should take into account parameters such as the patient's clinical context or the clinician's specialty. Moreover, the system must provide tools to customize the knowledge implemented within it and to monitor alert overrides.

B. **Support collaborative work, advocate a team approach, and make the system a team player**. The alerting system must encourage collaboration between the healthcare professional managing medications (e.g. physicians, pharmacists and nurses). Overall, alerts must deliver the same information to all clinicians, even if additional supplementary data can be presented as a function of the healthcare professional's role. The alerting system must help clinicians to understand how other healthcare professionals have already managed the alert.

C. **Fit with clinicians' workflow and their mental model**. The alerting system must comply with clinicians' needs and tasks. Alerts must be presented at the right moment in the decision-making process. Only the most severe alerts must interrupt the users; other alerts must be displayed more discreetly. Alerts must be concise, understandable and consistently structured so that users can easily find the relevant data. Once the alert has been satisfied, the clinicians must be able to resume their tasks easily.

D. **Display relevant data within the alert**. The system must provide clinicians with the information needed to make informed decisions. This includes the cause of the unsafe event (the medications involved), the description of the unsafe event, the severity/priority of the event, the mechanism of the interaction, the patient's clinical context, and evidence supporting the alert. Lastly, the system must suggest – but not impose – a means of remedying or monitoring the unsafe event.

E. **Make the system transparent for the user**. The alerting system must help clinicians to understand what the system can and cannot do and how it works, in order to prevent erroneous interpretation of its behavior. The user must have access to (i) the types of data that are checked, (ii) the formulas and rules applied, (iii) the list of the unsafe events that are targeted, and (iv) a description of the alerts' levels of severity.

F. **Include actionable tools within the alert**. The alert must provide several tools that help clinicians to easily and quickly translate their alert-informed clinical decision into actions: for example, buttons to modify/cancel/discontinue an order or override the alert, to order actions for monitoring an event, and to provide patient education. Other tools are recommended for managing the alert: pulling up the alert at a later time, sending the alert into a clinical note, removing the alert for a patient, and gaining access to the patient's medical records.

The final list of summarized usability design principles is given in Fig. 4. Table 2 provides a detailed version of the principles and corresponding flaws.

Discussion
Answers to study questions
The present study sought primarily to provide a specific, comprehensive, structured list of usability design principles for the medication alerting systems implemented in hospital or primary care settings. The secondary objective was to pair this list with the set of documented usability flaws, assess the match between the usability flaws that are known and the existing design principles, obtain illustrations of the existing violations of the principles, and present evidence that not applying usability design principles may be detrimental.

A total of 60 specific usability design principles for medication alerting systems were identified and organized hierarchically around 6 meta-principles: (A) improve the signal-to-noise ratio, (B) support collaborative work, (C) fit the clinicians' workflow and their mental model, (D) display relevant data within the alert, (E) make the system transparent for the user, and (F) include actionable tools within the alert. The

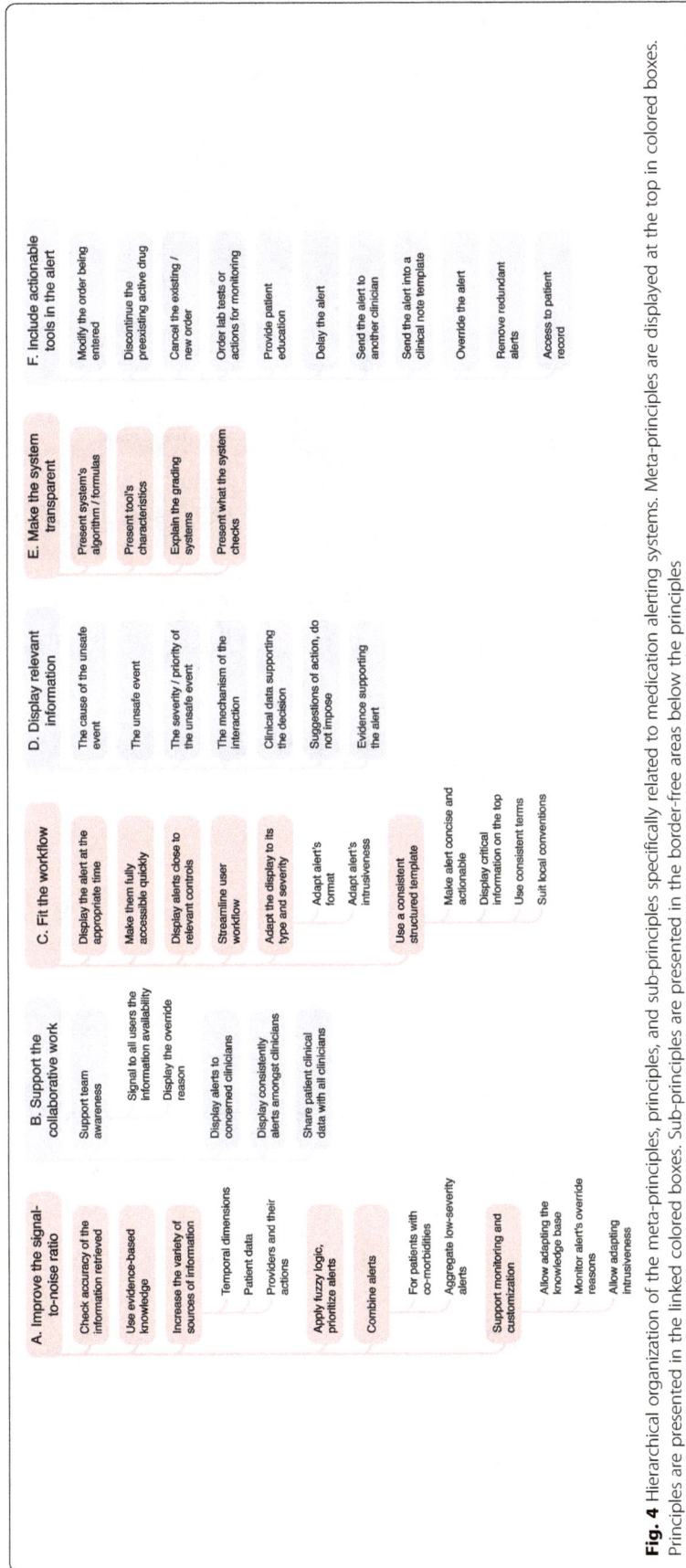

Fig. 4 Hierarchical organization of the meta-principles, principles, and sub-principles specifically related to medication alerting systems. Meta-principles are displayed at the top in colored boxes. Principles are presented in the linked colored boxes. Sub-principles are presented in the border-free areas below the principles

Table 2 Summarized usability design principles, and descriptions of the main corresponding flaws. Principles and sub-principles are presented respectively as first and second indents. Principles that have been added or extended to complete the matching process are given in italics. The oblique bars indicate the absence of corresponding flaws

Usability design principles	Summary of corresponding flaws
Meta-principle A:	
#1 Improve the signal-to-noise ratio by improving the sensitivity and the specificity of the alerting system in order to decrease the number of irrelevant alerts [1, 4, 19, 20, 23] (*e.g.*, system (non-medical) alerts, alerts with little evidence, low clinical relevance or redundant alerts, *alerts that require no action*).	There are too many alerts [8, 25–29] some are redundant [10, 25, 27, 30, 31] or irrelevant [11, 31], other do not need any action [29]. Potential events are over- or under-detected [10] due to sensitivity/specificity issues [32] or inappropriate triggering thresholds [11].
#2 Check the accuracy of the information retrieved from the CPOE (Computerized Physician Order Entry) /EHR (Electronic Health Record) [19], check whether they are outdated and / or reconciliated [1, 23].	Alerts are inconsistent with EHR data [10] especially with lists of patient's actual medications [10, 12, 32, 33] or with patient's diagnoses [34].
#3 Use adequate evidence-based alert knowledge base [19]. It should be regularly up-dated/maintained [1, 2] (see #13).	Medications interactions highlighted by the alerts are unknown in pharmaceutical reference books [27]. Knowledge supporting the alerts is not updated [34].
#4 Increase the variety of the sources of information used in the triggering model (e.g. several allergy bases [19]) and reconcile multiples entries [1]; when data are missing (degraded conditions), the system must continue to function [1].	/
#5 Consider temporal dimensions: interval between drugs' administration [23]: distinguish "now", "standing", and "future" orders, evolution of the unsafe event: increase the severity of the unsafe event if it gets worse [21], time lab tests are overdue [1, 19], *interval between the appearance of the unsafe event and the administration of drugs*.	The alert is irrelevant because the adverse effect it presents happens too fast to be manageable [29]. The system does not distinguish orders specified as "now" and those specified as "future" or "standing" [31].
#6 Consider patient clinical context [1, 19, 23, 24]: besides the specific drug regimen(s) (e.g. dose, route, duration of therapy, sequence of initiating co-therapy, timing of co-administration), add patient and laboratory data into the expected interaction (e.g. age, gender, body weight, mitigating circumstances, predisposing risks factors, drug serum level, renal function, co-morbidity, and previous experiences). *Consider the point during patient's stay at which the alert is presented.*	Medication order checking is not patient tailored [26, 35]: alerts may be valid but not applicable to patient clinical context [10, 31, 36]: e.g. pregnancy alerts for male patients and women of non-child-bearing age [32], no distinction between true allergies and side effects [10, 27]. An alert that is supposed to appear the last day of the stay (which is unforeseeable) appears every day [34].
#7 Consider actions already taken by the provider (e.g. dose adjustment) [21] **and provider-specific data** [1, 23] (e.g. clinical specialty: *some drugs may be used off-label*, others may be voluntarily duplicated triggering "duplicate orders" [19]).	Alerts appear while the corrective or monitoring actions have already been taken by the physicians [29]. Some corrective actions that are clinically relevant are not accepted by the system [36]. In some specialties, adverse events are intentional [29, 32] (e.g. psychiatry [32]); in other, drugs are used off-label (e.g. pediatrics [32]). Clinicians already know the alerts [25, 29].
#8 Include fuzzy logic-based algorithms, multi-attribute utility model and filters into the triggering model to change alerts' activation when certain conditions apply [1, 19, 20]. Define appropriately thresholds to trigger the alerts and to prioritize the alerts according to the patient's clinical context and the severity of the unsafe event [1, 4, 20, 23] (see #28).	Alerts triggering thresholds are too low [26]. Alerts are not ordered by severity level [22]. Non-significant, or low incidence, alerts are presented [11, 12, 29].
#9 Combine alerts [1]:	/
#10 Recommendations must be combined in a consistent way for patients with co morbidities [4].	/
#11 Aggregate low severity alerts in a single display to be reviewed all at once at a convenient point in the workflow [1, 20, 23].	Alerts are not grouped according to their severity [22].
#12 Support monitoring of the usage of alerts and their customization [1, 2, 19, 23, 24]	/

Table 2 Summarized usability design principles, and descriptions of the main corresponding flaws. Principles and sub-principles are presented respectively as first and second indents. Principles that have been added or extended to complete the matching process are given in italics. The oblique bars indicate the absence of corresponding flaws (Continued)

Usability design principles	Summary of corresponding flaws
#13 **Allow expert committees in each organization to adapt the knowledge-base and suggestions** for action to local practices and guidelines and to remove potential errors from the base. Customizations should persist across version upgrades [19, 23, 24].	Alerts are in conflicts with local and common practices [10, 27, 36].
#14 **Monitor alerts' override reasons**: alerts frequently overridden and of little value should be considered for removal or for a change of their presentation format (e.g. intrusiveness) [1, 2, 19, 23, 24]. However, do not eliminate or turn off relevant alerts even for specialists [24].	/
#15 **Allow institutional flexibility in determining interruptive vs. non-interruptive alerts** [23, 24].	/
Meta-principle B:	
#16 **Support the collaborative work.** Advocate a team approach [24], make the alerting system a team player [21].	The system does not inform physicians whether pharmacists review their justification of override and / or find them useful [10].
#17 **Provide functions to support the team awareness of the alert management** [21, 24]: (see #56).	/
#18 **Signal the availability of information to all users** [21] (even to non-prescribing clinicians).	/
#19 **Display override reasons** entered by a physician to nurses and pharmacists in order to allow them to understand the rationale for overriding [1, 19, 21, 23, 24].	Justifications and comments are displayed to no one [37].
#20 **Display alerts to concerned clinicians** and then to non-prescribing clinicians as a second check [24]. Redirect alerts that do not concern physicians to support staff [1].	Pharmacists receive alerts that concern physicians (e.g. drug interaction [38]). Physicians receive alerts related to drugs administration that concern nurses [11, 29]. Physiotherapists and nurses receive alerts related to the ordering of drugs while they do not prescribe [26].
#21 **Display consistently the basic alert content, i.e. the main elements of the alert, amongst all clinicians** [21, 24]. Nonetheless, the detailed presentation may differ based on clinicians' expertise (e.g. pharmacists may need more pharmacological data) [1, 23], on their role (privileges, responsibilities) and on the context of use [24]. Details may be presented upon request [21].	The way data are displayed is not adequate for all clinicians' types [10].
#22 **Share patient clinical information in the alert summary screen with all clinicians** (e.g. with pharmacists) [1, 4].	/
Meta-principle C:	
#23 **Fit the clinicians' workflow and their mental model** [1, 2, 4, 20].	Mental model implemented in the system does not fit users' one [12].
#24 **Display the alert at the appropriate time** during the decision making[1, 2, 24] or later during the medication management process [19].	Alerts appear out of the logical workflow [30], either too late in the ordering process [7, 8, 25, 31, 38, 39] or too early [7, 31].
#25 **Alerts must be displayed and fully accessible quickly**: screen transition time must be well under a second [1, 2], avoid scrolling and tabs [24].	Alerts appearance is delayed [12]: lags/down-times of 8 sec. [28] up to 15 sec. [10]. Clinicians must explore several parts of the alerts to get all relevant data [9]: they must scroll [10, 11, 22], explore several tabs [9, 40], or find information in tooltips [26] because short versions of alerts are not sufficiently informative [31].
#26 **Display alerts over the CPOE/EHR screen** in close proximity to the relevant controls and displays [20, 23].	Alerts are outside the region of the screen where clinicians are looking [26, 34].

Table 2 Summarized usability design principles, and descriptions of the main corresponding flaws. Principles and sub-principles are presented respectively as first and second indents. Principles that have been added or extended to complete the matching process are given in italics. The oblique bars indicate the absence of corresponding flaws (*Continued*)

Usability design principles	Summary of corresponding flaws
#27 Streamline users' workflow in response to alerts [22]. Make the resolution of alerts quick and easy (few steps) through screen operations [1, 22, 24]; cancel or reset alerts in response to the appropriate corrective action, do not require acknowledgment before a corrective action [20]. After the alert is resolved, resume the workflow [19] (see #49).	/
#28 Adapt the display of the alert to its type (medication alerts, system alerts) and its severity [19, 20, 23, 24].	Alerts of different severity levels and of different types are not distinguished [22].
#29 Adapt alert's format (e.g. color, symbol) and location on the screen [20, 24]. More severe alerts must be placed within the focal region of the user's visual field in order of importance while non severe alerts must be placed in side regions [1, 20, 23]. Distinguish system vs. medication alert messages [20].	Alerts are not distinguished by severity nor by type [10, 22, 32]. All alerts look the same [22]
#30 Adapt alert's intrusiveness [1, 4, 19, 21, 23, 24]. Interruptive alerts should be reserved for high severity warning and used judiciously: they should require an explicit response. Less important alerts must be displayed less intrusively (e.g. on-demand) as messages not requiring any actions. *Do not use pop-up alerts for system messages.*	High risk alerts are not seen when not intrusive [31]. On the contrary, low risk alerts that pop-up annoy users. Moreover, non-medication alerts are too intrusive [30] and contribute to desensitize the users [10, 27].
#31 Use a consistent structured alert template across the various systems used by the clinicians [23, 24].	Alerts combined but not structured cause visualization difficulties [10, 12, 27, 34]: users face difficulties to find specific data [11]. The lack of guidance bother users and their understanding [30, 35, 41]. Useful ondemand information available in EHR is not available in the alerts [22].
#32 Make the alert concise and actionable: the description of the problem should be shorter than 10 words [1, 19, 24, 24]; labels of button must be concise too [1] (see #49).	Alerts contain too much text or extraneous information [10, 25, 30, 41].
#33 Present the most critical information on the top-level of the alert: the unsafe event, its causes and its severity [1, 23, 24]. **Then display on-demand (linked) information** on background and secondary considerations (contextual information, mechanism of interaction and evidence[19, 24]. The suggestion of action could be presented either at the top level or on-demand [20, 24] (see #36.	No data are highlighted within the alert [9, 10], the alert is on a paragraph form [41].
#34 Use consistent terms, phrases, classifications, colors and definitions (e.g. for the severity) [1, 21, 22].	/
#35 Terminology and messages should suit local conventions [23] and be understandable and non-ambiguous [1, 23].	The message conveyed by the alert is not understandable [10, 12, 40]: the text is ambiguous [41]. Icons used are misinterpreted [28, 41] as well as buttons labels [35].
Meta-principle D: **#36 Display relevant data within the alert** [1, 20, 23, 24] (see #33). For the relevant tools to propose, see meta-principles F.	/
#37 The cause of the unsafe event *and its characteristics (e.g. dose)* [1, 19, 20, 23]. Use the medication name as ordered as well as generic drug names when identifying the interaction [24], do not focus on pharmacological / therapeutic classes [24].	Alert does not provide information on why it is triggered [10, 12, 27].
#38 The unsafe event (potential or currently happening) [19, 20, 23, 24]. Do not use generic term (e.g. risk), prefer concrete description [24]. Present the frequency or incidence of the unsafe event [24].	Alert does not inform on the unsafe event [9, 10, 12, 27].
#39 The severity / priority of the unsafe event [1, 20, 23, 24]: use color code and a signal word to inform on the severity [20].	Alert does not inform on the severity of the unsafe event [9, 10, 27].
#40 The mechanism of the interaction (possibly by embedded links) [23, 24].	Alert does not provide information on how the causes of the unsafe event conduct to the unsafe event [9].

Table 2 Summarized usability design principles, and descriptions of the main corresponding flaws. Principles and sub-principles are presented respectively as first and second indents. Principles that have been added or extended to complete the matching process are given in italics. The oblique bars indicate the absence of corresponding flaws *(Continued)*

Usability design principles	Summary of corresponding flaws
#41 Relevant data supporting the decision-making process and the suggestions of action [1, 4, 23, 24]: e.g. contextual information, modifying and predisposing factors (e.g. co-morbidity or lab-values). Provide a link to a summary of patient clinical data [23]. *Display data necessary to interpret values provided (e.g. thresholds).*	The alert does not provide essential patient information for the prescriber [10]. User can link to outside sources of information from elsewhere in the system, but there is no link within the alert [22]. Even when alerts provide patient biological results, the thresholds to interpret them are not presented [9].
#42 Suggest, do not impose. Make the system a clinician's partner [21]: provide clinically appropriate suggestions of action for mitigating the potential harm, do not impose [1, 19, 20, 23, 24]. Present possible ancillary orders such as monitoring/ surveillance actions, drug alternative (incl. Dose and frequency) and / or order modification or cancellation [1, 2, 23, 24]. Make the suggestions actionable [24] (see meta-principle F). In case of multiple suggestions, prioritize them and present their conditions of application [24]. Justify suggestions [21, 24]: check locally suggestions [24] and include link to institution-specific guidelines [19], make consensual suggestions [1, 19]. Monitor whether or not users followed through with the suggested action they started; if users fail notify them they did not finish the action they started [22].	Alerts do not provide suggestions of action [10, 22, 29, 41] nor alternative treatment options [9]. Alerts provide erroneous suggestions of action [35].
#43 Evidence supporting the alert (incl. Strength and source) using symbols/letter/ numbers [24]. Include a link to a more complete documentation (monograph, evidence, extended information, context) [1, 2, 19, 23, 24].	Alerts do not provide existing evidence or the evidence that supports the alert is poor and contradict clinicians' knowledge [10, 27, 29]. The alert does not present evidence references [9].
Meta-principle E:	
#44 Make the system transparent for the user. The system must not be a black box and its coverage must be accessible to its user [19]. Inform users when necessary data are missing (e.g. severity of the unsafe event) [24]. Make accessible:	The decision support is invisible to users [42]: capabilities and limitations of the system along with types of data that are checked are not shown to the users [10, 27, 42].
#45 The alerting algorithm / logic / formulas implemented within the system [1, 20, 23].	No alerts are appearing after ordering medications although clinicians expect one to come up for a patient [12]. The calculation formulas that the system applies are not understood by clinicians [7].
#46 A description of the characteristics of the tools included in the alert (e.g. duration of activation).	The system is not explicit about how to use and manage alerts effectively [31]: it does not make it clear that one can turn off some alerts [10] and for how much time [36].
#47 Explanations on the grading systems: levels of severity used by the alerting system (and their number by unsafe event) [20, 24], and explanations of their classification as unsafe events [20]).	The system does not explain the levels of severity that are used [22].
#48 The events that are checked by the alerting system [20] and *the type and format of data (e.g. free-text, origin of the data (other hospital data), name of drugs vs. Anatomical Therapeutic Chemical-ATC codes)*	The system does not explain which interactions are actually checked [10], which patients' data are analyzed [31], whether orders in free text are checked [10] and whether checking is based on drugs' names or on ATC codes [13].
Meta-principle F:	
#49 Include actionable tools within the alert to allow clinicians to take actions intuitively, easily and quickly [1, 2, 4, 19–24]; display those tools close to the suggestions they are related to [23] (see #27 and #32). The list of actionable tools should include:	There are dead ends in which clinicians face no reasonable options to proceed [28]; there are no useful actionable options [22].
#50 Modify the order being entered (or its dose) [1, 22–24]. For instance, propose formulary drugs lists [19] for formulary drug alerts. Allow ordering a drug suggested [23] or a new drug: in this case, clearly state that the existing drug will be discontinued if the new one is finalized [23], open a pre-populated ordering screen for the new drug [23].	The system does not guide users for switching a medication [41].
#51 Discontinue the preexisting active drug [22–24].	The system does not guide user for discontinuing a medication [41].
#52 Cancel the existing / new order [1, 22–24].	/

Table 2 Summarized usability design principles, and descriptions of the main corresponding flaws. Principles and sub-principles are presented respectively as first and second indents. Principles that have been added or extended to complete the matching process are given in italics. The oblique bars indicate the absence of corresponding flaws (*Continued*)

Usability design principles	Summary of corresponding flaws
#53 Order lab tests or actions for monitoring as justified by the alert [1, 24].	/
#54 Provide patient education [24].	/
#55 Delay the alert for a predetermined amount of time ("snooze" function) [24], *allow users to get the alert again.*	Alerts cannot be pulled up later, hindering alert resolution [10, 36]. Moreover, it is not possible to get the alert again [11].
#56 Send the alert to another clinician [24].	The system does not support the transmission of alerts to others clinicians [28].
#57 Send the alert into the clinical note template	The system does not allow clinicians to send the alerts into a template for patient's record [28, 41].
#58 Override the alert (meaning continue ordering, ignoring the alert) [22–24]. Most severe unsafe events must be more difficult to override (e.g. require a second confirmation, or even no possibility of overriding [23]) than less severe ones. Alerts must require the reason for override [24] (especially the most critical ones, optional otherwise [23]. Avoid text entries, propose a list of 3–4 (max 5 items) selectable coded reasons; reasons must be 1–2 word long [19, 23, 24].	The system does not provide appropriate options for justifying overrides [28]. The system is not explicit about the necessity to enter a justification [37]; moreover, free-text entries are not effective in the override justification logic [10] and entering data to justify overrides is seen as time burden [10, 36].
#59 Allow providers to remove redundant alerts for a patient who has previously tolerated a drugs combination (after more than one override) or when providers feel they have sufficient practice and knowledge about this alert or when the alert is outdated for a specific patient [1, 23].	The system does not provide users the possibility to remove irrelevant alerts that therefore continue to appear [28].
#60 Allow users access easily patient's record from the alert screen to change erroneous data (e.g. allergy) or to add new data. Do not require entering additional data in the alert [1, 19].	The system asks the users to enter data in the alert and then in the patient record, leading to wasting time and double documentation [28].

9 analyzed publications contributed to this list to different extents; we consider that the collation of several sets of usability design principles found in the literature expands the variety of topics represented in each individual set.

The match between the summarized usability design principles and the list of documented usability flaws was quite good: 34 principles were directly matched, and the context of application was extended for 9 principles. Nonetheless, 15 principles did not match any of the documented usability flaws. In view of the hierarchical organization of the principles, some principles are also not matched because their meta-principle or one or more of their sub-principles are matched - thus artificially reducing the quality of the match. We also identified limited gaps in the principles found in the literature; two new principles had to be created.

From a qualitative point of view, a few instances of usability flaws appear to contradict the corresponding usability design principles. For instance, some principles recommend including non-prescribers (e.g. pharmacists and nurses) in the alert management process, in order to promote collaboration between healthcare professionals (e.g. #20). However, it has been reported that nurses are annoyed by medication alerts that interrupt their work [26]. The balance between promoting collaboration between healthcare professionals and not disrupting non-prescribers' tasks is delicate. Overall, instances of usability flaws must be used so that the corresponding design principles are not taken too literally.

Study strengths

The results of the present study represent an improvement with respect to the current literature. We did not change the principles extracted from the literature. By combining and summarizing the extracted principles, they are now clearly identified, listed, and organized hierarchically into a comprehensive, consistent, and structured hierarchy. Furthermore, the process of matching the principles to the usability flaws allows one to identifying evidence to show that not applying these principles has negative consequences. Each principle is now associated with the best available evidence of its violation. As far as we know, the present study is the first to have drawn up this type of list.

In addition to providing evidence, the matching process also provided concrete illustrations of violations of usability design principles. The illustrations may help people designing and evaluating alerting systems to identify the "usability mistakes" that should not be made or to catch these mistakes during the evaluation phases. In fact, the illustrations provide a clearer understanding of the design principles to be applied.

Study limitations

The retrieval of the usability design principles might have biased the representativeness of the principles and the flaws. We considered only publications reporting general sets of design principles, rather than evaluations giving system-specific usability recommendations. Grey literature was excluded. Moreover, most of the analysis was performed by one investigator, with a second investigator independently crosschecking the results. Together, these biases might have caused us to miss a few relevant principles. Consequently, the principles that we extended or created in the present study may have already been described in other publications (e.g. as system-specific recommendations on usability). Likewise, some usability flaws might have been missed during the systematic review [17] due to publication and reporting biases: it might have been possible to match principles not matched in the present study with usability flaws documented outside our review [17]. Despite these limitations, the match between the usability design principles and the usability flaws was quite good and ensured that the principles and flaws retrieved were representative. This good level of matching might be due (at least in part) to the inclusion of Zachariah's publication [22] and reports written by closely linked authors in both sets of publications (i.e. the set used to establish the list of principles and the set used to establish the list of flaws, e.g. [4, 20, 23]). In the present study, the risk of self-matching bias was considered to be acceptable because our objective was to obtain the most comprehensive possible list of design principles and corresponding flaws. On the contrary, not including a publication in one set because its authors had also worked on a publication included in the other set could have led us to ignore relevant usability design principles and/or usability flaws.

The frequency of appearance of the design principles was analyzed in order to establish the level of support for the design principles (i.e. the number of publications they were found in). However, we do not interpret this number as an indicator of which principles should be prioritized. Firstly, reporting and publishing biases and differences in the focus of the publications analyzed may have biased the frequency of appearance. Even without these biases, prioritizing the principles would imply that we are able to predict the severity of the consequences of the related usability flaws. However, the severity depends on many other factors, such as the system's other features and other flaws, and the context of use. This is one reason why most sets of design principles - whether developed for interactive systems (e.g. Nielsen's [43] and Scapin's [44] sets) or for a specific type of technology (e.g. the ones included in our analysis) - do not prioritize

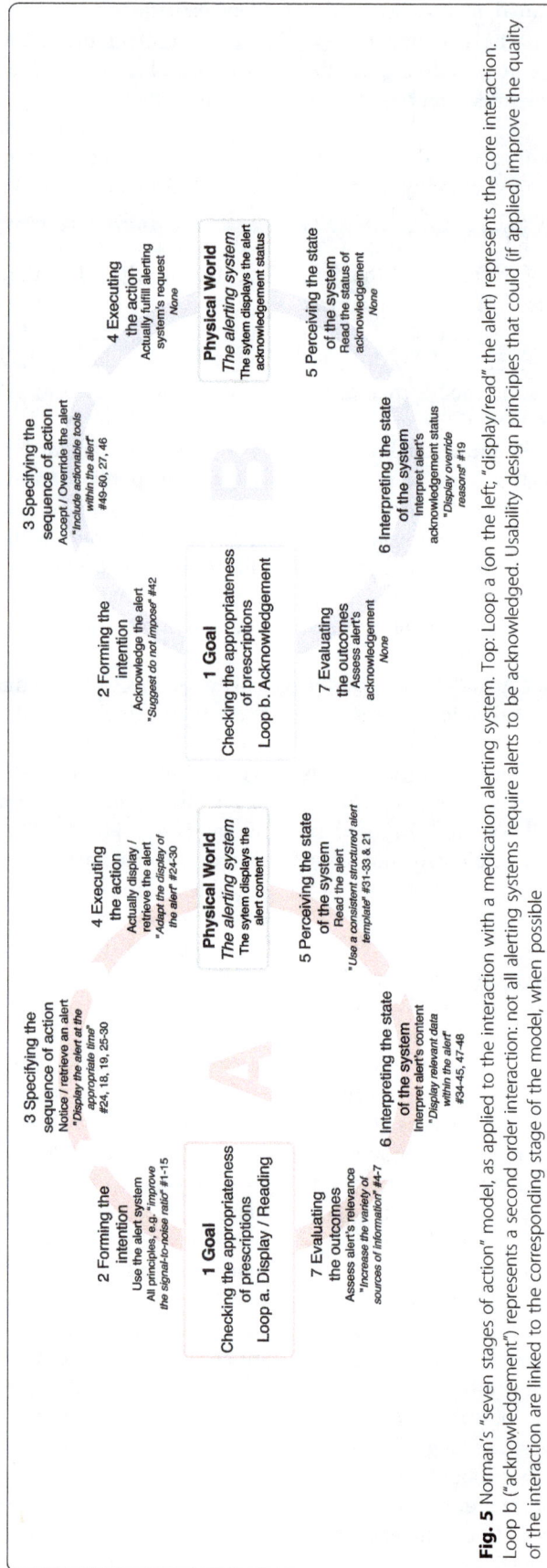

Fig. 5 Norman's "seven stages of action" model, as applied to the interaction with a medication alerting system. Top: Loop a (on the left; "display/read" the alert) represents the core interaction. Loop b ("acknowledgement") represents a second order interaction: not all alerting systems require alerts to be acknowledged. Usability design principles that could (if applied) improve the quality of the interaction are linked to the corresponding stage of the model, when possible

principles. Design principles can be prioritized by a person who is aware of the alerting system's characteristics and context of use.

In the present study, we addressed the evidence in favor of usability design principles by examining the violation of these principles. Evidence to suggest that applying design principles is beneficial has not yet been considered, due to reporting bias in the literature. Even though our present evidence is not based on instances of successful design, it may be convincing enough to persuade designers to apply usability design principles. Once researchers have begun to report on the positive usability characteristics of medication alerting system, the present analysis will have to be updated.

The significance of the present results for a user interacting with a medication alerting system

Usability design principles are related to various components of the alerting system: the triggering model, the knowledge implemented, the cognitive model implemented in the system, the information displayed, and the tools proposed within the alert. Applying these usability design principles might improve the clinician-alerting system interaction and the collaboration between clinicians. According to Norman's "seven stages of action" model [45], the user's interaction with a system encompasses two stages: the action stage translates a goal into an action sequence, and the evaluation stage compares the changes perceived in the world with the initial goal of the action (see Fig. 5). A clinician interacts with an alerting system in order to check the appropriateness of the prescriptions (step 1). Two "action and evaluation loops" may then be described. The main loop is "display/read" the alert. The second "acknowledgement" loop depends on the alerting system model; in some models, acknowledgment is not required.

For the "display/read" loop (loop a, Fig. 5, left), improving the overall usability of the alerting system by applying the whole set of design principles may facilitate the interaction and increase the clinician's intention to use the alerting system (step 2). More specifically, the whole "improving the signal-to-noise ratio" meta-principle may help to improve the relevance of the alerts, decrease alert fatigue, and thus increase the clinician's will to use the alerting system. In step 3, principles such as "signal the availability of information to all users" (#18) and "display the alert at the appropriate time" (#24) could make it easier to notice and retrieve alerts. In step 4, applying the "fit the clinician's workflow" meta-principle may help the clinician to display the alerts. Once alerts are displayed, clinicians have to read and interpret them (in steps 5 and 6). Applying the "use a consistent structured alert template", "display relevant data", and "make the system transparent" principles (#31,

#36, and #44, respectively) may make the alerts more readable and help the clinicians to interpret them. Lastly, "extend[ing] the sources of information used in the triggering model" (#4) may make it easier for clinicians to assess the alerts' relevance (step 7).

Once alerts are interpreted, physicians may have to acknowledge them (loop b, Fig. 5, right). Applying the "suggest - do not impose" principle (#42) may increase the probability with which a clinician acknowledges the alert and perform corrective actions (step 2). Next, "includ[ing] actionable tools within the alerts" (#49) may make it easier and quicker to specify and execute corrective actions (e.g. modify the order; step 3). If a physician overrides an alert and enters the reason why, "display[ing] override reason" (#19) might help other clinicians to interpret the alert's acknowledgement status (step 6) and decide whether or not the alert has been properly assessed.

In summary, applying this set of usability design principles might improve both the action and evaluation stages of a user's interaction with the alerting system - mainly in the "display/read" loop but also in the "acknowledgement" loop. Some principles go beyond Norman's model, which relates to an individual's interaction with the alerting system and not interactions between clinicians or the clinicians' workflow. Adhering to the "fit the clinicians' workflow" meta-principle might decrease the risk of rejection. Moreover, if the "support collaborative work" meta-principle were to be applied, the alerting system could truly help clinicians to gain the same mental representation of the prescription being checked; this would help them to coordinate their actions and improve patient safety.

Generalizability of the study

The list of usability flaws used in the matching process might increase over time, depending on whether new publications report usability flaws. Moreover, technology evolves rapidly, and the related principles might change accordingly. For instance, the principles presented here are formulated for medication alerting systems implemented on laptop and/or desktop computers. However, as mobile health technologies are refined and expanded, alerting systems will be progressively installed on mobile devices. This might modify the applicability of the usability design principles listed here. It will therefore be essential to update this work regularly and take account of the latest trends and developments. However, the maintenance of this knowledge may be time-consuming, and represents a challenge for human factors specialists in the field of medical informatics. Manufacturers should be associated with this process.

Some design principles insist on the need for promoting collaboration between clinicians (#16) but ignore the key person in the medication management process - the patient. Only principle #54 mentions the patient (being able to "provide patient education"). However, as for other information technologies, the implementation of an alerting system changes the nature of the patient-clinician interaction [46]. It is important to ensure that poor usability has not damaged the patient-clinician interaction. On the contrary, increased usability should underpin patient-clinician discussion, empower the patient [47], and ensure that care remains patient-centered. The current literature on the usability of medication alerting systems does not consider the patient as a stakeholder in medication management. Future research on the usability of medication alerting system should integrate patients as stakeholders in medication management, so as to adapt or extend usability design principles to their specific features.

Although the structured design principles target only medication alerting systems implemented in hospital or primary care settings, some principles may be applied to other kinds of alerting systems. For instance, part of the "fit the clinicians' workflow" meta-principle could also be applied to laboratory result alerting systems. Nonetheless, the evidence that underpins the principles presented here is valid for medication alerting systems only.

In addition to the results, the method used to build this set of evidence-based usability design principles could also be applied to evidence-based usability design principles for other kinds of technology. However, this method is very time-consuming, and requires in-depth knowledge of the usability of the technology in question if the data are to be analyzed correctly.

Turning the results into a usable, practical tool for designers and evaluators

The present set of evidence-based usability design principles for medication alerting systems must be made accessible to and usable by designers and evaluators. At present, the principles are presented as a printable table (Table 2) that might not be ideal for optimal use. We intend to use the table to develop tools that present the evidence-based knowledge in a way that suits the needs of the various system designers and evaluators (usability experts, computer scientists, etc.) in various contexts of use (design, evaluation, procurement processes, etc.). With that aim in mind, we have started to identify the needs of medication alerting system designers and evaluators [48]. Accordingly, we developed (i) a checklist that measure the appropriate use of evidence-based principles in the design of medication alerting systems, and (ii) a set of interactive design instructions illustrated by visual representations of good and bad usability practices, in order to help designers make informed design decisions.

This list of usability design principles should help designers to make evidence-based usability design decisions. Nonetheless, and even though we believe that the list is helpful, it is not intended to be used as a stand-alone system or to replace the requirement for expertise in usability and design. Firstly, the present list does not include general design principles for unspecified interactive systems; it must therefore be used in combination with sets of general usability design principles for interactive systems (e.g. [43, 44]). Secondly, several principles require insights into the users' cognitive tasks and their decision-making processes in order to adjust (for instance) an alert's format and the moment at which it appears (e.g. #24). Hence, work system and cognitive work analyses [49] must be performed so the principles are applied in an optimal way. Thirdly, principles moderate each other; they must not be applied alone or in an unquestioning manner. Human factors specialists and designers must use their expertise to determine which principles must be applied and how they must be applied, given the characteristics of the alerting system and the setting in which it is implemented in (hospital vs. primary care, for example). In summary, this structured list of usability design principles must be used as a support for expertise and not as a substitute for it.

Applying some of the principles listed here may present specific technical and organizational challenges when seeking to tailor alerts. For instance, the "prioritize the alerts according to patient's clinical context and the severity of the unsafe event" (#8) principle requires access to valid data on the patient's clinical context, stay, and treatment. However, these data are often not standardized or structured enough to be used in the alerting system's set of rules [50]. Further research is needed to overcome these challenges.

Ultimately, presenting designers and evaluators with evidence-based knowledge may help to decrease the occurrence of unforeseen and potentially harmful usability-induced use errors. Nonetheless, one must be aware that improving the usability of an existing system or ensuring that the usability of a system under development is optimal is no guarantee of success. Other issues arising during the development of a medication alerting system (e.g. an error-ridden knowledge base, a poor implementation process, unsuitable settings, etc.) can ruin even optimal levels of usability. Even though it is necessary to consider usability during the design, development, and evaluation of medication alerting systems, one must never neglect the relevant technical, social, and managerial factors that also contribute to the system's success or failure.

Conclusions

In the present study, we developed an evidence-based, structured, specific, comprehensive list of usability design principles for medication alerting systems, and then illustrated them with the corresponding usability flaws. This list should help designers and usability experts to gain a better understanding of usability design principles. We expect that the list can be used during the design and evaluation processes of medication alerting systems, in order to prevent usability issues that could have a counterproductive impact on clinicians (e.g. alert fatigue) and potentially harmful outcomes for patients (e.g. errors in medication dosing). Although operational barriers may complicate the deployment and maintenance of the evidence-based usability design principles presented in the present study, our results show that the approach is feasible. Indeed, our approach could be transferred to other health information technologies for the generation of specific lists of evidence-based usability design principles. In this way, designers and evaluators could be provided with tools to help them avoid usability design issues in health information technology and thus decrease the likelihood of unforeseen and potentially harmful usability-induced use errors.

Additional files

Additional file 1: Appendix 1. List of usability design principles identified in the 9 papers and the corresponding usability design principles summarized (for definitions, please refer to Table 2). (DOCX 248 kb)

Additional file 2: Appendix 2. The 9 papers' contributions to the summarized principles. Crosses show that a given principle is mentioned in a paper. The right-hand-most column gives the number of papers mentioning a given principle. The bottom two rows present the number of principles mentioned by each paper and the proportion of the full list of principles mentioned by each paper. It should be noted that the percentages are based on the 58 principles summarized in step 1. Principles #46 and #57 were created after the matching process and therefore were not included here. (DOCX 56 kb)

Additional file 3 Appendix 3. Results of the matching between instances of usability flaws (from Marcilly et al. [17]) and the usability design principles summarized in the present study. (DOCX 82 kb)

Abbreviations
ATC: Anatomical Therapeutic Chemical; CPOE: Computerized Physician Order Entry; EHR: Electronic Health Record

Acknowledgements
The authors would like to thank the staff at the University of Lille 2 library for their very efficient work in retrieving the required publication. The author would like to thank Melissa Baysari for her feedback on the wording of Table 2, Emmanuel Castets and Pierre-François Gautier for the figures' design. Finally, the authors would like to thank the reviewers and editors for their constructive comments.

Authors' contributions
RM designed the study, retrieved the data, performed the analysis and wrote the paper. EA helped to design the study, provided methodological support and supported the writing of the paper by reading it several times and providing advice to improve the report of the study. ER supported the writing of the paper by reading it several times and validating it. Additionally, ER checked English spelling and grammar. JN provided a methodological support and supported the writing of the paper by reading it several times and providing advice to improve the report of the study. MCBZ retrieved the data, performed the analysis and supported the writing of the paper by reading it several times and providing advice to improve the report of the study.
All authors approved the present version of the paper.

Competing interests
The authors declare that they have no competing interests.

Author details
[1]Univ. Lille, INSERM, CHU Lille, CIC-IT / Evalab 1403 - Centre d'Investigation clinique, EA 2694, F-59000 Lille, France, Maison Régionale de la Recherche Clinique, 6 rue du professeur Laguesse, 59000 Lille France. [2]Institute of Medical Informatics, UMIT – University for Health Sciences, Medical Informatics and Technology, 6060 Hall in Tirol, Austria. [3]eHealth Services Research Group, School of Engineering and ICT, University of Tasmania, Private Bag 87, Hobart, Tasmania 7001, Australia. [4]General Electric Healthcare Partners, 92772, Boulogne Billancourt cedex, France.

References
1. Horsky J, Schiff GD, Johnston D, Mercincavage L, Bell D, Middleton B. Interface design principles for usable decision support: a targeted review of best practices for clinical prescribing interventions. J Biomed Inform. 2012; 45:1202–16.
2. Bates DW, Kuperman GJ, Wang S, Gandhi T, Kittler A, Volk L, Spurr C, Khorasani R, Tanasijevic M, Middleton B. Ten commendments for effective clinical decision support: making the practice of evidence-based medicine a reality. J Am Med Inform Assoc. 2003;10:523–30.
3. Jaspers MW, Smeulers M, Vermeulen H, Peute LW. Effects of clinical decision-support systems on practitioner performance and patient outcomes: a synthesis of high-quality systematic review findings. J Am Med Inform Assoc. 2011;18:327–34.
4. Sittig DF, Wright A, Osheroff JA, Middleton B, Teich JM, Ash JS, Campbell E, Bates DW. Grand challenges in clinical decision support. J Biomed Inform. 2008;41:387–92.
5. Campbell EM, Guappone KP, Sittig DF, Dykstra RH, Ash JS. Computerized provider order entry adoption: implications for clinical workflow. J Gen Intern Med. 2009;24:21–6.
6. Marcilly R, Ammenwerth E, Roehrer E, Pelayo S, Vasseur F, Beuscart-Zephir MC. Usability flaws in medication alerting systems: impact on usage and work system. Yearb Med Inform. 2015;10:55–67.
7. Horsky J, Kaufman DR, Patel VL. Computer-based drug ordering: evaluation of interaction with a decision-support system. Stud Health Technol Inform. 2004;107:1063–7.
8. Ash JS, Sittig DF, Campbell EM, Guappone KP, Dykstra RH. Some unintended consequences of clinical decision support systems. AMIA Annu Symp Proc. 2007:26–30.
9. Duke JD, Bolchini DA. Successful model and visual design for creating context-aware drug-drug interaction alerts. AMIA Annu Symp Proc. 2011: 339–48.
10. Russ AL, Zillich AJ, McManus MS, Doebbeling BN, Saleem JJ. Prescribers' interactions with medication alerts at the point of prescribing: a multi-method, in situ investigation of the human-computer interaction. Int J Med Inform. 2012;81:232–43.
11. van der Sijs H, van Gelter T, Vulto A, Berg M, Aarts J. Understanding handling of drug safety alerts: a simulation study. Int J Med Inform. 2010;79:361–9.
12. Russ AL, Saleem JJ, McManus MS, Zillich AJ, Doebbling BN. Computerized medication alerts and prescriber mental models: observing routine patient care. Proc Human Factors Ergon Soc Annu Meet. 2009;53:655–9.
13. Hartmann Hamilton AR, Anhoj J, Hellebek A, Egebart J, Bjorn B, Lilja B. Computerised physician order entry (CPOE). Stud Health Technol Inform. 2009;148:159–62.
14. International Standardization Organization Ergonomics of human system interaction - part 210: human centered design for interactive systems (rep N °9241-210). Geneva: international standardization Organization; 2010.
15. Marcilly R, Peute L, Beuscart-Zephir MC. From usability engineering to evidence-based usability in health IT. Hat evidence supports the use of computerized alerts and prompts to improve clinicians' prescribing behavior? Stud Health Technol Inform. 2016;222:126–38.
16. Marcilly R, Beuscart-Zephir MC, Ammenwerth E, Pelayo S. Seeking evidence

to support usability principles for medication-related clinical decision support (CDS) functions. Stud Health Technol Inform. 2013;192:427–31.

17. Marcilly R, Ammenwerth E, Vasseur F, Roehrer E, Beuscart-Zephir MC. Usability flaws of medication-related alerting functions: a systematic qualitative review. J Biomed Inform. 2015;55:260–71.

18. Nielsen J. Enhancing the explanatory power of usability heuristics. CHI '94 proceedings of the SIGCHI conference on human factors in. Comput Syst. 1994:152–8.

19. Kuperman GJ, Bobb A, Payne TH, Avery AJ, Gandhi TK, Burns G, Classen DC, Bates DW. Medication-related clinical decision support in computerized provider order entry systems: a review. J Am Med Inform Assoc. 2007;14: 29–40.

20. Phansalkar S, Edworthy J, Hellier E, Seger DL, Schedlbauer A, Avery AJ, Bates DW. A review of human factors principles for the design and implementation of medication safety alerts in clinical information systems. J Am Med Inform Assoc. 2010;17:493–501.

21. Pelayo S, Marcilly R, Bernonville S, Leroy N, Beuscart-Zephir MC. Human factors based recommendations for the design of medication related clinical decision support systems (CDSS). Stud Health Technol Inform. 2011; 169:412–6.

22. Zachariah M, Phansalkar S, Seidling HM, Neri PM, Cresswell KM, Duke J, Bloomrosen M, Volk LA, Bates DW. Development and preliminary evidence for the validity of an instrument assessing implementation of human-factors principles in medication-related decision-support systems–I-MeDeSA. J Am Med Inform Assoc. 2011;18(Suppl 1):i62–72.

23. Horsky J, Phansalkar S, Desai A, Bell D, Middleton B. Design of decision support interventions for medication prescribing. Int J Med Inform. 2013;82: 492–503.

24. Payne TH, Hines LE, Chan RC, Hartman S, Kapusnik-Uner J, Russ AL, et al. Recommendations to improve the usability of drug-drug interaction clinical decision support alerts. J Am Med Inform Assoc. 2015;22:243–1250.

25. Baysari MT, Westbrook JI, Richardson KL, Day RO. The influence of computerized decision support on prescribing during ward-rounds: are the decision-makers targeted? J Am Med Inform Assoc. 2015;18:754–9.

26. Kortteisto T, Komulainen J, Makela M, Kunnamo I, Kaila M. Clinical decision support must be useful, functional is not enough: a qualitative study of computer-based clinical decision support in primary care. BMC Health Serv Res. 2012;12:349–57.

27. Russ AL, Zillich AJ, McManus MS, Doebbeling BN, Saleem JJA. Human factors investigation of medication alerts: barriers to prescriber decision-making and clinical workflow. AMIA Annu Symp Proc. 2009:548–52.

28. Saleem JJ, Patterson ES, Militello L, Render ML, Orshansky G, Asch SM. Exploring barriers and facilitators to the use of computerized clinical reminders. J Am Med Inform Assoc. 2005;12:438–47.

29. van der Sijs H, Aarts J, van Gelter T, Berg M, Vulto A. Turning off frequently overridden drug alerts: limited opportunities for doing it safely. J Am Med Inform Assoc. 2008;15:439–48.

30. Feldstein A, Simon SR, Schneider J, Krall M, Laferriere D, Smith DH, Sittig DF, Soumerai SB. How to design computerized alerts to safe prescribing practices. Jt Comm J Qual Saf. 2004;30:602–13.

31. Krall MA, Sittig DF. Clinician's assessments of outpatient electronic medical record alert and reminder usability and usefulness requirements. Proc AMIA Symp. 2002:400–4.

32. Weingart SN, Massagli M, Cyrulik A, Isaac T, Morway L, Sands DZ, Weissman JS. Assessing the value of electronic prescribing in ambulatory care: a focus group study. Int J Med Inform. 2009;78:571–8.

33. Russ AL, Saleem JJ, McManus MS, Frankel RM, Zillich AJ. The workflow of computerized medication ordering in primary care is not prescriptive. Proc Human Factors Ergon Soc Annu Meet. 2010;54:840–4.

34. Wipfli R, Betrancourt M, Guardia A, Lovis CA. Qualitative analysis of prescription activity and alert usage in a computerized physician order entry system. Stud Health Technol Inform. 2011;169:940–4.

35. Khajouei R, Peek N, Wierenga PC, Kersten MJ, Jaspers MW. Effect of predefined order sets and usability problems on efficiency of computerized medication ordering. Int J Med Inform. 2010;79:690–8.

36. Patterson ES, Nguyen AD, Halloran JP, Asch SM. Human factors barriers to the effective use of ten HIV clinical reminders. J Am Med Inform Assoc. 2004;11:50–9.

37. Chused AE, Kuperman GJ, Stetson PD. Alert override reasons: a failure to communicate. AMIA Annu Symp Proc. 2008:111–5.

38. Koppel R, Metlay JP, Cohen A, Abaluck B, Localio AR, Kimmel SE, Strom BL. Role of computerized physician order entry systems in facilitating medication errors. JAMA. 2005;293:1197–203.

39. Khajouei R, de Jongh D, Jaspers MW. Usability evaluation of a computerized physician order entry for medication ordering. Stud Health Technol Inform. 2009;150:532–6.

40. Saleem JJ, Patterson ES, Militello L, Anders S, Falciglia M, Wissman JA, Roth EM, Asch SM. Impact of clinical reminder redesign on learnability, efficiency, usability, and workload for ambulatory clinic nurses. J Am Med Inform Assoc. 2007;14:632–40.

41. Trafton J, Martins S, Michel M, Lewis E, Wang D, Combs A, Scates N, Tu S, Goldstein MK. Evaluation of the acceptability and usability of a decision support system to encourage safe and effective use of opioid therapy for chronic, noncancer pain by primary care providers. Pain Med. 2010;11:575–85.

42. Chan J, Shojania KG, Easty AC, Etchells EE. Usability evaluation of order sets in a computerised provider order entry system. BMJ Qual Saf. 2011;20:932–40.

43. Nielsen J. Usability Engineering Boston: Academic Press; 1993.

44. Scapin DL, Bastien JMC. Ergonomic criteria for evaluating the ergonomic quality of interactive systems. Behav Inf Technol. 1997;6:220–31.

45. Norman DA. The Design of Everyday Things. New-York: Basic Book; 1988.

46. Pearce C. Computers, patients, and doctors—theoretical and practical perspectives. In: Shachak A, Borycki EM, Reis SP, editors. Health Professionals' Education in the Age of Clinical Information Systems, Mobile Computing and Social Networks: Academic Press, Elsevier; 2017.

47. Náfrádi L, Nakamoto K, Schulz PJ. Is patient empowerment the key to promote adherence? A systematic review of the relationship between self-efficacy, health locus of control and medication adherence. PLoS One. 2017;12

48. Marcilly R, Monkman H, Villumsen S, Kaufman D, Beuscart-Zéphir M-C. How to present evidence-based usability design principles dedicated to medication-related alerting systems to designers and evaluators? Results from a workshop. Stud Health Technol Inform. 2016;228:609–13.

49. Vicente KJ. Cognitive work analysis. Mahwah, NJ: Lawrence Erlbaum Associates; 1999.

50. Riedmann D, Jung M, Hackl WO, Stuhlinger W, van der SH, Ammenwerth E. Development of a context model to prioritize drug safety alerts in CPOE systems. BMC Med Inform Decis Mak. 2011;11:35.

9

Using data-driven sublanguage pattern mining to induce knowledge models: application in medical image reports knowledge representation

Yiqing Zhao[1,2], Nooshin J. Fesharaki[1], Hongfang Liu[2] and Jake Luo[1*] ⓘ

Abstract

Background: The use of knowledge models facilitates information retrieval, knowledge base development, and therefore supports new knowledge discovery that ultimately enables decision support applications. Most existing works have employed machine learning techniques to construct a knowledge base. However, they often suffer from low precision in extracting entity and relationships. In this paper, we described a data-driven sublanguage pattern mining method that can be used to create a knowledge model. We combined natural language processing (NLP) and semantic network analysis in our model generation pipeline.

Methods: As a use case of our pipeline, we utilized data from an open source imaging case repository, *Radiopaedia.org*, to generate a knowledge model that represents the contents of medical imaging reports. We extracted entities and relationships using the Stanford part-of-speech parser and the "Subject:Relationship:Object" syntactic data schema. The identified noun phrases were tagged with the Unified Medical Language System (UMLS) semantic types. An evaluation was done on a dataset comprised of 83 image notes from four data sources.

Results: A semantic type network was built based on the co-occurrence of 135 UMLS semantic types in 23,410 medical image reports. By regrouping the semantic types and generalizing the semantic network, we created a knowledge model that contains 14 semantic categories. Our knowledge model was able to cover 98% of the content in the evaluation corpus and revealed 97% of the relationships. Machine annotation achieved a precision of 87%, recall of 79%, and F-score of 82%.

Conclusion: The results indicated that our pipeline was able to produce a comprehensive content-based knowledge model that could represent context from various sources in the same domain.

Keywords: Knowledge modeling, Sublanguage analysis, Natural language processing, Semantic network, Big data analysis, Medical imaging, Text mining, Information extraction

Background

A *knowledge model* is a formalized representation of information in a given domain. The graphical representation of a knowledge model consists of semantic categories as nodes and semantic relationships as edges. A knowledge model can be employed in order to transform unstructured text data into a computable logical format. For example, Weng et al. developed EliXR, a model for formalizing clinical research eligibility criteria [1]. In this model, a frame-based (based on pre-defined event frame e.g. drug exposure + frequency + dosage) and ontology-dependent template (e.g. extract drug name using ontology) were used to extract information into 20 clinically relevant semantic types (e.g., medication, dosage) from eligibility criteria. The knowledge model was able to cover a 99.8% of the content with average labeling error rate of 5.9%. Bashyam et al. developed a system that provided an overview of the patient's imaging

* Correspondence: jakeluo@uwm.edu
[1]Department of Health Informatics and Administration, Center for Biomedical Data and Language Processing, University of Wisconsin-Milwaukee, 2025 E Newport Ave, NWQ-B Room 6469, Milwaukee, WI 53211, USA
Full list of author information is available at the end of the article

data in a model with four dimensions: time, space, existence, and causality [2]. In a similar manner, Coden et al. proposed a Cancer Disease Knowledge Representation Model (CDKRM), which was able to automatically extract information from free-text pathology reports [3] by incorporating Natural Language Processing (NLP), machine learning, and domain-specific rules. In general, the described knowledge models significantly facilitate the process of retrieving information through structuring the free-text medical documents.

Furthermore, recent studies have shown a great potential for using knowledge model components as machine learning features. To clarify, we mentioned this to demonstrate the significance of generating a knowledge model (the end product of our work). But our method doesn't involve any machine learning step. For example, Yetisgen-Yildiz et al. [4, 5] developed a pipeline to automatically extract semantic components from radiology reports. They first constructed a knowledge model (with an ontology of 11 section categories) of radiology reports sections to identify section boundaries using rule-based approach. Then features (both syntactic and semantic) for each section were extracted and fed into a classification algorithm in order to automatically identify critical clinical recommendations. The pipeline achieved an F-score of 0.75. In a study [6], thromboembolic diseases described in radiology reports were detected using NLP and machine learning techniques. In this study, NLP techniques were used to extract concepts of thromboembolic diagnosis and incidental findings, which were then employed as features of a supervised machine learning algorithm. The proposed conceptual model achieved performance improvement in all cases with F-score of 0.98, 1.00, and 0.80 for pulmonary embolism identification, deep-vein thrombosis, and incidental clinically relevant findings, respectively.

It has been also shown that the knowledge model plays a significant role in setting up a knowledge base when the text mining techniques are used [7–9]. Moreover, with the growing need for integration of data sources (e.g. written protocol, EHR data, published case report) in order to establish a comprehensive knowledge base, a domain-specific knowledge model becomes essential for uniform content representation. In addition, the importance of knowledge model as a fundamental component of developing clinical decision support systems has been studied previously [10, 11]. Some existing efforts that address this need include: 1) setting up a Common Data Model (CDM) or the use of Resource Description Framework (RDF) to represent elements and relationships in a text [10, 12–14]. 2) using ontologies as knowledge models to build automatic information retrieval systems [8, 15–17]. However, building automatic information retrieval systems based on CDMs is difficult since the automatic mapping of entities to those data models can be totally challenging, and thus, the

current efforts usually involve a significant amount of manual labeling in the first step of developing a system [14, 18, 19]. On the other hand, although ontologies have been widely used for knowledge representation, their complex hierarchy and insufficient relations between concepts have restricted the potential of using them to mine the most clinically relevant knowledge automatically and precisely. Moreover, an ontology building is a time-consuming process – usually expert-based and heuristic [15, 20, 21].

To address the unmet need (for integration of data sources to establish a comprehensive knowledge base), we proposed a data-driven sublanguage pattern mining method to induce a context-based knowledge model. According to Zellig Harris's sublanguage principle, restricted domains (e.g., biomedical) have unique syntactic patterns and a limited number of semantic types [22, 23]; therefore, the language grammar can be revealed and subsequently, the semantic relations can be identified as syntactic and/or semantic patterns. A combination of NLP and semantic network analysis techniques make it possible to reveal a sublanguage pattern model in a domain-specific content [24, 25]. In contrast to the above top-down approaches (CDM, RDF, ontology, etc), our method employed a novel, bottom-up, context-based approach that combines both syntactic analysis and data-driven semantic network analyses in order to explore semantic relations in a specific corpus. In this paper, we utilized an open source medical image report data repository as a use case. However, the pipeline can be extended to other domain-specific knowledge models as well.

Methods

The proposed method has four major steps: corpus development, syntactic processing, semantic processing, and knowledge model generation. Functionally speaking, the entire pipeline is able to complete tasks of entity recognition, relation extraction, semantic category assignment and semantic network analysis. Sublanguage patterns were detected with semantic network analysis and a comprehensive knowledge model was then constructed based on the sublanguage patterns. Figure 1 shows the data-driven pipeline for knowledge model generation of the image reports.

Corpus development

Radiopaedia.org [26] contains a large variety number of medical imaging case reports, along with physicians' in-depth case analyses and discussions. The data covers cases in 19 different body systems (e.g., breast, cardiac, spine) with 14 different modalities (e.g., CT, MRI). Using data in Radiopaedia.org, we built a corpus by parsing (with JSoup Package [27]) the data consisting of textural notes of clinical images such as body system, user-defined keywords, patient demographics, image modalities, clinical findings,

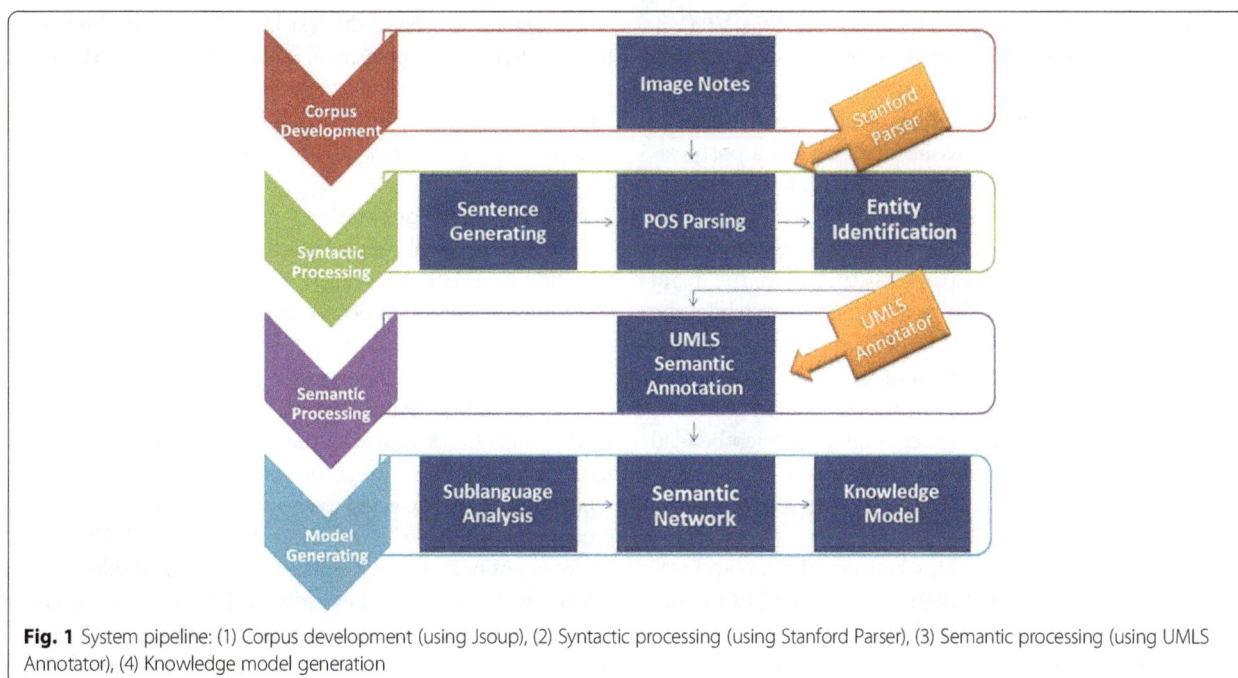

Fig. 1 System pipeline: (1) Corpus development (using Jsoup), (2) Syntactic processing (using Stanford Parser), (3) Semantic processing (using UMLS Annotator), (4) Knowledge model generation

and case discussion. The extracted data contained 23,410 physician-remarked medical image reports as of Feb 7, 2017. The first case published on Radiopaedia.org was May 7, 2008. Thus, the collected corpus represents a wide range of contemporary radiology case reports with different modalities, age groups, ethnic groups and body systems.

Syntactic processing

Sublanguage patterns can be revealed through identification of semantic relations based on language grammar. So, syntactic processing such as Hearst's lexico-syntactic analysis is an important step of sublanguage pattern mining, which provides users with "is-a" relationships by extracting the hypernymic/hyponymic relations from the text [28, 29] despite diverse syntactic variations. However, this method has limited ability to reveal other relationships such as location, causality, and indication while these relationships are important in medical imaging domain [30, 31]. Representing sentences with predicate-argument structures (PAS) combined with shallow semantic parsing are usually used for more complicated patterns within a medical text [32, 33]. These methods always require annotated corpora for training supervised machine-learning systems; however, there are very limited annotated clinical narrative corpora within the clinical domain, many of which may not be easily adapted to the medical imaging domain. As a result, we extracted and examined "Subject:Relationship:Object" (SRO) structures [34, 35] from imaging notes to generate a semantic network and to formulate a knowledge model. SRO structures are considered the core units for representing the content of each note. We examined "Subject/Object"

pairs in a process similar to Hearst's examination of hypernymic/hyponymic pairs, but with more comprehensive relationships between entities.

We reorganized each imaging note into short sentence segments by period, comma, colon, "and", "which", and so on. Next, we used the Stanford part-of-speech (POS) parser version 3.5.2 [36, 37] to analyze the syntactic structure of each sentence to extract the "Subject:Relationship:Object" parsing schema. Given this schema, we first identified the verb phrases (VP) or prepositional phrases (PP) in each parse tree and then determined whether each phrase was an embedded structure. A parse tree [38] is an ordered, rooted tree that represents the syntactic structure of an English sentence according to some context-free grammar using grammatical tags for each word or phrase together with the relationships between words and phrases. An embedded structure is defined as a verb phrase or prepositional phrase that contains other VP or PP within its structure. We also extracted maximal (longest) noun phrases (NP) and adjective phrases (ADJP) as entities, and marked them as a Subject or Object. Adverbs were separately extracted as modifiers of either Subject, Relationship or Object in the "Subject:Relationship:Object" schema.

We generalized four types of embedded structures: (1) NP + VP:(Verb+VP:(Verb +NP)), such as "A has become B". This structure usually relates to the passive voice or past tense. The verb is extracted as a combination of two words e.g., "have become", so that we could keep the tense of relation in our schema. (2) NP + VP:(Verb +PP:(Prep +NP)), such as "A present with B". In this structure, the main relation was extracted as the entire phrasal verbs "present with" in order to keep the phrasal verbs intact. (3) NP+ VP:(VB + VP:(Verb +PP:(Prep+NP)), such as "A is associated with B". This structure is a combination of the first two. (4) NP + VP:(Verb +NP + PP:(Prep+NP)), such as "A demonstrated a patient with previous history". This is a postpositive structure; the main relation was extracted only by using the verb, but the Object is considered to be the combination of NP + PP (in this case, "patient with previous history"). This is a postpositive structure, and the main relation is extracted only by using the verb, while the Object is a combination of NP and PP (in this case, "patient with previous history"). This is a novel step, as most previous studies only deal with simple syntactic patterns, but not the nested ones, which could lose embedded syntactic relations between words and phrases.

Semantic annotation

After extracting the relationships between the medical imaging entities, we annotated each entity in the SRO structure with its semantic labels. In this paper, "entity" refers to semantically taggable phrases. We used the Unified Medical Language System (UMLS) and SRO as our semantic reference and labeling structure, respectively. The UMLS is a knowledge source that integrates biomedical concepts from various controlled vocabularies, classifications, and other biomedical ontologies [39]. This semantic labeling method is completely different from previous ones that were based on a set of manually defined event templates [40].

A UMLS semantic tagger was used to assign a semantic type to each NP or ADJP (entities). The details of the tagger have been described in [41]. While most previous methods tagged all nouns/adjectives in an identified noun phrase [42, 43], we assigned only one tag to each NP/ADJP by extracting the maximal one. The tag is defined to

be the semantic type of the last UMLS-recognizable entity in an NP/ADJP. For example, our method assigned the semantic annotation of *Observation* for the whole phrase "right breast pain" instead of a list of three separate annotations – *Location + Body Part + Observation.*

Knowledge model generation

To reveal the sublanguage pattern, we summarized the semantic types occurring in the corpus and visualized entity relationships using a co-occurrence-based semantic network. Co-occurrence incidence is defined as two semantic types, the Subject and Object, respectively, in one relation. Based on the induced semantic network, we discovered the network concentrates primarily on the top 40 semantic types, indicating a strong sublanguage pattern in the radiology case report corpus. We selected top 40 semantic types because increasing the number of semantic types beyond 40 doesn't improve entity coverage significantly (~ 98.1% if selected top 50) but will introduce complexity in the model significantly. Moreover, semantic types ranking 41 or beyond are typically not related to medical image domains and could have semantic type mapping errors.

We selected the top 40 semantic types that have the highest contents coverage (98% of overall UMLS-recognizable entities), which were further regrouped according to both the UMLS semantic hierarchy and the domain-specific semantic network (Fig. 2). We also added four conceptually important semantic types according to expert's advice (despite its low frequency in our corpus; marked with "*" in Table 1). The rationale and results of semantic regrouping have been discussed in the Discussion section. A Semantic types are the original semantic labels defined in the UMLS system; the semantic categories defined in this study are then generated by regrouping semantic types. Finally, we

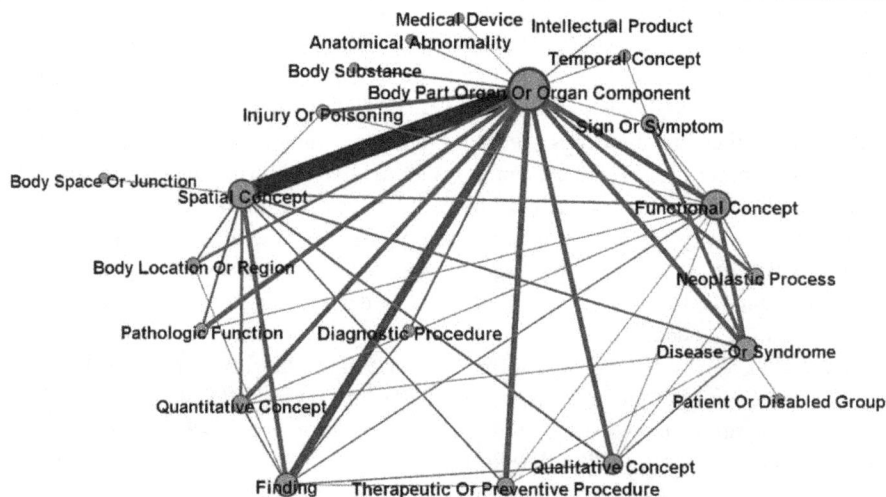

Fig. 2 Co-occurrence network of top 40 semantic types (subgraph). The thickness of the edge demonstrates weight (the number of co-occurrence incidences); a thicker edge means more co-occurrence incidences exist in the relation. The size of the nodes indicates connectivity (the number of other nodes connected to it). The network graph represents the complexity of the semantic co-occurrence pattern of semantic types in imaging notes

Table 1 Regrouping of UMLS semantic types to form 14 semantic categories (four conceptually important semantic types are marked with "*")

New Semantic Category	Included UMLS Semantic Types	Type Counts
Abnormality	Anatomical Abnormality, Acquired Abnormality, Congenital Abnormality	3
Body Part	Body Part Organ or Organ Component, Body Substance, Body System*, Tissue, Cell, Gene or Genome, Receptor*	7
Classification	Classification	1
Functional Concept	Functional Concept	1
Location	Spatial Concept, Body Location or Region, Body Space or Junction	3
Medical Activity	Diagnostic Procedure, Therapeutic or Preventive Procedure, Laboratory Procedure, Health Care Activity, Research Activity, Activity	6
Medical Device and Object	Medical Device, Manufactured Object	2
Observation	Finding, Sign or Symptom, Injury or Poisoning, Laboratory or Test Result, Phenomenon or Process	5
Pathology	Disease or Syndrome, Neoplastic Process, Mental or Behavioral Dysfunction, Cell or Molecular Dysfunction, Pathologic Function	5
Physiology	Cell Function, Organ or Tissue Function, Organism Function*, Physiologic Function	4
Qualitative Concept	Qualitative Concept	1
Quantitative Concept	Quantitative Concept	1
Substance	Pharmacologic Substance, Substance, Biologically Active Substance, Biomedical or Dental Material*	4
Temporal Concept	Temporal Concept	1

formulated a knowledge model using nine induced semantic categories and five original semantic types (Table 1).

We examined the top 100 mostly co-occurred relationships based on the weight of a relationship edge (total co-occurred incidences from the entire corpus) in the semantic network. We chose to include 100 top weighted relationships (e.g., "Location:Body Part", "Observation:-Body Part") and 13 conceptually important relationships (e.g., "Substance: Observation"). Addition of 13 conceptually important relationships involved empirical input but it is essential to complement previous automatic entity extraction and analysis when generating a knowledge model. Subsequently, the proposed weight-based selection simplified the complex network by removing the co-occurred relationships with no obvious semantic relations, yet still revealed the structure of the sublanguage pattern.

To label the relationships, we selected 1000 "Subject/Object" instances within each of the 113 relationships in the knowledge model to make sure that all the relationships were covered. In addition, we made sure of at least five instances for each relationship. In total, we randomly selected 1000 "Subject/Object" instances from a pool of "Subject/Object" pairs generated from the 23,410 cases. Two physicians (JZ, Singapore General Hospital, Department of Internal Medicine; HZ, Greenfield Dental, Milwaukee, Wisconsin) were asked to assign specific relationship tags to each "Subject/Object" pair. The relationship tags were named explicitly based on the conceptual logic indicated by the "Relationship" (verb or preposition) in each SRO

structure in a medical context; top examples are shown in Table 2. Later, we evaluated another 894 "Subject/Object" pairs from 83 randomly selected image reports.

Evaluation design
Knowledge model
The knowledge model was evaluated by using a corpus of 83 randomly selected image reports; including 43 image reports from Radiopaedia.org, 10 imaging case reports from the *Journal of Radiology Case Reports* [44], 15 case reports from the *BJR Case Report* [45], and 15 case reports from *RadioGraphics* [46]. Here we used data from four different sources in order to test the generalizability of our model, which was built from a single source. The corpus contained 402 sentence segments, 1718 noun phrases, and 894 "Subject/Object" pairs. Two independent raters with a clinical background (JZ and HZ) were asked to assign semantic annotations and relationship tags to each "Subject/Object" pair. Each rater received an instruction manual (see Additional file 1) that defined the scope and the meaning of induced semantic categories and the relationships among them. The manual also included examples to help raters assign semantic categories to identified noun phrases. The raters annotated the relationships in each SRO structure based on the manual; if they encountered any relationship not identified in the manual, they were asked to label the missed relationship with new category labels. We examined the raters' tagging results and the default relationship tags

Table 2 Ten most frequently co-occurred "Subject/Object" relationships identified from the corpus of 23,410 image reports

Co-occurrence Pair	Example	Count
Location:Body Part	frontal view:of(Situated_at):vertebral body; lower outer quadrant:of(Modifies):right breast	19,625
Observation:Body Part	erythema:of(Occurs_in):left breast; mass lesion(Occurs_in):in:left breast	15,219
Pathology:Body Part	B-cell lymphoma:of(Occurs_in):breast; fibroadenoma:with(Modifies):tissue	14,904
Medical Activity:Body Part	ultrasound: in(Acts_on):left breast; CT scans: of(Acts_on):skull	13,479
Observation:Pathology	x-ray findings:as(Indicative_of):pleural effusions; all features:of(Indicative_of):fibroadenoma	13,439
Functional Concept:Pathology	outcome:of(Describes):breast cancer; case:of(Related_to): previous DCIS	12,394
Pathology:Pathology	Haemangiomas:are(Be): benign vascular tumors; complications:include(Has):vessel thrombosis	12,119
Medical Activity:Pathology	drainage:confirmed(Shows):breast abscess; mastectomy:for(Acts_on):breast malignancy	11,924
Medical Activity:Observation	Chest x-ray:performed for(Deals_with):chest pain; biopsy:of(Acts_on):small lesion	11,890
Observation:Observation	breast lump:with(Shows):occasional pain; features:of(Shows):benign lesion	11,882

offered by the formalized knowledge model. The relationship coverage is calculated as follows:

Knowledge model relationship coverage

$$= \frac{\#\text{of raters' tags covered by the knowledge model}}{\text{Total Relationship Counts}}$$

Machine annotation

For evaluation of machine annotation, currently, there is no gold standard to semantically model and evaluate radiology case reports. To generate a reference standard for evaluation, the 1676 noun phrases (excluding 42 noun phrases not covered by the knowledge model) were reviewed by two independent raters using the methods described in the previous section. On the other hand, the automatic machine annotation of semantic categories for the 1676 noun phrases was generated by the pipeline described previously. Later, the consensus results of the two raters were used as a reference standard to evaluate the machine annotations of semantic categories. Precision, recall, and F-score have been defined, respectively, as follows:

$$\text{Precision} = \frac{\text{TP}}{\text{TP} + \text{FP}};$$

$$\text{Recall} = \frac{\text{TP}}{\text{TP} + \text{FN}};$$

$$\text{F-score} = 2 * \frac{\text{Precision} * \text{Recall}}{\text{Precision} + \text{Recall}}$$

The agreement was calculated by comparing the manual annotation of the raters. If the raters select the same label to annotate relationship, or same semantic category to annotate phrases, the annotation was considered as agreed. Otherwise, it was considered a disagreed annotation.

$$\text{Agreement} = \frac{\text{Agreed}}{\text{Agreed} + \text{Disagreed}}.$$

Results

Semantic network analysis

The extracted semantic entities from the results of the syntactic processing stage included 289,782 noun phrases (NP) and adjective phrases (ADJP). The results of using 135 UMLS semantic types for semantic annotation demonstrated that the majority (80.32%) of the radiology cases in the corpus covered by the top 22 (16.3%) UMLS semantic types (Fig. 3). The resulting semantic network at this level was consisting of 135 nodes (semantic types) and 3492 distinct co-occurrence pairs, while 352,356 total co-occurrence incidences (each fall under 3492 distinct co-occurrence relationships) were extracted at the entity instance level.

We conducted a network analysis and extracted the top 100 important network relationships based on the weight (the number of co-occurrence incidences on the edges). This network indicated a strong sublanguage pattern among medical image reports, because (1) A small subset of semantic types was used to (top 40 + 4 expert chosen) cover a large amount of corpus (98%), and (2) there were many repeated relationships in the medical imaging reports' entities. This led us to further generalize the semantic network into a knowledge model.

Semantic type regrouping

To achieve high-quality semantic classification for entities [47] and to simplify the concept-relation representation [48], the semantic types in the network were regrouped into 14 semantic categories based on the hierarchical structure of UMLS [20, 49] and their position in the semantic network (Table 1). Among the 14 categories, five common UMLS types were reused without regrouping, including "Functional Concept", "Qualitative

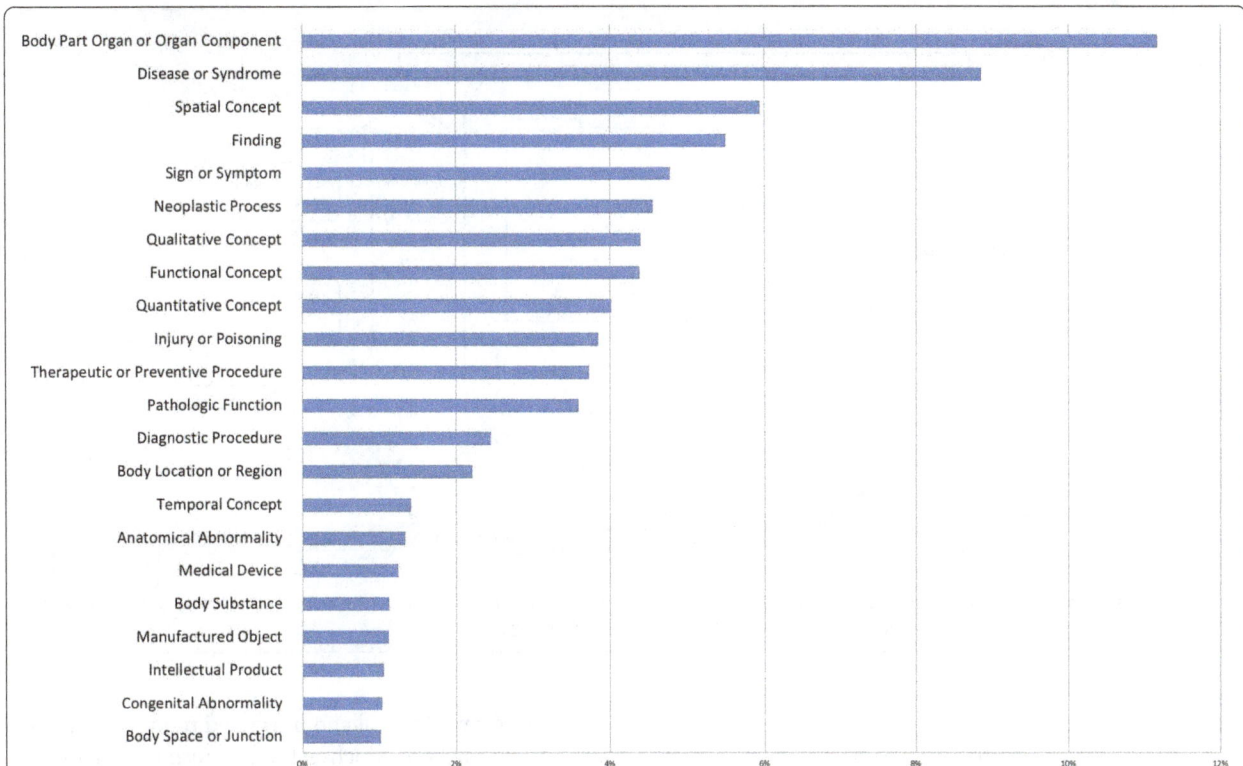

Fig. 3 Summary of different semantic types (among 289,782 NP and ADJP, top 22). Majority (80.32%) of the radiology case corpus covered by the top 22 (16.3%) UMLS semantic types

Concept", "Quantitative Concept", "Temporal Concept", and "Classification". Regrouping the semantic types led to nine new semantic categories specific to image reports (Table 1). The top ten most frequent co-occurred "Subject/Object" relationships based on regrouped semantic types are shown in Table 2. The final knowledge model has 113 semantic relationships.

Knowledge model

By linking the semantic categories with semantic relationships, we generalized a UMLS-based knowledge model for representing semantic information in medical image reports. The generated knowledge model is shown in Fig. 4; the significant relationships in the co-occurrence network are shown with the dotted lines, while the core semantic categories that are intrinsically closely related (determined by domain experts) and are significant in the knowledge model are presented in the dotted boxes. The significance of relationships and semantic categories were determined based on the total number of occurrence in the corpus.

Figure 5 shows the semantic categories and relationships created for two sentences; "Serial IVU films showing widely separated pubic bones with absent symphysis" and "Complex L-transposition of the great arteries with cardiac pacemaker". This image also shows how the created categories and relationships contribute to the generation of sub-sections of the overall knowledge model. The knowledge model provides a simple yet expressive view of content in the image reports, which can be used to facilitate future information retrieval and knowledge representation of medical image reports.

Coverage evaluation of knowledge model

The initial inter-rater agreement was 92% for semantic annotation and 95% for relationship tags. After the raters' discussion, the agreement reached 100%. The results showed that the use of 14 knowledge model semantic categories led into representing the semantics of 98% of the NP/ADJP, while 113 knowledge model relationships were required for annotation of 97% of the Subject/Object pair relationships. Additionally, 3% of the uncovered relationships involved some rare semantic types outside of the 14 semantic categories, such as "Biomedical Occupation or Discipline" and "Organism".

Evaluation of machine annotation

Based on our evaluation, machine annotation achieved an overall precision of 87%, recall of 79%, and F-score of 0.8299 (detailed evaluation results are listed in Table 3). Error analysis will be provided in the Discussion section.

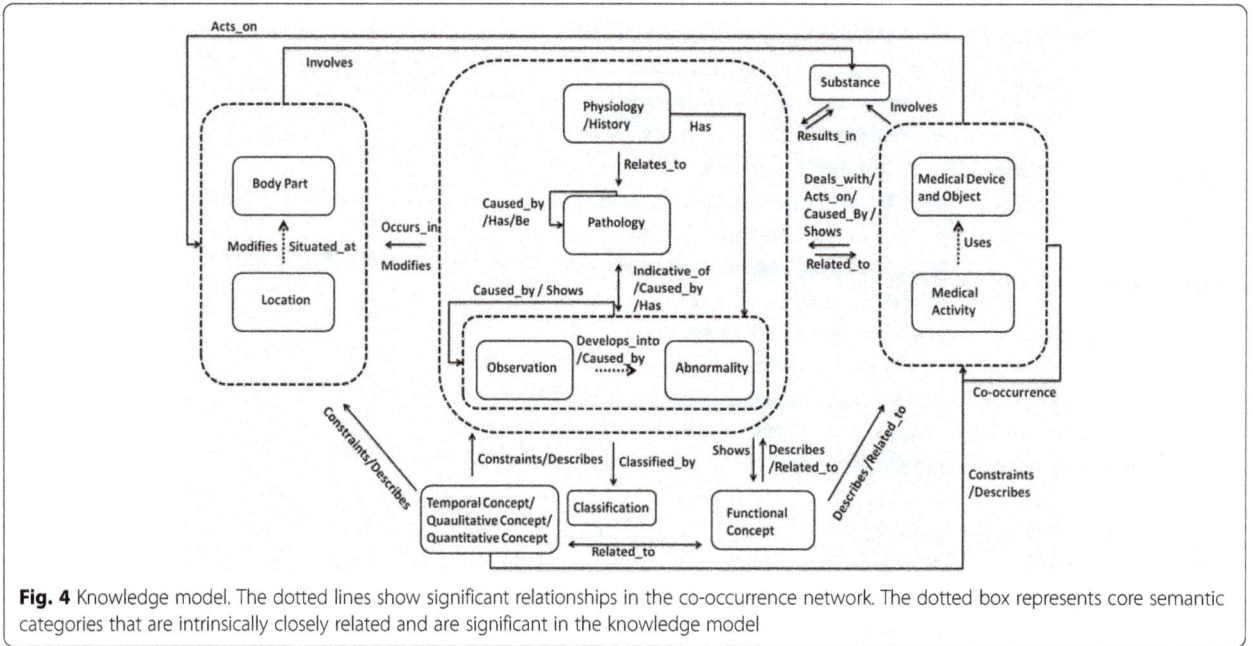

Fig. 4 Knowledge model. The dotted lines show significant relationships in the co-occurrence network. The dotted box represents core semantic categories that are intrinsically closely related and are significant in the knowledge model

Discussion

In the medical domain, there are many complex relationships between entities, such as a clinical observation related to a certain pathology, or an observed disease co-occur with its comorbidities; therefore, we need a comprehensive knowledge model to support structured formalization of medical knowledge. A knowledge model (also referred to as an information model), is an important prerequisite for extracting information. The model has two components: (1) Semantic annotations that conceptualize entities in the imaging notes, and (2) relationships that link the discrete

entities to form a logi/cal and integrated model. The advantage of our method, which extracts information based on the knowledge model, is discussed in the following sections. We also discuss the advantages of using semantic pattern mining to generate a knowledge model as follows;

Compared to frame-based method for building knowledge model

Compared with previous studies that combined syntactic and semantic analysis and a pre-defined topic frame or event template to model information in a corpus [50–52],

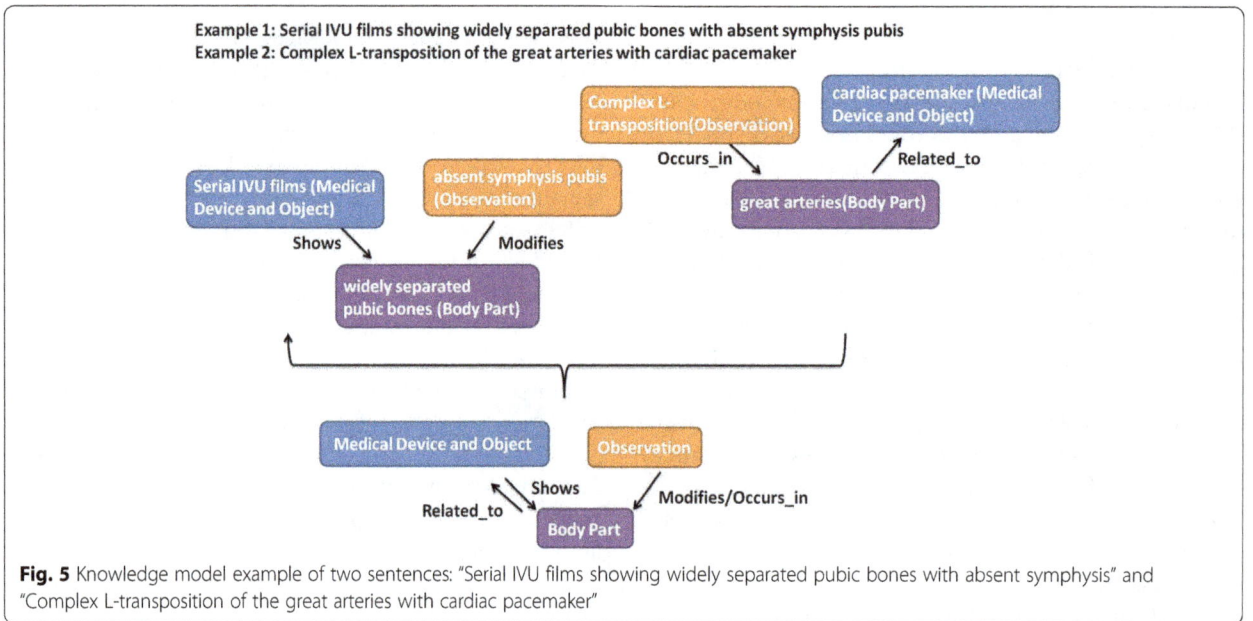

Fig. 5 Knowledge model example of two sentences: "Serial IVU films showing widely separated pubic bones with absent symphysis" and "Complex L-transposition of the great arteries with cardiac pacemaker"

Table 3 Evaluation of semantic annotation performance

Semantic Categories	True Positive (TP)	True Negative (TN)	False Positive (FP)	False Negative (FN)	Precision	Recall	F-Score
Abnormality	16	1660	4	12	80.0%	57.1%	0.6667
Body Part	238	1438	38	26	86.2%	90.2%	0.8815
Classification	12	1664	0	6	100.0%	66.7%	0.8000
Functional Concept	90	1586	14	12	86.5%	88.2%	0.8738
Location	230	1446	54	58	81.0%	79.9%	0.8042
Medical Activity	22	1654	14	26	61.1%	45.8%	0.5238
Medical Device and Object	8	1668	14	0	36.4%	100.0%	0.5333
Observation	168	1508	16	62	91.3%	73.0%	0.8116
Pathology	202	1474	4	50	98.1%	80.2%	0.8821
Physiology	16	1660	4	4	80.0%	80.0%	0.8000
Qualitative Concept	172	1504	22	60	88.7%	74.1%	0.8075
Quantitative Concept	78	1598	4	4	95.1%	95.1%	0.9512
Substance	24	1652	12	24	66.7%	50.0%	0.5714
Temporal Concept	56	1620	2	0	96.6%	100.0%	0.9825
Overall	1332	22,132	202	344	86.8%	79.5%	0.8299

our knowledge model is able to provide a higher coverage of both semantic categories annotated and semantic relationships involved. In Friedman's work [51], NPs were parsed into entities of problem and modifier (location, observation). For example, "Status post myocardial infarction" was framed as [problem, myocardial infarction, [status, post]]. Modifiers were generated around the core of the noun phrases "problem, myocardial infarction". This approach had a limited scope since it was only able to distinguish the modifiers into "location" and "observations". Here we didn't compare our result directly with the Friedman study because 1) Friedman's study did not report the coverage but only reported precision, recall, specificity, and sensitivity; 2) even though we also evaluated machine annotation performance using precision and recall, it is difficult to compare our task with previous studies since their tasks were disease specific and domain specific; 3) most frame-based templates were manually drafted, making it less likely to represent the true characteristics of a corpus for a specific domain. Our approach contributes to a data-driven and content-based perspective for generating knowledge model. The data-driven and content-based method is able to produce a knowledge model with higher coverage and more domain-specific representation. Thus, our knowledge model was able to cover 98% of the content in image notes corpus and reveal 97% of the relationships.

Compared to machine learning-based method for building knowledge model

Several studies have explored the extraction of semantic relationships between entities using machine learning methods [53, 54]. Nevertheless, both methods require knowledge models to guide information extraction. For example, when training machine-learning algorithms (e.g., conditional random fields, SVM) to extract entities and their relationships in free-text, we first need to define a target model (e.g., entity labels, schema) to support machine annotation and relationship mapping. Previous studies often used knowledge models that were manually defined by experts focusing only on a specific domain, such as mammography and chest radiographic reports [55, 56]. By using a semantic network, we employed a novel approach that combines syntactic analysis with data-driven network analysis to explore semantic relations in a specific corpus. Compared with prior works that mostly involved syntactic analysis plus a rule-based or a supervised learning method to generate topic frames, our approach could potentially adapt to another corpus with reduced manual efforts.

Compared to ontology-based method for building knowledge model

RadMiner [57] uses ontologies to represent the relationships between semantic entities. It can semantically analyze radiology reports using a clinical terminology called *Lexicon of Standardized Radiological Terms* (RadLex) [58]; however, concepts in the ontology model have complex relationships which are usually not well represented in the ontology itself. By a using context-based semantic network, we could better represent (higher coverage of) relationships between entities compared with other methods. By using UMLS, we also developed a knowledge model with a higher coverage than RadMiner, which uses RadLex.

RadMiner supports structured reporting of image findings and indexing of teaching cases. Despite its high coverage of anatomical structures, one study [59] showed that only 2.32% of phrases in a de-identified radiology report were exactly mapped to RadLex, while 50.53% of phrases were only partially mapped; in contrast, 10.40 and 85.95% of phrases were exactly and partially mapped to UMLS. Another study [60] demonstrated the lower coverage of RadLex for representing clinical language in imaging reports, especially for disease condition and non-radiology procedures; however, disease condition and non-radiology procedures comprise a significant percentage of content in image reports and case reports. Compared with RadMiner, our work provided a higher level and more comprehensive knowledge model comprising 14 semantic categories. We regrouped the most frequent UMLS semantic types into 14 semantic categories to reduce complexity results from the UMLS hierarchy or radiology language while still achieving a high coverage of radiology content.

Subject:Relationship:Object structure

One advantage of using the SRO structure is that it can retain the relationships at the phrase level and reveal only the closest semantic relation in one sentence, thereby significantly reducing the chance for misinterpretation ("noises"). For example, if we analyze the sentence "There are foci of intensely increased radiotracer uptake in T9" at a sentence level, we will generate six co-occurrence relationships: "There/ foci, There/ intensely increased radiotracer uptake, There/T9, foci/T9, foci/ intensely increased radiotracer uptake, intensely increased radiotracer uptake/ T9". In contrast, if we analyze the sentence with the SRO structure, we will generate three relationships: "There:are:-foci", "foci:of: intensely increased radiotracer uptake in T9", "intensely increased radiotracer uptake:in: T9". These three relationships and their corresponding Subject and Object can be represented concisely.

Content-based semantic type regrouping

We are aware of the complexity of UMLS hierarchical structure. Some recent studies have focused on reducing the complexity of radiology report content from an ontology perspective [21, 61, 62]. A pilot study [61] investigated the possibility of using 19 different vocabulary sources in UMLS to index XML-structured image reports. This study confirmed the enhancement of indexing precision of radiology reports by choosing the optimal subsets of UMLS vocabularies. In order to achieve high-quality semantic classification [47] and simplify concept relation representation [48], we regrouped the 40 most frequently occurring semantic types in our corpus into 14 major semantic categories. One of our main contributions in this work was a new regrouping strategy that incorporated a method, previously proposed by McCray et al. [20], and our domain specific adaptation. McCray's method aggregated UMLS semantic types based on the inherent

structure of UMLS. Our domain specific adaptation was based on the structure of the semantic network (Fig. 3).

Clinically relevant granularity of noun phrases

Another novelty of our method was that we parsed maximal NP/ADJPs instead of base NP/ADJPs. Mapping entities according to base NP/ADJPs would result in returning a large amount of false positive results due to unsuitable granularity level. Our method, by keeping noun phrases intact and examining maximal NP/ADJPs instead of splitting one long NP/ADJPs into base NP/ADJPs and modifiers, was able to be regarded as a phrase-level information retrieval tool that filled the gap between word-level information retrieval (most of the prior work) and sentence-level information retrieval. Our method provided an efficient tool for tasks that would favor minimal query input but need a broader scope for information retrieval.

Error analysis

Based on our evaluation results, we concluded that there would be five major causes for errors with machine annotation.

(1) Some of the errors were caused by considering the tag of the last noun as the semantic type for the whole noun phrase. For example, "absent symphysis pubis" was considered "Observation" based on the examples in the annotation manual; however, as "symphysis pubis" was tagged as "Location", it was then considered to be a "Location" concept instead of "Observation".

(2) Ambiguity in the meaning of words in a medical imaging context caused incorrect classification for UMLS semantic types. For example, "defect" was tagged as "Functional Concept" by the UMLS tagger, but actually, it is closer to an "Abnormality" in this context. In fact, the UMLS is known to associate numerous concepts with questionable semantic types.

(3) Annotation error might also be caused by using a UMLS tagger trained on a general EHR corpus instead a more confined domain of medical image reports [41].

(4) UMLS didn't recognize typological errors and abbreviations. The low precision in "Medical Activity" was mostly caused by this type of error. For example "MRI TOF" was tagged as "MRI[Medical Activity] TOF[Abnormality]" instead of "MRI[Medical Activity] TOF[Medical Activity]", because UMLS was not able to recognize the abbreviation of "TOF" as a Medical Activity.

(5) Parsing error contributed to our overall error rate. Even though Stanford parser assumed to be less dependent on training corpus [63], it was shown previously that changing the word frequencies according to the medical context in the training corpus would improve parsing performance [64].

Limitations and future work

One limitation of our work was that the relationships in the network were manually reviewed and labeled. Since our work mainly focused on the pipeline for generating a knowledge model, automatic relationship labeling was beyond our scope. However, it will be an interesting work for the future. In the future, we may be able to develop an annotated corpus based on our existing annotation of semantic entities and relationships, and then build an automated system to annotate relationships in image reports domain.

Another limitation is that our pipeline is not currently deployed in any framework (e.g. UIMA). Nor is it packaged into an installable software. However, since we have listed all the components of this work as a step-by-step diagram and have mentioned external software or packages we used in each step, the pipeline can be reproduced.

Other limitations come from our utilizing existing tools for parsing and annotating corpus. The tools are not trained on our specific domain, which may result in errors, as mentioned in the "Error Analysis" section. To reduce parsing errors, our future work will include retraining the parser and tailoring to the medical imaging domain. To solve the problems with incorrect semantic annotation, we can consider two approaches for future improvement: (1) Incorporate RadLex and FMA [65], which provides better semantic type assignment over Body Part, or incorporate other ontologies that have more comprehensive terminologies in "Medical Activity" and "Substance", two low-performing UMLS semantic categories. (2) Reexamine and correct semantic types assignment errors based on specific domain context and avoid issues brought up by ambiguous and ill-defined UMLS semantic types, such as Functional Concept. (3) Future work to reduce errors caused by abbreviations or medical metaphors includes incorporating a list of common abbreviations/metaphors used in a radiology setting during the data processing step and adding spell-check modules to ensure better tagging quality.

At this time we cannot evaluate the precision and recall for the relationships, because we do not have an automated machine annotation for the semantic relationships; we can only automate the semantic annotation for the entities. The next step in our work is to create a machine annotation method for semantic relationships between the entities.

Conclusions

We proposed a data-driven approach that used NLP and semantic network analysis to construct a knowledge model. We used medical image domain as a use case to demonstrate our system. The resulting knowledge model of medical image reports included 14 semantic categories and 113 semantic relationships. The evaluation using medical image reports from four different sources showed that the knowledge model created using a single source, Radiopaedia.org, was generalizable. The machine-tagging evaluation of 1676 entities achieved an overall precision of 87%, recall of 79%, and F-score of 82%. The knowledge model was able to cover 98% of the content in the evaluation corpus and revealed 97% of the relationships. This indicates that our knowledge model is comprehensive and covers a majority of concepts and relationships in medical image reports. Our pipeline to develop knowledge models demonstrated great potential of facilitating and improving information retrieval.

Abbreviations
ADJP: Adjective Phrases; CDM: Common Data Model; EHR: Electronic Health Records; FMA: Foundational Model of Anatomy; NLP: Natural Language Processing; NP: Noun Phrases; PAS: Predicate-argument structures; PP: Prepositional Phrases; RadLex: Lexicon of Standardized Radiological Terms; RDF: Resource Description Framework; SRO: Subject:Relationship:Object; SVM: Support Vector Machines; UMLS: Unified Medical Language System; VP: Verb Phrases

Acknowledgements
The knowledge model was conceptualized with the support from Jiping Zhou from Singapore General Hospital, Department of Internal Medicine, and Hai Zhang from Greenfield Dental, Milwaukee, Wisconsin.

Funding
This study was made possible by the UWM Research Foundation and GE Healthcare Catalyst Grant. The work was conducted at the Center for Biomedical Data and Language Processing in collaboration with the Department of Health Informatics and Administration, College of Health Sciences, University of Wisconsin-Milwaukee. The funders had no role in study design, data collection and analysis, decision to publish, or preparation of the manuscript. Its contents are solely the responsibility of the authors and do not necessarily represent the official views of the funders.

Authors' contributions
JL conceived and designed the study, supervised the conduct of the study and data collection, created the framework of data analysis and evaluation, participated in drafting the manuscript. YZ performed corpus building, syntactic processing, semantic annotation, and network analysis, participated in evaluation and drafted the manuscript. YZ, NF, HL, and JL participated in the network analysis, carried out the evaluation and revised the manuscript. All authors have read and approved the manuscript.

Competing interests
The authors declare that they have no competing interests.

Author details
[1]Department of Health Informatics and Administration, Center for Biomedical Data and Language Processing, University of Wisconsin-Milwaukee, 2025 E Newport Ave, NWQ-B Room 6469, Milwaukee, WI 53211, USA. [2]Division of Biomedical Statistics and Informatics, Mayo Clinic, Rochester, 205 3rd Ave SW, Rochester, MN 55905, USA.

References
1. Weng C, Wu X, Luo Z, Boland MR, Theodoratos D, Johnson SB. EliXR: an approach to eligibility criteria extraction and representation. J Am Med Inform Assoc. 2011;18(Supplement 1):i116–24.
2. Bashyam V, Hsu W, Watt E, Bui AA, Kangarloo H, Taira RK. Problem-centric organization and visualization of patient imaging and clinical data 1. Radiographics. 2009;29(2):331–43.

3.   Coden A, Savova G, Sominsky I, Tanenblatt M, Masanz J, Schuler K, Cooper J, Guan W, De Groen PC. Automatically extracting cancer disease characteristics from pathology reports into a disease knowledge representation model. J Biomed Inform. 2009;42(5):937–49.

4.   Yetisgen-Yildiz M, Gunn ML, Xia F, Payne TH. A text processing pipeline to extract recommendations from radiology reports. J Biomed Inform. 2013; 46(2):354–62.

5.   Yetisgen-Yildiz M, Gunn ML, Xia F, Payne TH. Automatic identification of critical follow-up recommendation sentences in radiology reports. In: *AMIA Annual Symposium Proceedings: 2011*: American medical informatics association; 2011; 1593.

6.   Pham A-D, Névéol A, Lavergne T, Yasunaga D, Clément O, Meyer G, Morello R, Burgun A. Natural language processing of radiology reports for the detection of thromboembolic diseases and clinically relevant incidental findings. BMC bioinformatics. 2014;15(1):266.

7.   Perera S, Henson C, Thirunarayan K, Sheth A, Nair S. Data driven knowledge acquisition method for domain knowledge enrichment in the healthcare. In: *Bioinformatics and Biomedicine (BIBM), 2012 IEEE International Conference on: 2012*: IEEE; 2012. p. 1–8.

8.   Paiva L, Costa R, Figueiras P, Lima C. Discovering semantic relations from unstructured data for ontology enrichment: Asssociation rules based approach. In: *Information Systems and Technologies (CISTI), 2014 9th Iberian Conference on: 2014*: IEEE; 2014. p. 1–6.

9.   Lin K, Wu M, Wang X, Pan Y. MEDLedge: a Q&a based system for constructing medical knowledge base. In: *Computer Science & Education (ICCSE), 2016 11th International Conference on: 2016*: IEEE; 2016. p. 485–9.

10. Samwald M, Freimuth R, Luciano JS, Lin S, Powers RL, Marshall MS, Adlassnig K-P, Dumontier M, Boyce RD, An RDF. OWL knowledge base for query answering and decision support in clinical pharmacogenetics. Studies in health technology and informatics. 2013;192:539.

11. Musen MA, Middleton B, Greenes RA. Clinical decision-support systems. In: Biomedical informatics: Springer; 2014. p. 643–74.

12. Clunie DA. DICOM structured reporting: PixelMed publishing; 2000.

13. FitzHenry F, Resnic F, Robbins S, Denton J, Nookala L, Meeker D, Ohno-Machado L, Matheny M. Creating a common data model for comparative effectiveness with the observational medical outcomes partnership. Applied clinical informatics. 2015;6(3):536.

14. Mehrabi S, Wang Y, Ihrke D, Liu H. Exploring gaps of family history documentation in EHR for precision medicine-a case study of familial hypercholesterolemia ascertainment. AMIA Summits on Translational Science Proceedings. 2016;2016:160.

15. Khelif K, Dieng-Kuntz R, Barbry P. An ontology-based approach to support text mining and information retrieval in the biological domain. J UCS. 2007; 13(12):1881–907.

16. Pletscher-Frankild S, Palleja A, Tsafou K, Binder JX, Jensen LJ. DISEASES: text mining and data integration of disease–gene associations. Methods. 2015; 74:83–9.

17. Wei C-H, Kao H-Y, Lu Z. PubTator: a web-based text mining tool for assisting biocuration. Nucleic Acids Res. 2013;41(W1):W518–22.

18. Wang Y, Desai M, Ryan PB, DeFalco FJ, Schuemie MJ, Stang PE, Berlin JA, Yuan Z. Incidence of diabetic ketoacidosis among patients with type 2 diabetes mellitus treated with SGLT2 inhibitors and other antihyperglycemic agents. Diabetes Res Clin Pract. 2017;128:83–90.

19. Lambert CG, Mazurie AJ, Lauve NR, Hurwitz NG, Young SS, Obenchain RL, Hengartner NW, Perkins DJ, Tohen M, Kerner B. Hypothyroidism risk compared among nine common bipolar disorder therapies in a large US cohort. Bipolar Disord. 2016;18(3):247–60.

20. McCray AT, Burgun A, Bodenreider O. Aggregating UMLS semantic types for reducing conceptual complexity. Studies in health technology and informatics. 2001;84(0 1):216.

21. Soysal E, Cicekli I, Baykal N. Design and evaluation of an ontology based information extraction system for radiological reports. Comput Biol Med. 2010;40(11):900–11.

22. Harris Z. Discourse and sublanguage. Sublanguage: studies of language in restricted semantic domains. 1982:231–6.

23. Friedman C, Kra P, Rzhetsky A. Two biomedical sublanguages: a description based on the theories of Zellig Harris. J Biomed Inform. 2002;35(4):222–35.

24. Pustejovsky J, Anick P, Bergler S. Lexical semantic techniques for corpus analysis. Computational Linguistics. 1993;19(2):331–58.

25. Grishman R, Kittredge R. Analyzing language in restricted domains: sublanguage description and processing: Psychology Press; 2014.

26. Radiopaedia [http://radiopaedia.org/].

27. jsoup: Java HTML Parser.

28. Hearst MA. Automatic acquisition of hyponyms from large text corpora. In: *Proceedings of the 14th conference on Computational linguistics-Volume 2: 1992*: Association for Computational Linguistics; 1992. p. 539–45.

29. Hearst MA. Automated discovery of WordNet relations. *WordNet: an electronic lexical.* database. 1998:131–53.

30. Dhungana UR, Shakya S. Hypernymy in WordNet, its role in WSD, and its limitations. In: *Computational Intelligence, Communication Systems and Networks (CICSyN), 2015 7th International Conference on: 2015*: IEEE; 2015. p. 15–9.

31. Potok TE, Patton RM, Sukumar SR. SYSTEM AND METHOD OF CONTENT BASED RECOMMENDATION USING HYPERNYM EXPANSION. US Patent. 2017; 20(170):262–528.

32. Pradhan SS, Ward WH, Hacioglu K, Martin JH, Jurafsky D. Shallow semantic parsing using support vector machines. In: HLT-NAACL: 2004; 2004. p. 233–40.

33. Palmer M, Gildea D, Kingsbury P. The proposition bank: an annotated corpus of semantic roles. Computational linguistics. 2005;31(1):71–106.

34. Hindle D. Noun classification from predicate-argument structures. In: *Proceedings of the 28th annual meeting on Association for Computational Linguistics: 1990*: Association for Computational Linguistics; 1990. p. 268–75.

35. Parsons T. Events in the semantics of English, vol. 5: Cambridge. Ma: MIT Press; 1990.

36. De Marneffe M-C, MacCartney B, Manning CD. Generating typed dependency parses from phrase structure parses. In: Proceedings of LREC: 2006; 2006. p. 449–54.

37. Chen D, Manning CD. A fast and accurate dependency parser using neural networks. In: Proceedings of the 2014 conference on empirical methods in natural language processing (EMNLP): 2014; 2014. p. 740–50.

38. Ágel V. Dependency and valency: an international handbook of contemporary research, vol. 1: Walter de Gruyter; 2006.

39. McCray AT. The UMLS semantic network. In: *Proceedings/Annual Symposium on Computer Application in Medical Care Symposium on Computer Applications in Medical Care: 1989*: American medical informatics association; 1989. p. 503–7.

40. Jacobs PS, Krupka GR, Rau LF: Lexico-semantic pattern matching as a companion to parsing in text understanding. In: HLT: 1991; 1991.

41. Luo Z, Duffy R, Johnson S, Weng C. Corpus-based approach to creating a semantic lexicon for clinical research eligibility criteria from UMLS. AMIA Summits on Translational Science Proceedings 2010. 2010:26–30.

42. Cheng LT, Zheng J, Savova GK, Erickson BJ. Discerning tumor status from unstructured MRI reports—completeness of information in existing reports and utility of automated natural language processing. J Digit Imaging. 2010;23(2):119–32.

43. Chapman WW, Bridewell W, Hanbury P, Cooper GF, Buchanan BG. A simple algorithm for identifying negated findings and diseases in discharge summaries. J Biomed Inform. 2001;34(5):301–10.

44. Journal of Radiology Case Reports [http://www.radiologycases.com/index.php/radiologycases].

45. BJR Case Report [http://www.birpublications.org/journal/bjrcr].

46. RadioGraphics [http://pubs.rsna.org/journal/radiographics].

47. Fan J-W, Xu H, Friedman C. Using contextual and lexical features to restructure and validate the classification of biomedical concepts. BMC bioinformatics. 2007;8(1):264.

48. Burgun A, Bot G, Fieschi M, Le Beux P. Sharing knowledge in medicine: semantic and ontologic facets of medical concepts. In: *Systems, Man, and Cybernetics, 1999 IEEE SMC'99 Conference Proceedings 1999 IEEE International Conference on: 1999*: IEEE; 1999. p. 300–5.

49. Chen Z, Perl Y, Halper M, Geller J, Gu H. Partitioning the UMLS semantic network. Information Technology in Biomedicine, IEEE Transactions on. 2002;6(2):102–8.

50. Friedlin J, McDonald CJ. A natural language processing system to extract and code concepts relating to congestive heart failure from chest radiology reports. In: *AMIA Annual Symposium Proceedings: 2006*: American Medical Informatics Association. 2006:269.

51. Friedman C, Shagina L, Lussier Y, Hripcsak G. Automated encoding of clinical documents based on natural language processing. J Am Med Inform Assoc. 2004;11(5):392–402.

52. Dligach D, Bethard S, Becker L, Miller T, Savova GK. Discovering body site and severity modifiers in clinical texts. J Am Med Inform Assoc. 2014;21(3): 448–54.

53. Bundschus M, Dejori M, Stetter M, Tresp V, Kriegel H-P. Extraction of semantic biomedical relations from text using conditional random fields. BMC bioinformatics. 2008;9(1):1.

54. Luo Z, Johnson SB, Lai AM, Weng C. Extracting temporal constraints from clinical research eligibility criteria using conditional random fields. In: AMIA annual symposium proceedings: 2011; 2011. p. 843–52.

55. Bozkurt S, Gülkesen KH, Rubin D. Annotation for information extraction from mammography reports. In: ICIMTH: 2013; 2013. p. 183–5.

56. Bell DS, Pattison-Gordon E, Greenes RA. Experiments in concept modeling for radiographic image reports. J Am Med Inform Assoc. 1994;1(3):249.

57. Gerstmair A, Daumke P, Simon K, Langer M, Kotter E. Intelligent image retrieval based on radiology reports. Eur Radiol. 2012;22(12):2750–8.

58. Langlotz CP. RadLex: a new method for indexing online educational materials 1. Radiographics. 2006;26(6):1595–7.

59. Wang L, Vall D. Assessing the ability of RadLex to represent the common clinical language in imaging reports. In: *Radiological Society of North America 2011 Scientific Assembly and Annual Meeting*. Chicago IL; November 26–December 2; 2011.

60. Hong Y, Zhang J, Heilbrun ME, Kahn CE Jr. Analysis of RadLex coverage and term co-occurrence in radiology reporting templates. J Digit Imaging. 2012; 25(1):56–62.

61. Huang Y, Lowe HJ, Hersh WR. A pilot study of contextual UMLS indexing to improve the precision of concept-based representation in XML-structured clinical radiology reports. J Am Med Inform Assoc. 2003;10(6):580–7.

62. Taira RK, Soderland SG, Jakobovits RM. Automatic structuring of radiology free-text reports 1. Radiographics. 2001;21(1):237–45.

63. Zhang Y, Jiang M, Wang J, Xu H. Semantic role labeling of clinical text: comparing syntactic parsers and features. In: *AMIA Annual Symposium Proceedings: 2016*: American medical informatics association; 2016; 1283.

64. Huang Y, Lowe HJ, Klein D, Cucina RJ. Improved identification of noun phrases in clinical radiology reports using a high-performance statistical natural language parser augmented with the UMLS specialist lexicon. J Am Med Inform Assoc. 2005;12(3):275–85.

65. Foundational Model of Anatomy ontology [http://sig.biostr.washington.edu/projects/fm/AboutFM.html].

Effect of clinical decision rules, patient cost and malpractice information on clinician brain CT image ordering

Ronald W. Gimbel[1]*[iD], Ronald G. Pirrallo[2], Steven C. Lowe[3], David W. Wright[4], Lu Zhang[1], Min-Jae Woo[1], Paul Fontelo[5], Fang Liu[5] and Zachary Connor[1,3]

Abstract

Background: The frequency of head computed tomography (CT) imaging for mild head trauma patients has raised safety and cost concerns. Validated clinical decision rules exist in the published literature and on-line sources to guide medical image ordering but are often not used by emergency department (ED) clinicians. Using simulation, we explored whether the presentation of a clinical decision rule (i.e. Canadian CT Head Rule - CCHR), findings from malpractice cases related to clinicians not ordering CT imaging in mild head trauma cases, and estimated patient out-of-pocket cost might influence clinician brain CT ordering. Understanding what type and how information may influence clinical decision making in the ordering advanced medical imaging is important in shaping the optimal design and implementation of related clinical decision support systems.

Methods: Multi-center, double-blinded simulation-based randomized controlled trial. Following standardized clinical vignette presentation, clinicians made an initial imaging decision for the patient. This was followed by additional information on decision support rules, malpractice outcome review, and patient cost; each with opportunity to modify their initial order. The malpractice and cost information differed by assigned group to test the any temporal relationship. The simulation closed with a second vignette and an imaging decision.

Results: One hundred sixteen of the 167 participants (66.9%) initially ordered a brain CT scan. After CCHR presentation, the number of clinicians ordering a CT dropped to 76 (45.8%), representing a 21.1% reduction in CT ordering ($P = 0.002$). This reduction in CT ordering was maintained, in comparison to initial imaging orders, when presented with malpractice review information ($p = 0.002$) and patient cost information ($p = 0.002$). About 57% of clinicians changed their order during study, while 43% never modified their imaging order.

Conclusion: This study suggests that ED clinician brain CT imaging decisions may be influenced by clinical decision support rules, patient out-of-pocket cost information and findings from malpractice case review.

Keywords: Clinical decision making, CT brain, Mild head trauma, Patient cost information, Simulation research, Malpractice information, Canadian CT head rule, Emergency department clinicians, Evidence-based medicine

* Correspondence: rgimbel@clemson.edu
[1]Department of Public Health Sciences, Clemson University, 501 Edwards Hall, Clemson, SC 29634-0745, USA
Full list of author information is available at the end of the article

Background

Minor head trauma is a common condition treated by emergency department (ED) clinicians [1, 2]. Over one million computed tomography (CT) scans are conducted annually in the United States for these patients, with less than 10% demonstrating findings that change medical management [3–5]. The need for brain CT in patients with minor head trauma has been thrust into the national spot light because of concerns about the long-term danger of low-dose radiation exposure and the desire to decrease unnecessary health care costs [4, 6].

There are numerous reasons why clinicians may order advanced medical imaging for patients despite clinical evidence suggesting otherwise. These issues include, but are not limited to, unfamiliarity or mistrust of clinical decision rules [5, 7] and estimation of radiation burden [8–11], fear of malpractice lawsuits [12–14], and lack of knowledge of the cost of medical imaging.

With respect to minor head trauma, several validated evidence-based clinical decision rules have been published to help guide clinicians in ordering brain CTs [3, 5, 15]. While these rules differ with respect to sensitivity and specificity, they provide a medically and legally justified pathway to support decision making. Despite this, evidence suggests that many clinicians do not follow clinical decision rules unless reinforced by practice policy and/or integrated into clinical work flow [12, 16].

It is well documented in the literature that "clinician fear of a malpractice suit" exists, and influences clinical decision making [3, 12, 14, 17]. Fear of a lawsuit has led to increased CT ordering, despite the existence and validation of clinical decision rules [16, 18].

Finally, substantial literature reveals that clinicians are unfamiliar with cost implications of testing to patients, payers, and health systems [19–21]. However, evidence suggests that clinician awareness of testing cost may influence their decision making, especially toward less-costly testing options [21–23]. One abstract even shows that insured medical patients are more likely to receive a brain CT in cases of minor head injuries than patients without health insurance [16].

This study expands our previous research on how information influences clinician decision making in medical image ordering for adult and pediatric patients in the primary care environment [23, 24]. In our earlier work, we incorporated simulation-based methodology to explore how clinician medical image ordering behavior might be influenced by the introduction of clinical decision rules, estimated radiation exposure information, and estimated cost. We analyzed the temporal effect of information presentation to clinicians and the relationship between clinician demographics and medical image ordering behavior.

Goals of the investigation

In our current study, we seek to explore whether presentation of the Canadian CT Head Rule (CCHR), findings from a medical-legal review of malpractice cases related to lack of CT ordering in head trauma victims, and estimated patient out-of-pocket cost for CT imaging might influence clinician ordering in response to clinical vignettes in the simulated emergency department environment. Our goal was to further inform practicing emergency department clinicians and the medical informatics community as they collaborate to build clinical decision support systems that aid clinical decision making.

Methods

Study design and setting

This was a multi-center, double-blinded, with balanced ([1:1]) randomization, parallel-group study conducted in the United States with the Departments of Emergency Medicine, Greenville Health System (Greenville, SC) and Emory Healthcare (Atlanta, GA). The study was approved by the Institutional Review Boards of both health systems. There were no changes to the methods after the simulation trial had commenced. As this was a web-accessible simulation study, participants could participate in the study anywhere connectivity allowed. Participants could access the simulation study via a computer or portable device (e.g. tablet) that was internet-accessible.

Selection of participants

Study participation was limited to clinicians, with image ordering capability for patients, and employed in the emergency department of one of the two health systems. Clinicians included attending physicians, resident physicians, physician assistants and nurse practitioners Randomization occurred when the clinicians indicated their occupational profession (see above). Specifically, an electronic balancer allocated each participant (by occupational profession) to one of two groups. The two groups were the LEGAL-COST group or the COST-LEGAL group, both described below, which differed in the temporal order in which they were presented information in the study. The study was double-blinded in that neither the investigators nor the participants were aware of the order in which legal and cost information would be presented. For clarity, both groups received all information which differs from a traditional interventional trial with intervention and control groups.

Recruitment

An electronic email invitation from each department's academic leadership was sent to all ED clinicians and EM residents. Reminder emails were sent to all at approximately 14 days and 21 days after the initial invitation. Leadership was blinded to participation, assuring voluntary participation without fear of repercussion.

Interventions

Our intervention consisted of two clinical vignettes, follow-up decision screens and collection of demographic data (Additional file 1). Both clinical vignettes were jointly developed by the emergency medicine and radiology clinician study authors. The cases were designed to provide sufficient information for the clinician to make a determination regarding need for CT imaging. Both cases were designed to fall below the threshold, as outlined in the CCHR, for requiring CT imaging. To further unify the cases both patients had known normal renal function and no allergy to contrast.

Following an electronic-based informed consent process, participants were presented with clinical vignette #1 which described a 58-year-old female (simulation patient) who presents to the Emergency Department after falling on ice hitting her head on the sidewalk (Additional file 1). Following the case presentation, the clinicians were prompted to make a medical image ordering decision for this patient among three options: CT brain (without and with contrast), CT (without contrast), or no imaging.

After their initial imaging decision, the clinicians were presented with the brain CT ordering criteria based on the CCHR [1, 15]. We included a hyperlink to three manuscripts (2 abstracts, 1 full-text) supporting the criteria for clinicians who desired to review further material [15, 25, 26]. The clinicians were provided a first opportunity to modify their initial imaging order.

After their opportunity to modify based on the CCHR, the next topic presented was estimated out of pocket costs regarding the expense of the ED visit with and without imaging. The costs were based on actual local ED charges with the average patient out-of-pocket expense after insurance for a brain CT identified as $843. This was derived from actual data (year 2015) calculated from a Level 1 Trauma Center in the Southeast United States. Following presentation of this information, clinicians were provided a second opportunity to modify their initial imaging order.

The third topic presented was a collection of findings from a malpractice case law review (years 1972–2014) covering situations where the clinician did not order a brain CT for a minor head trauma. Participants were provided with an additional hyperlink to the original published article for review [3]. The malpractice law review was included as an evidence source that addresses "clinician fear of malpractice lawsuit if not ordering a brain CT for minor head trauma". Following presentation of this information, clinicians were provided a third and final the opportunity to modify their initial imaging order.

After all of the information was presented, constituting the breadth of the intervention, vignette #2 was presented to assess how clinicians might apply their new knowledge for similar scenarios moving forward. Vignette #2 describes a 62- year old female (simulation patient) who had a witnessed slip and fall at home (Additional file 1). Following this case presentation, the clinicians were given a single opportunity to make a medical image ordering decision among three options: CT brain (without and with contrast), CT (without contrast), or no imaging. Thus, a total of 5 clinical decisions were recorded for each participant based on 2 cases.

Demographic and general survey data were gathered from participants. Demographic data included age, gender, role (i.e. practicing clinician, trainee), and years of clinical practice. Two exploratory questions on the participant's economic attitudes required responses presented on a Likert-like 1–7 scale. The first was "Making better use of my resources makes me feel good"; participants were asked to agree or disagree with the statement. The second was "I believe in being careful in how I spend my money"; participants were asked to agree or disagree with the statement. Both of these questions were derived from the consumer-oriented literature where the focus was on measurement of consumer frugality [27].

Our study concluded with an option for participants to earn a no-cost one Category 1 AMA physician continuing medical education (CME) credit. Participants were redirected from our study website to the Continuing Medical Education Office of the Greenville Health System. There participants reviewed summary material from our study, were provided the opportunity to review full-text reference papers, then complete a post-education survey assessing comprehension to receive CME credit.

Methods and measurements

As presented in Fig. 1, and described above, participants made image ordering decisions at five points in the study. The decisions were made by the participants within the simulation study and recorded in our server-based analysis database in descriptive form (e.g. no imaging, brain CT without contrast) in Microsoft Excel® format. A copy of the database was distributed to researchers at Clemson University where the descriptive data were properly coded for analysis by two researchers (MW, RG). The coded file was then imported into SAS, v.9.4 (Cary, NC).

Following the second image ordering decision point the participants were asked how they signed orders and prescriptions (i.e. as a physician, nurse practitioner, physician assistant, or other). Based on the response, participants were stratified by clinician type and balanced randomized [1:1] to one of two parallel arms (i.e. LEGAL-COST group

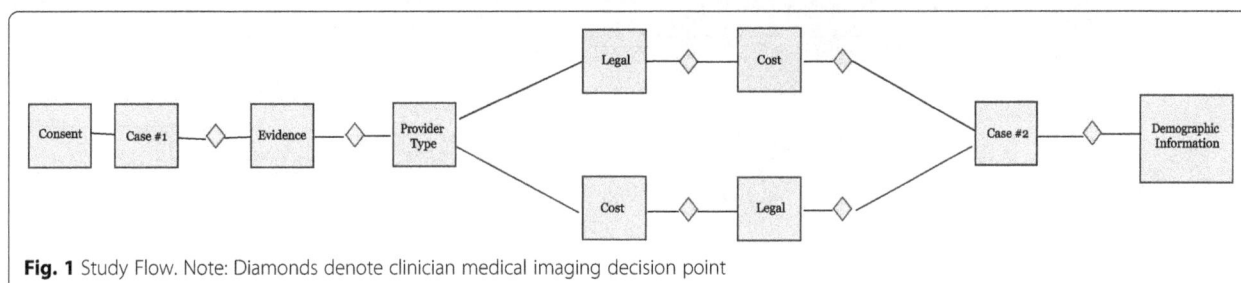

Fig. 1 Study Flow. Note: Diamonds denote clinician medical imaging decision point

or the COST-LEGAL group). Stratification was used to ensure the clinician types were equally distributed and thereby ensuring the two arms were homogeneous. The difference between the two arms was the temporal presentation of supplemental decision information. The LEGAL-COST group was presented information on malpractice case law then patient out-of-pocket cost information. The COST-LEGAL group was presented information on patient out-of-pocket cost information then malpractice case law information. The participant study flow is shown in Fig. 1.

Outcomes

The primary outcome measure for the study was the physicians' selection of imaging tests after receiving CCHR information, malpractice case review information, and patient out-of-pocket expense information. We also measure the physicians' selection of imaging tests immediately following clinical vignette #1 and after presentation of clinical vignette #2.

Analysis

Data were recorded in our intervention server, housed at the National Institutes of Health, in a Microsoft Excel spreadsheet. The data were downloaded and analyzed using SAS, ver. 9.4 (Cary, NC). In our study, because clinicians' ordering image vs. not ordering image was the main comparison of interest, CT brain modalities (with or without contrast) were grouped together and compared with the no imaging order group. To compare the clinicians' change in image ordering, McNemar test was employed and a multiple comparison adjustment was performed using Bonferroni correction. For the comparison of the demographic or other professional characteristics among different clinician groups, Chi-square test was employed to compare the proportions of categorical variables; if more than 20% of the cells had sample size less than 5, Fisher Exact test was applied instead. Analysis of Variance (ANOVA) test was used to compare the mean (standard deviation) of continuous variables.

A sample size of 155 will achieve 80% power to detect a difference in the proportion of selecting CT imaging if 30% of clinicians choose CT order in the absence of evidence and change to no imaging order when the

evidence is presented and 15% of clinicians choose no imaging order in the absence of evidence and changed to CT order when the evidence is presented.

Results

Characteristics of study subjects

Participants in the study included 150 emergency medicine physicians, 12 nurse practitioners, and 5 physician assistants allocated to one of 2 groups; the LEGAL-COST group ($n = 82$) and the COST-LEGAL group ($n = 85$). There was one clinician missing the initial imaging order and another five clinicians missing the 3rd order. These participants were included in the study sample and analyzed. All other data items were complete.

Approximately 90% of the participants were practicing clinicians with 10% being trainees; balanced among the 2 groups. Gender was balanced with slightly more males than females participating in both groups. Approximately two thirds of participants had > 5 years of clinical practice experience; included in the group were the > 40% with > 10 years of clinical practice. Just over half of the participants were ≤40 years of age (Table 1). There were no significant differences between the 2 groups with respect to demographics (Table 1) or initial image ordering decisions to clinical vignette #1 (Table 2).

Main results

Clinician image ordering decisions are presented in Table 2. For clinical vignette #1, 116 of the 167 participants (66.9%) initially order a CT image. After presentation of the CCHR, with option to access abstracts or full-text manuscript supporting the rule, the number of clinicians ordering a CT image dropped to 76 (45.8%), which represents a 21.1% statistically significant ($P = 0.002$) reduction in CT ordering in favor of no medical imaging. It is noteworthy that only 7.8% ($n = 13$) of the 167 participants accessed either ≥1 abstract ($n = 6$) or full-text manuscript ($n = 7$) indexed to the decision screen prior to making their imaging decision.

Following the CCHR-related imaging decisions, clinicians were presented with either LEGAL (LEGAL-COST group) or COST (COST-LEGAL group) information. In the LEGAL-COST group, after receiving information about malpractice judgements against clinicians who did

Table 1 Participant demographics

	LEGAL-COST group ($n = 82$)	COST-LEGAL group ($n = 85$)	P-value*	Both groups ($n = 167$)
Clinician type			0.92	
Physician	73 (89.0%)	77 (90.6%)		150 (89.8%)
Nurse Pract.	6 (7.3%)	6 (7.1%)		12 (7.2%)
Physician Assist.	3 (3.7%)	2 (2.4%)		5 (3.0%)
Role			0.74	
Practicing clinician	73 (89.0%)	77 (90.6%)		150 (89.8%)
Trainee	9 (11.0%)	8 (9.4%)		17 (10.2%)
Years of Practice			0.31	
Less than 5 years	32 (39.0%)	24 (28.2%)		56 (33.5%)
5–10 years	17 (20.7%)	23 (27.1%)		40 (24.0%)
More than 10 years	33 (40.3%)	38 (44.7%)		71 (42.5%)
Gender			0.23	
Male	49 (59.8%)	43 (50.6%)		92 (55.1%)
Female	33 (40.2%)	42 (49.4%)		75 (44.9%)
Age (year)			0.40	
< 30	6 (7.3%)	10 (11.8%)		16 (9.6%)
31–40	40 (48.8%)	34 (40.0%)		74 (44.3%)
41–50	14 (17.1%)	21 (24.7%)		35 (20.9%)
51+	22 (26.8%)	20 (23.5%)		42 (25.2%)

*P-value was calculated using Chi-square test except for the comparison of clinician type, P-value was calculated using Fisher exact test (more than 20% of cells with sample size less than 5)
Notes: LEGAL-COST indicates exposure to legal then cost information; COST-LEGAL indicates exposure to cost then legal information

not order a CT of the brain in mild trauma cases, the number of clinicians ordering a CT image was 38 (49.4%) and the difference was significant ($P = 0.05$) when compared to their initial order, and but not significant when compared to their previous image order that followed presentation of the CCHR. After presentation of patient out-of-pocket expense information, the number of clinicians ordering a CT was 39 (47.6%) where the difference was significant ($P = 0.01$) when compared with

their initial order but not significant when compared to their previous image order that followed presentation of malpractice judgement information.

In the COST-LEGAL group, after presentation of patient out-of-pocket expense information, the number of clinicians ordering a CT image was 41 (48.2%) and the difference was significant ($P = 0.002$) when compared to their initial order, but not significant when compared to their previous image order that followed presentation of

Table 2 Proportion of computed tomography ordering in clinician medical image order decisions

		Case #1				Case #2
		Initial choice (Initial order)	CCHR (2nd order)	Legal (3rd order for Legal-Cost group; or 4th order for Cost-Legal group)	Cost (4th order for Legal-Cost group; or 3rd order for Cost-Legal group)	Final choice (5th order)
Both groups	n (%)	116 (66.9%)	76 (45.8%)	85 (52.5%)	80 (47.9%)	109 (65.7%)
($n = 167$)	P-value*		Initial vs. CCHR: 0.002	Initial vs. Legal: 0.002	Initial vs. Cost: 0.002	Initial vs. Final: 1.00
LEGAL-COST[a]	n (%)	56 (68.3%)	36 (43.9%)	38 (49.4%)	39 (47.6%)	50 (61.0%)
($n = 82$)	P-value*		Initial vs. CCHR: 0.003	Initial vs. Legal: 0.05 CCHR vs. Legal: 0.8	Initial vs. Cost: 0.01 Legal vs. Cost: 1.00	Initial vs. Final: 1.00
COST-LEGAL[b]	n (%)	60 (71.4%)	40 (47.6%)	47 (55.3%)	41 (48.2%)	59 (70.2%)
($n = 85$)	P-value*		Initial vs. CCHR: 0.002	Initial vs. Legal: 0.05 Cost vs. Legal: 1.00	Initial vs. Cost: 0.002 CCHR vs. Cost: 1.00	Initial vs. Final: 1.00

Abbreviations: CCHR Canadian CT Head Rule
*P-values were calculated using McNemar test and a multiple comparison adjustment was performed using Bonferroni correction
[a]LEGAL-COST indicates exposure to legal then cost information
[b]COST-LEGAL indicates exposure to cost then legal information

the CCHR. After receiving information about malpractice judgements, the number of clinicians ordering a CT was 47 (55.3%) and the difference was significant ($P = 0.05$) when compared with their initial order but not significant when compared to their previous image order that followed presentation of patient out-of-pocket expense information.

When comparing the clinician's initial decision regarding medical imaging ordering in response to clinical vignette #1 to their decision in response to clinical vignette #2, the differences were not significant. It is noteworthy that the clinical scenarios in both vignette's, albeit not precisely the same case, were within the criteria for no medical imaging necessary when applied to the CCHR. In clinical vignette #2, approximately two thirds of clinicians ordered a CT for their patients which is consistent with their response to clinical vignette #1 (Table 2).

Comparing the initial medical imaging decision and the three subsequent imaging decision options for clinical vignette #1, 49 (30.4%) of clinicians always ordered a CT image, 20 (12.4%) of clinicians never ordered a CT image, and 98 (57.2%) changed their CT image order at least once (Table 3). Of 36 participants who changed their imaging order more than once, 27 (16.2%) changed their order at least twice, 6 (3.6%) changed their order at least three times, and 3 (1.8%) modified their imaging order four times (data not shown in the table).

The majority of clinicians who always ordered CT imaging had accumulated > 10 years in clinical practice and scored lower on both the use of resource and care with money questions as compared with clinicians never ordering CT or those that changed their imaging order,

but the difference did not achieve statistical significance (Table 3). In contrast, the majority who never ordered a CT image had accumulated < 10 years in clinical practice and scored higher on both the use of resource and care with money questions as compared to clinicians who always ordered a CT image or those that changed their imaging order (Table 3).

When aggregating data from both groups comparing CT image ordering and response to the "use of resource question", those participants who indicated a 7 score (strongly agree) on the "use of resource question" did not have a significantly different CT ordering behavior from those with a question score of 1–6 for clinical vignette #1. However, this shifted in clinical vignette #2 where the two groups were significantly different ($p = 0.02$); those scoring a 7 were more likely not to order a CT image while those scoring 1–6 were more likely to order CT image (Table 4). When aggregating data from both groups comparing CT image ordering and response to the "being careful in spending money" question, there were no statistical differences recognized (Table 4).

Limitations

Our study was based in a simulation environment. The sounds, interruptions, clinical pressures, and triage triggers of emergency department workflow were absent. Furthermore, participants were not responsible for following policies or other considerations in the clinical scenarios. It is possible that the clinicians may have manipulated their medical imaging decisions in search of the "right answer" and did not truly consider the implication of new information in their clinical care. The clinicians may not have conceptualized that the

Table 3 Clinician demographics and imaging decisions (by CT ordering behavior group)

	Clinicians who always ordered CT ($n = 49$)	Clinicians who never ordered CT ($n = 20$)	Clinicians who changed CT order ($n = 98$)	P-value[a]	Total ($n = 167$)
Provider type, %				0.70	
Physician	89.8	95.0	88.8		89.8
NP/PA	10.2	5.0	11.2		10.2
Gender, %				0.75	
Male	59.2	50.0	54.1		55.1
Female	40.8	50.0	45.9		44.9
Years of clinical practice, %				0.09	
< 5	26.5	40.0	35.7		33.5
5–10	18.4	40.0	23.5		24.0
> 10	55.1	20.0	40.8		42.5
Resource question, mean (SD)	6.00 (1.13)	6.45 (0.69)	6.17 (0.95)	0.22	6.16 (0.98)
Money question, mean (SD)	5.73 (1.18)	6.30 (0.73)	6.00 (1.06)	0.11	5.96 (1.08)

[a]Chi-square test was employed to compare the proportion of categorical variable; Analysis of Variance (ANOVA) test was employed to compare the means of continuous variable
Notes: CT, computed tomography; NP, nurse practitioner; PA, physician assistant; SD, standard deviation; mean response to resource question and money question based on 1–7 Likert-like scaled response

Table 4 Comparison of clinician response to attitudinal survey questions on resource utilization and spending money to CT ordering behavior

Survey question	Case #1 (initial order)			Case #2 (5th order)		
	CT	No image	P-value*	CT	No image	P-value*
Better use of my resources makes me feel good						
strongly agree (7)	51 (44.4%)	23 (46.0%)	0.84	42 (38.5%)	33 (57.9%)	0.02
< strongly agree (1–6)	64 (55.7%)	27 (54.0%)		67 (61.5%)	24 (42.1%)	
I believe in being careful in how I spend my money						
strongly agree (7)	40 (34.78%)	24 (48.0%) 26	0.11	38 (34.9%)	26 (45.6%)	0.18
< strongly agree (1–6)	75 (65.22%)	(52.0%)		71 (65.1%)	31 (54.4%)	

*P-value was calculated from Chi-square test

decision screens and variables (i.e. evidence, cost, legal) were fully applicable in clinical scenario #2 in the same manner as scenario #1. This study includes participants from 2 southern US states that have different state tort and liability malpractice reforms and environments that may not be applicable to other US practice locations.

Discussion

Evidence from our simulation-based study suggests that ED clinician decision making may be influenced by clinical decision rules, patient out-of-pocket cost information, and findings from malpractice case review.

Some (49 of 167; 29.3%) selected CT imaging for their simulated patient and were impervious to all information presented. It is possible that these clinicians believed the CT scan was the best test for the patient and were not influenced to change their ordering behavior. The majority of these clinicians were male, recorded > 10 years of clinical practice, and scored the lowest response on our use of resource and care in use of money questions.

The largest group of clinicians (98 of 167; 58.7%) modified their medical imaging order at least once for clinical vignette #1 when presented clinical decision rule, cost, and malpractice care review information. Of these clinicians about one third (36 of 98; 36.7%) modified their imaging order more than once.

An unexpected finding in our research was clinician medical image ordering in response to clinical vignette #2. The second case was similar to the first clinical vignette in that in neither case, when applied to the clinical decision rule, would a CT image be indicated for the patient. It appears that when presented with a new case the clinicians reverted to their original medical image ordering behavior. This may be due to the limitations of a simulation-based study or possibly due to their interpretation of vignette #2 differently than anticipated. Our study was not designed or powered to address why clinicians did not change their ordering behavior in response to clinical vignette #2.

Conclusion

Our research contributes to the body of evidence on clinician decision making and key information that may influence medical image ordering behavior. The findings suggest that clinicians may respond to key information if presented within the context of their clinical workflow. In our study, we provided links to source documents and evidence supporting the information. Clinicians are typically decisive in their decision making with their patients. Medical informaticians and health information technologists should be extremely thoughtful in their information presentation when designing clinical decision support systems and other tools.

Abbreviations
AMA: American Medical Association; ANOVA: Analysis of variance; CCHR: Canadian CT Head Rule; CME: Continuing medical education; CT: Computed tomography; ED: Emergency department; EM: Emergency medicine

Acknowledgements
The authors acknowledge the professional and much appreciated support of Clemson University Research Associate Karen Edwards, MS who coordinated the bulk of logistics and communication related to Institutional Review Board approval at each site.

Funding
Grant support (2015001097) for the research was provided by the Health Sciences Center, Greenville Health System, Greenville, SC, USA. The funder had no role in the design of the study and collection, analysis, and interpretation of data and in writing the manuscript. This research was supported by the Intramural Research Program of the National Institutes of Health (NIH), National Library of Medicine (NLM) and Lister Hill National Center for Biomedical Communications (LHNCBC).

Authors' contributions
RG, RP, SL, DW and ZC conceived the study and designed the trial. RP, SL, DW, and ZC developed the clinical vignettes and supporting data, then

verified the clinical vignettes fit within the decision rule parameters. LZ and MW provided statistical powering and an analysis strategy for the study, led data collection from the portal, then conducted data analysis. Both LZ and MW also assisted RG on interpretation of findings. RG, RP, SL, PF, DW, and FL supervised the conduct of the trial and data collection. PF and FL designed the intervention interface, information security, and data retrieval strategy. RP and DW undertook recruitment of clinicians and data collection. RG drafted the article, and all authors contributed substantially to its revision and approved final version. RG take responsibility for the paper as a whole.

Competing interests

The authors declare that they have no competing interests.

Author details

[1]Department of Public Health Sciences, Clemson University, 501 Edwards Hall, Clemson, SC 29634-0745, USA. [2]Department of Emergency Medicine, Greenville Health System, Greenville, SC, USA. [3]Department of Radiology, Greenville Health System, Greenville, SC, USA. [4]Department of Emergency Medicine, Emory University, Atlanta, GA, USA. [5]Lister Hill National Center for Biomedical Communication, National Library of Medicine, Bethesda, MD, USA.

References

1. Bouida W, Marghli S, Souissi S, Ksibi H, Methammem M, Haguiga H, Khedher S, Boubaker H, Beltaief K, Grissa MH, et al. Prediction value of the Canadian CT head rule and the New Orleans criteria for positive head CT scan and acute neurosurgical procedures in minor head trauma: a multicenter external validation study. Ann Emerg Med. 2013;61(5):521–7.
2. Stiell IG, Lesiuk H, Wells GA, McKnight RD, Brison R, Clement C, Eisenhauer MA, Greenberg GH, MacPhail I, Reardon M, et al. The Canadian CT head rule study for patients with minor head injury: rationale, objectives, and methodology for phase I (derivation). Ann Emerg Med. 2001;38(2):160–9.
3. Lindor RA, Boie ET, Campbell RL, Hess EP, Sadosty AT. Failure to obtain computed tomography imaging in head trauma: a review of relevant case law. Acad Emerg Med. 2015;22:1493–8.
4. Melnick ER, Szlezak CM, Bentley SK, Dziura JD, Kotlyar S, Post LA. CT overuse for mild traumatic brain injury. Jt Comm J Qual Patient Saf. 2012;38:483–9.
5. Morton MJ, Korley FK. Head computed tomography use in the emergency department for mild traumatic brain injury: integrating evidence into practice for the resident physician. Ann Emerg Med. 2012;60(3):361–7.
6. Sharp AL, Nagaraj G, Rippberger EJ, Shen E, Swap CJ, Silver MA, McCormick T, Vinson DR, Hoffman JR. Computed tomography use for adults with head injury: describing likely avoidable emergency department imaging based on the Canadian head CT rule. Acad Emerg Med. 2017;24(1):22–30.
7. Cabana MD, Rand CS, Powe NR, Wu AW, Wilson MH, Abboud PAC, Rubin HR. Why don't physicians follow clinical practice guidelines?: a framework for improvement. J Am Med Assoc. 1999;282(15):1458–65.
8. Borgen L, Stranden E, Espeland A. Clinicians' justification of imaging: do radiation issues play a role? Insights Imaging. 2010;1:193–200.
9. Arslanoglu A, Bilgin S, Kubali Z, Ceyhan MN, Ilhan MN, Maral I. Doctors' and intern doctors' knowledge about patients' ionizing radiation exposure doses during common radiological examinations. Diag Interv Radiol. 2007;13:53–5.
10. Lee RK, Chu WCW, Graham CA, Rainer TH, Ahuja AT. Knowledge of radiation exposure in common radiological investigations: a comparison between radiologists and non-radiologists. Emerg Med J. 2012;29:306–8.
11. Puri S, Hu R, Quazi RR, Voci S, Veazie P, Block R. Physicians' and midlevel providers' awareness of lifetime radiation-attributable cancer risk associated with commonly performed CT studies: relationship to practice behavior. AJR Am J Roentgenol. 2012;199(6):1328–36.
12. Derrick BJ, Quaas JW, Wiener DE, Polan RM, Chawla M, Mazori D, Newman DH. Head CT utilization for minor head injury: what motivates patients to present to the emergency department for evaluation, and why to emergency physicians choose to evaluate them with CT? Ann Emerg Med. 2014;58(4S):S248.
13. Lehnert BE, Bree RL. Analysis of appropriateness of outpatient CT and MRI referred from primary care clinics at an academic medical center: how critical is the need for improved decision support. J Am Coll Radiol. 2010;7:192–7.
14. McBride JF, Wardrop RMI, Paxton BE, Mandrekar J, Fletcher JG. Effect on examination ordering by physician attitude, common knowledge, and practice behavior regarding CT radiation exposure. Clin Imaging. 2012;36:455–61.
15. Harnan SE, Pickering A, Pandor A, Goodacre SW. Clinical decision rules for adults with minor head injury: a systematic review. J Trauma. 2011;71(1):245–51.
16. Dickinson J, Fortin E, Fisher J, Qiu S, Irvin CB. Privately insured medical patients are more likely to have a head CT. Ann Emerg Med. 2014;64(4S):S88.
17. Rosenthal DI, Weilburg JB, Schultz T, Miller JC, Nixon V, Dreyer KJ, Thrall JH. Radiology order entry with decision support: initial clinical experiences. J Am Coll Radiol. 2006;3(10):799–806.
18. Rohacek M, Albrrecht M, Kleim B, Zimmerman H, Exadaktylos A. Reasoons for ordering computed tomorgraphy scans of the head in patients with minor brain injury. Inquiry. 2012;43:1415–8.
19. Schilling UM. Cost awareness among Swedish physicians working at the emergency department. Eur J Emerg Med. 2009;16(3):131–4.
20. Allan GM, Lexchin J. Physician awareness of diagnostic and nondrug theraputic costs: a systematic review. Int J Technol Assess Health Care. 2008;24(2):158–65.
21. Sehgal RT, Gorman P. Internal medicine physicians' knowledge of health care charges. J Grad Med Educ. 2011;3(2):182–7.
22. Covington MF, Agan DL, Liu Y, Johnson JO, Shaw DJ. Teaching cost-conscious medicine: impact of a simple educational intervention on appropriate abdominal imaging at a community-based teaching hospital. J Grad Med Educ. 2013;5(2):284–8.
23. Gimbel RW, Fontelo P, Stephens MB, Olsen CH, Bunt C, Ledford CJW, Cook CAL, Liu F, Burke HB. Radiation exposure and cost influence physician medical image decision making: a randomized controlled trial. Med Care. 2013;51(7):628–32.
24. Bunt CW, Burke HB, Towbin AJ, Hoang A, Stephens MB, Fontelo P, Liu F, Gimbel RW. Point-of-care estimated radiation exposure and imaging guidelines can reduce pediatric radiation burden. J Am Board Fam Med. 2015;28(3):343–50.
25. Stiell IG, Wells GA, Vandemheen K, Clement C, Lesiuk H, Laupacis A, McKnight RD, Verbeek R, Brison R, Cass D, et al. The Canadiant CT head rule for patients with minor head injury. Lancet. 2001;357(9266):1391–6.
26. Stiell IG, Clement C, Rowe BH, Schull MJ, Brison R, Cass D, Eisenhauer MA, McKnight RD, Bandiera G, Holroyd B, et al. Comparison of the Canadian CT head rule and the New Orleans criteria in patients with minor head injury. JAMA. 2005;294(12):1511–8.
27. Lastovicka JL, Bettencourt LA, Hughner RS, Kuntze RJ. Lifestyles of the tight and frugal: theory and measurement. J Consum Res. 1999;26(1):85–98.

A pre-post study testing a lung cancer screening decision aid in primary care

Daniel S. Reuland[1*], Laura Cubillos[2], Alison T. Brenner[2], Russell P. Harris[1], Bailey Minish[3] and Michael P. Pignone[4]

Abstract

Background: The United States Preventive Services Task Force (USPSTF) issued recommendations for older, heavy lifetime smokers to complete annual low-dose computed tomography (LDCT) scans of the chest as screening for lung cancer. The USPSTF recommends and the Centers for Medicare and Medicaid Services require shared decision making using a decision aid for lung cancer screening with annual LDCT. Little is known about how decision aids affect screening knowledge, preferences, and behavior. Thus, we tested a lung cancer screening decision aid video in screening-eligible primary care patients.

Methods: We conducted a single-group study with surveys before and after decision aid viewing and medical record review at 3 months. Participants were active patients of a large US academic primary care practice who were current or former smokers, ages 55–80 years, and eligible for screening based on current screening guidelines. Outcomes assessed pre-post decision aid viewing were screening-related knowledge score (9 items about screening-related harms of false positives and overdiagnosis, likelihood of benefit; score range = 0–9) and preference (preferred screening vs. not). Screening behavior measures, assessed via chart review, included provider visits, screening discussion, LDCT ordering, and LDCT completion within 3 months.

Results: Among 50 participants, knowledge increased from pre- to post-decision aid viewing (mean = 2.6 vs. 5.5, difference = 2.8; 95% CI 2.1, 3.6, $p < 0.001$). Preferences across the overall sample remained similar such that 54% preferred screening at baseline and 50% after viewing; however, 28% of participants changed their preference (to or away from screening) from baseline to after viewing. We assessed screening behavior for 36 participants who had a primary care visit during the 3-month period following enrollment. Eighteen of 36 preferred screening after decision aid viewing. Of these 18, 10 discussed screening, 8 had a test ordered, and 6 completed LDCT. Among the 18 who preferred no screening, 7 discussed screening, 5 had a test ordered, and 4 completed LDCT.

Conclusions: In primary care patients, a lung cancer screening decision aid improved knowledge regarding screening-related benefits and harms. Screening preferences and behavior were heterogeneous.

Keywords: Cancer screening, Shared decision making, Primary care, Medicare, Pulmonary diseases

* Correspondence: dreuland@med.unc.edu
[1]Department of General Medicine and Clinical Epidemiology, University of North Carolina School of Medicine, Cecil G Sheps Center for Health Services Research, University of North Carolina at Chapel Hill, 725 Martin Luther King Jr. Blvd, CB 7590, Chapel Hill, NC 27599, USA
Full list of author information is available at the end of the article

Background

Lung cancer is the leading cause of cancer death in the United States (US) [1]. The National Lung Screening Trial (NLST) showed that annual low-dose computed tomography (LDCT) can reduce mortality from lung cancer in a high-risk population [2]. However, despite evidence for mortality reduction, LDCT screening can also lead to harms. For example, more than 95% of screen-detected nodules are ultimately determined to be benign (i.e. false positives) after follow-up evaluation, which can be costly and invasive [2]. Further, screening can also lead to the detection and unnecessary treatment of cancers that would not have affected the patient clinically in his/her lifetime (overdiagnosis) [3, 4].

Based on NLST findings and other evidence [5, 6], the US Preventive Services Task Force (USPSTF) found that there was sufficient support for the net benefit of screening to recommend annual screening with LDCT for patients ages 55–80 with 30 or more pack-years smoking history who have smoked in the past 15 years [4]. Because of the tradeoffs between benefits and harms involved, guidelines recommend a thorough process of informed and shared decision-making occur prior to commencing annual screening. [4, 7] However, experts remain concerned that widespread implementation of screening could happen without patients being appropriately informed [8]. These concerns are supported by accumulating evidence that US patients generally overestimate the benefits and are poorly informed about the potential harms of cancer screening [9–14]. These concerns informed a 2015 Centers for Medicare & Medicaid Services (CMS) coverage decision requiring that a "shared decision-making visit" involving the use of a patient decision aid be conducted before screening would be covered for CMS beneficiaries [15, 16].

Decision aids are evidence-based tools designed to facilitate informed and shared decision-making about complex treatments or screening choices [17]. A lung cancer screening decision aid may be a helpful adjunct in conveying the complex information about benefits and harms of screening. However, few lung cancer screening decision aids have been tested and, to our knowledge, none have been studied in a primary care setting, where cancer screening decisions typically take place [18–20]. Moreover, little is known about whether decision aids help screening-eligible patients develop a realistic understanding of the likelihood of benefitting from screening or improve their understanding of important but difficult to understand screening-related harms, such as false positives and overdiagnosis [18, 19].

Methods

We report the findings from a single-group primary care clinic-based study of a video decision aid on lung cancer screening in a cohort of screening-eligible primary care patients. We had three main study aims: first, to assess the effect of the decision aid on knowledge of the benefits and harms of screening and on screening preferences; second, to describe screening behavior within 3 months of viewing a screening decision aid; and third, to examine relationships between screening knowledge, preferences, and screening test ordering during subsequent primary care encounters.

Setting and participants

The study setting was an academic internal medicine practice serving approximately 13,000 patients. We identified active patients who were current or former smokers ages 55–80. We excluded patients with lung cancer, cancer treatment with chemotherapy or radiation within 18 months, recent hemoptysis or unexplained weight loss, or any chest CT within 18 months. Study staff reviewed electronic health records (EHR) and further excluded those who clearly did not meet USPSTF smoking history requirements (i.e. fewer than 30 pack-years or quit more than 15 years ago). Primary providers reviewed lists of their potentially eligible patients and excluded those deemed inappropriate for screening based on comorbidities. Approved patients were mailed a recruitment packet containing a study invitation letter and an opt-out card.

Patients then received a recruitment telephone call where an eligibility survey was administered to confirm screening eligibility based on USPSTF guidelines. Eligible patients who agreed to participate were scheduled for a study visit at the clinic. Upon arrival and consent, participants completed a baseline survey, viewed the video decision aid, and completed a follow-up survey. Screening behaviors were assessed via EHR review at 3 months. Participants received a $40 gift card. Data were collected from October 2015–October 2016 and analyzed from October 2016–February 2017.

Intervention

We previously developed and refined the decision aid based on feedback from screening-eligible patients from the community ($n = 11$) and providers from the academic medical center (n = 11) [21]. The decision aid was designed to meet requirements specified by CMS and relevant standards set by the International Patient Decision Aid Standards Collaboration, and to be accessible to those with low literacy [15, 22]. Written text was read aloud, and technical terms and concepts were explained using narration, graphics, and animations. We pre-tested the decision aid and measures with 10 screening-eligible participants before beginning the pre-post phase of the study.

Content included the rationale for screening, eligibility criteria, a description of the LDCT procedure, and a dynamic icon array (pictogram) that sequentially depicted estimates for benefits and harms of screening among 1000 individuals screened annually for 3 years (Fig. 1). Estimates were based on NLST trial data as presented in materials developed by the National Cancer Institute and the Veterans Health Administration (VHA) [2, 20, 23, 24]. Benefits presented in the pictogram were lung cancer deaths averted (3 per 1000 screened). Harms presented included false positives, need for biopsy that did not find cancer, serious complications from biopsies, and overdiagnosis. Other potential screening harms, presented qualitatively (not in the pictogram) included radiation exposure, anxiety and distress, and costs related to follow-up tests and procedures. The video concluded with an implicit values clarification exercise prompting the viewer to weigh the potential benefits and harms of screening and discuss them with his/her doctor. Participants viewed the 6-min video at the clinic on a tablet computer (available online https://goo.gl/1f7XIY).

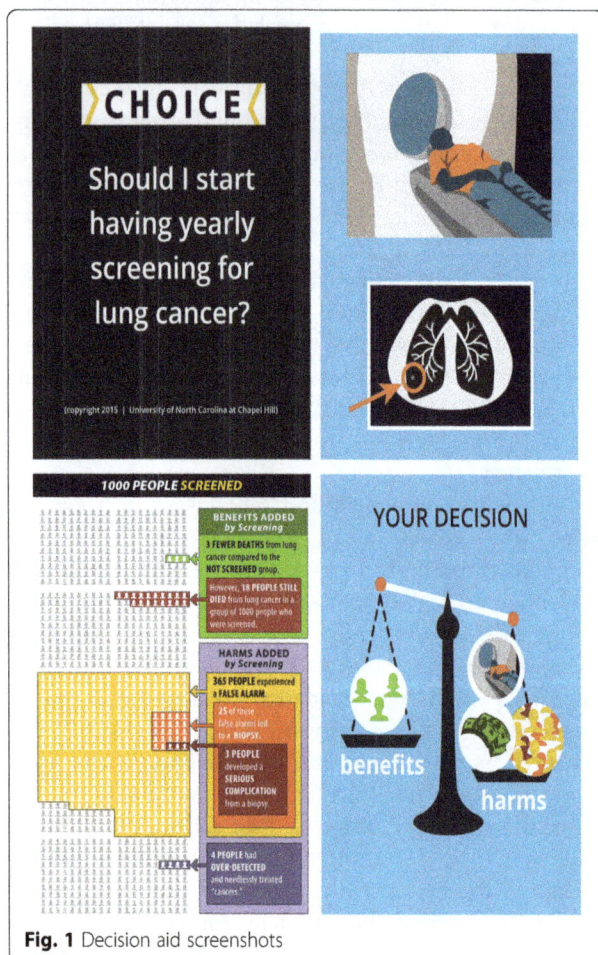

Fig. 1 Decision aid screenshots

Measures

Knowledge

We measured screening-related knowledge before and after decision aid viewing (items shown in Results, Table 2). Knowledge of benefit was assessed using a single item asking about the number of lung cancer deaths averted per 1000 individuals screened. Response options including contiguous estimates ranging from 0 up to 1000. Because our primary goal was to convey the "gist" concept that the number of individuals who benefit is small relative to the number of individuals screened, we treated responses that were within an order of magnitude of the value presented in the decision aid, i.e. up to 30 per 1000, as correct. Knowledge of harms was assessed using seven items adapted from a previously-published overdiagnosis knowledge scale [25] and one item about false positives. Knowledge items were categorized as either correct or incorrect, with "don't know" responses treated as incorrect. A knowledge score was calculated (0–9 points) by summing the correct answers.

Preference

Screening preference was assessed through a single 5-point Likert item adapted from a previous study asking participants how much they agreed with the statement "I plan to have a lung cancer screening test in the near future" (strongly agree to strongly disagree) [26].

Clinical screening behavior and LDCT findings

For patients who had a primary care visit, we assessed whether there was EHR documentation of each of the following: screening-related discussion, LDCT order, and LDCT completion. For completed CTs, we also recorded the LungRADS nodule classification based on the radiologist's report [27].

Decision aid acceptability

We assessed decision aid acceptability using a published scale measuring perception of decision aid length, balance, and suitability for decision-making [28].

Statistical analyses

We characterized the study population with descriptive statistics. We tested for pre-post changes in knowledge using a paired t-test for total score and McNemar's chi-squared tests for individual items. We dichotomized the preference item, defining "preference for screening" as "agree" or "strongly agree" responses. We calculated the proportions who changed their preference before and after decision aid viewing. We calculated proportions for screening behavior measures and LDCT findings among participants who had a provider visit after viewing the decision aid (and thus an opportunity for screening discussion and test ordering). We examined the relationship between (post-decision aid) knowledge and screening preference using logistic regression controlling for baseline preference. We also calculated the proportion of visits with a "preference concordant" decision, defined as either: preferring screening and having LDCT ordered, OR not preferring screening and not having an LDCT ordered. Analyses were conducted using STATA (Release-13, College Station, TX).

Results

Enrollment (see Fig. 2): We mailed 716 recruitment letters and reached 378 patients by telephone. Among 215 patients who completed the initial eligibility assessment, 135 were found ineligible. Common reasons for declining to complete the eligibility assessment included poor health, lack of time, and transportation challenges. Among the 80 patients initially found eligible for the study, 18 either declined participation or did not attend the study visit. Of the 62 (78%) eligible patients who participated, 10 completed the pre-test phase and thus were ineligible to participate in the main pre-post phase. Two additional participants were later found to be ineligible during the follow-up chart review phase of the study (because of recent chest CTs) and were excluded from analysis. The final analytic sample included 50 participants.

Sample characteristics (Table 1) include: mean age of 63 years; 48% female; 58% White; 30% Black; 12% other race; 50% high school education or less; 46% current smokers; average of 52 pack-years smoked; 40% COPD; and 56% had Medicare (alone or with another insurance).

Screening knowledge and preferences

Knowledge score (9-point scale) increased after viewing the decision aid from 2.6 to 5.5 (difference = 2.8; 95% confidence interval [CI] 2.1, 3.6, $p < 0.001$) (Table 2). Before decision aid viewing, the most common response was that 401–700 individuals benefit per 1000 screened. After decision aid viewing, the most common response category was 1–5 per 1000. In the overall sample, 27 (54%) participants preferred screening at baseline and 25 (50%) preferred screening after viewing.

Of the 27 participants who preferred screening pre-decision aid viewing, 8 (30%) changed and did not prefer screening after viewing. Of the 23 participants who did

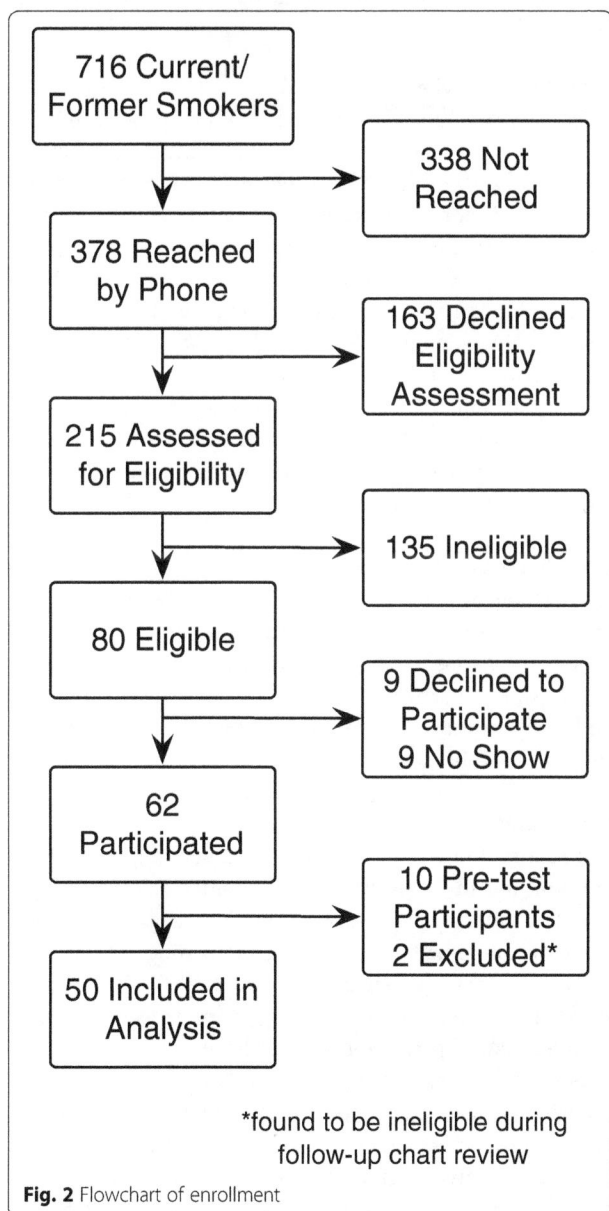

Fig. 2 Flowchart of enrollment

716 Current/ Former Smokers

338 Not Reached

378 Reached by Phone

163 Declined Eligibility Assessment

215 Assessed for Eligibility

135 Ineligible

80 Eligible

9 Declined to Participate 9 No Show

62 Participated

10 Pre-test Participants 2 Excluded*

50 Included in Analysis

*found to be ineligible during follow-up chart review

Table 1 Participant Characteristics ($n = 50$)

	Average or %
Age	63
Sex (% Female)	48%
Race/Ethnicity	
White	58%
Black	30%
Other	12%
Education	
≤ 12 years	50%
Smoking status (% current)	46%
Pack-years smoked[a]	52
COPD	40%
Insurance Status	
No insurance	8%
Private insurer (only)	28%
Medicare (only)	30%
Medicaid (only)	8%
Medicare, plus other insurer	26%

[a](average packs per day * years smoked)

Table 2 Changes in knowledge and intent to initiate lung cancer screening before and after viewing the decision aid ($n = 50$)

	Pre	Post	Difference (95% CI), p-value
Potential Harms of Screening			
Who do you think is more likely to be diagnosed with lung cancer? *People who are screened for lung cancer.[a] People who are NOT screened for lung cancer*	36%	62%	26% (8%, 44%), p < 0.001
ALL lung cancers will eventually cause illness and death if they are not found and treated. *True/False[a]/Don't Know*	6%	54%	48% (31%, 65%), p < 0.001
When screening finds lung cancer, doctors can tell whether the cancer will ever cause harm. *True/False[a]/Don't Know*	16%	62%	46% (62%, 30%), p < 0.001
Even lung cancers that may not cause any health problems are likely to be treated. *True[a]/False/Don't Know*	66%	80%	14% (4%, 32%), p = 0.09
Screening tests lead some people to get cancer treatments that they do not need. *True[a]/False/Don't Know*	18%	76%	58% (40%, 76%), p < 0.001
Screening tests find harmless lung cancers about as often as they prevent death from lung cancer. *True[a]/False/Don't Know*	24%	52%	28% (9%, 47%), p < 0.001
Which of these 2 statements best describes over-detection from screening? *Screening finds a cancer that would never have caused trouble[a] Screening finds an abnormality but extra tests show it is not cancer*	16%	28%	12% (3%, 27%), p = 0.08
An abnormal result from lung cancer screening always means the person has lung cancer. *True/False[a]/Don't Know*	66%	88%	22% (5%, 39%), p < 0.001
Chances of Benefitting from Screening			
For the next question, please think about 1000 current and former smokers who are getting screened every year for lung cancer. Out of 1000 people who get a chest CT scan, about how many will have their lives prolonged? *0 1-5[a] 6-10[a] 11-30[a] 31–100 101–200 201–400 401–700 701–1000 Don't Know*	18%	48%	30% (12%, 48%), p < 0.001
Average Knowledge Score (0–9 points)	2.6	5.5	2.8 (2.1,3.6), p < 0.001

[a]Correct response(s)

not prefer screening pre-decision aid, 6 (26%) preferred screening post-decision aid.

We observed an inverse relationship between post-decision aid knowledge and screening preference (odds ratio = 0.73; 95% CI 0.54, 0.98; $p = 0.03$). For each point increase in post-decision aid knowledge score there was an estimated 27% reduction in the odds of preferring screening.

Decision aid acceptability

Most participants ($n = 48$, 96%) reported that the decision aid was "useful in making a decision about getting screened for lung cancer." Most participants ($n = 29$, 58%) felt that the decision aid was balanced, 16 (32%) indicated that it was slanted toward getting screened, and 5 (10%) indicated that it was slanted toward no screening.

Screening behavior

Thirty-six participants had a clinic visit in the 3 months following study enrollment (Fig. 3), among whom 21 (58%) had concordance between test preference and test ordering. Among 18 participants preferring screening after decision aid viewing, 10 (56%) discussed screening, 8 (44%) had a test ordered, and 6 (33%) completed LDCT. Among the 18 not preferring screening, 7 (39%) discussed screening, 5 (28%) had a test ordered, and 4 (22%) completed LDCT. Discordance was greatest for the 18 participants who indicated they preferred screening, of whom 10 did not subsequently have an LDCT ordered. Notably, in 8 of these 10 cases, there was no apparent screening discussion with the provider.

LDCT findings

Among the 10 completed LDCTs, 7 were LungRADS category 1 (normal result) and 2 were category 2 (small nodules, benign appearance). One was category 4a (suspicious findings); this participant preferred screening in the study and the recommended 3-month follow-up scan showed resolution of the nodule.

Discussion

We report findings from testing a lung cancer screening decision aid in 50 primary care patients. We found that decision aid viewing was associated with greater knowledge of the benefits and harms of screening. At baseline, we found that participants tended to greatly overestimate the chances of benefitting from screening. After viewing, participants tended to have a more realistic understanding of the chances of benefitting. We also found that decision aid viewing led to improved understanding of two important but conceptually complex screening-related harms: false positives and overdiagnosis. To our knowledge, this study is the first to

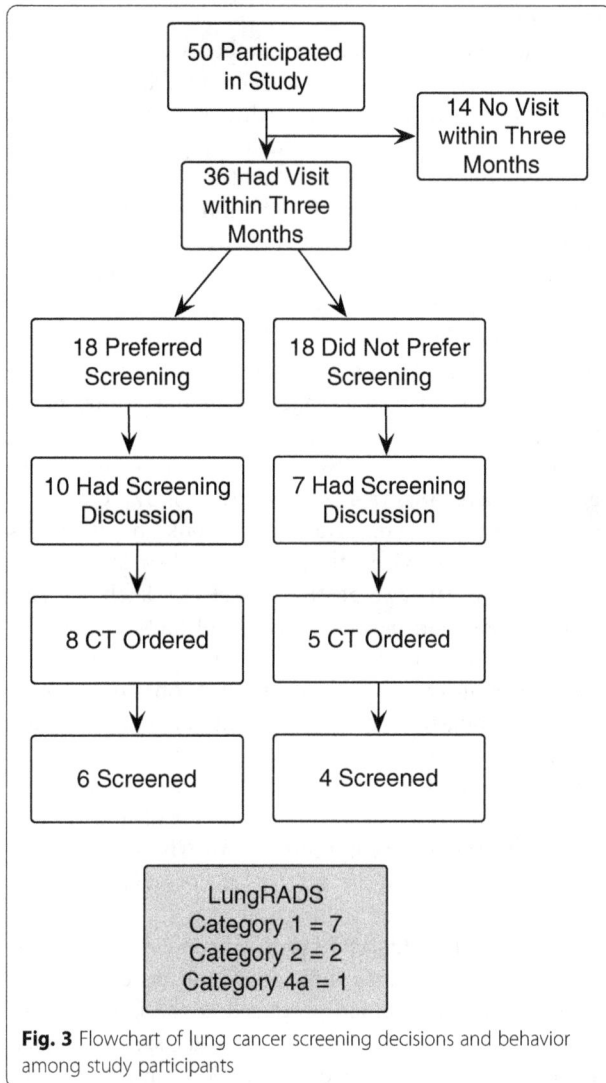

Fig. 3 Flowchart of lung cancer screening decisions and behavior among study participants

respectively) [18, 19]. All participants in our study were eligible for screening based on current USPSTF guidelines.

We found that baseline (pre-decision aid) screening preferences were heterogeneous, with roughly half of participants falling into each of our two preference groups (preferring screening vs. not). Although decision aid viewing was not associated with net changes in the proportions in each of these preference groups in the overall study sample, about one-quarter of participants in each group actually changed their screening preference after decision aid viewing (in opposite directions). Our findings suggest that we cannot assume screening-eligible primary care patients will be uniformly inclined toward or away from screening. Moreover, our results also suggest that a non-trivial proportion of primary care patients may change their preferences as they become more informed about screening.

Our results are consistent with the findings of Kinsinger et al.'s VHA pragmatic screening demonstration pilot [29] in that we observed heterogeneity in screening behavior. Among participants who preferred screening and saw a provider within 3 months of decision aid viewing, about half discussed LDCT scanning with their provider and about a third completed an LDCT. We also found that some participants who did not prefer screening after decision aid viewing ended up completing an LDCT. Kinsinger et al. similarly found that 50% of eligible patients completed screening [29]. While the VHA demonstration program developed and utilized paper-based decision support materials (from which we adapted our video decision aid), no data are available regarding the manner and extent to which they were used.

Our findings that 50% of patients preferred screening post-decision aid and 28% completed screening (among patients with post-decision aid primary care encounters), contrasts with findings from what is, to our knowledge, the only other study to assess screening completion in individuals receiving a lung cancer screening decision aid. That study, conducted by Mazzone et al. in patients attending a tertiary screening program, found that 95% of participants completed screening after undergoing a shared decision making visit [20]. We hypothesize that the overwhelming majority of patients who attend a dedicated lung cancer screening program assume that the purpose of referral to such a program is to complete screening, rather than to decide about screening. When considering Mazzone's findings alongside our results, it suggests that the time frame during which screening-eligible patients actually make decisions about screening is before they attend a dedicated screening program. Tertiary lung cancer screening programs are now being implemented in the US, and many claim to be able to conduct shared decision making. Our findings add to the

demonstrate that viewing a decision aid can help attenuate biased perceptions about the benefits and harms of lung cancer screening.

Our study complements and extends a limited body of empiric evidence about lung cancer screening decision aids. Previous studies were conducted in populations recruited from the community [19], or referral settings such as a tobacco cessation clinic [18] or a dedicated, sub-specialty screening program [20]. Our study was conducted in a primary care setting and allowed providers to exclude patients they believed to be poor screening candidates based on co-morbidity concerns. Thus, despite being relatively small, our study mimicked a systematic, practice-based approach to screening. Furthermore, two of three prior studies tested lung cancer screening decision aids in mixed populations that included relatively small numbers of screening eligible patients ($n = 14$ and $n = 11$,

discourse regarding the appropriate implementation context for medical decision making about lung cancer screening.

We found that the more knowledge participants had about benefits and harms of screening, the less likely they were to prefer screening. The fact that we did not observe differences in screening behavior suggests the need for additional research aimed at understanding how we can help ensure that patients receive care that is consistent with their preferences. This will likely require interventions beyond providing patient decision aids.

Our study examined decision aid effects on knowledge about two important harms of screening: overdiagnosis and false positives. We chose these outcomes because: 1) overdiagnosis and false positive tests can cause substantial harms in screened populations; 2) CMS explicitly requires that information about overdiagnosis and false positives be included in lung cancer screening decision aids; and 3) these harms may not be recognized or understood by patients making medical decisions about cancer screening [9, 15, 25]. Other knowledge domains are also probably relevant to decisions about lung cancer screening [8]. Further research is needed to assess the validity of measures of decision-relevant knowledge and to better understand knowledge thresholds at which patients may be considered adequately informed to make medical decisions about cancer screening.

We found relatively low concordance (58%) between (post-decision aid) preferences and LDCT ordering during subsequent provider visits. It appears that a major driver of discordance was that many patients who preferred screening and did not have an LDCT ordered did not actually have an opportunity to discuss screening with their provider. This finding points to an important problem in implementation of patient decision support in health care. Decision aids are intended not to replace but to inform discussions between patients and providers about medical decisions [30, 31]. However, competing demands and lack of adequate provider time to deliver preventive services are important barriers to effective communication and decision-making [16]. Further, lung cancer screening is especially complex given both the risk for lung cancer in this population and the chances of serious complications as a consequence of screening. Thus, further research is needed to understand how best to structure lung cancer screening decision support interventions in the primary care medical home to ensure that there is adequate time for patients and providers to discuss and deliberate. Moreover, more research is needed to understand the role that domains other than knowledge and stated preferences play in the complex picture of lung cancer screening behavior.

Limitations

Our study has limitations. First, because of the one-group, pre-post study design we were unable to compare the effects of the decision aid with usual care. Second, this was a single site study and many patients declined initial eligibility assessment. Additionally, patients received an incentive to participate and were required to attend a separate study visit, both of which can affect participant behavior and sample representativeness. Thus, the degree to which the findings are generalizable to other screening-eligible populations is unclear. Nevertheless, our participants were similar to NLST participants in terms of average age (63 in our study, 62 in NLST), pack-years smoked (52 vs. 56, respectively), percent current smokers (46% vs. 48%, respectively), and percent female (48% vs 41%, respectively) [32]. Our sample reflects a more disadvantaged population than was studied in the NLST in that they were less likely to be white (58% vs 91%, respectively) and less likely to have received education beyond high school (50% vs 70%, respectively) [33]. Third, knowledge was assessed immediately following completion of the decision aid and may not reflect long-term retention of lung cancer screening information. Finally, our behavior assessments were relatively crude in that we did not differentiate between chest CT scans discussed and ordered for diagnostic reasons (i.e. to evaluate symptoms) vs. for true screening.

Another consideration is that the decision aid we tested was not targeted to lung cancer risk. Ideally, information about benefits and harms of screening would be tailored to the patient's individual lung cancer risk, as occurs in the decision aid produced at the University of Michigan [33]. However, brief video decision aids such as ours or the one developed by Volk and colleagues [18] do not require high-level reading capability, entry of patient-specific data, or other interaction by the patient. Such a format offers potential advantages in terms of implementation, and may be better suited for low-literacy populations. Studies are needed to examine tradeoffs associated with using simpler versus more complex, tailored decision aids for lung cancer screening, particularly given the prevalence of low education and low literacy in the US screening-eligible population.

Conclusions

We found that, among primary care patients who are eligible for lung cancer screening based on USPSTF guidelines, viewing a lung cancer screening decision aid improved screening-related knowledge. It gave patients a more realistic perception of the likelihood of benefit. It also gave them a greater understanding of the nature of important screening-related harms. Our findings, although preliminary, suggest that a non-trivial proportion of screening-eligible patients may change their screening preferences after decision aid viewing. In contrast to findings in a referral population at a tertiary, sub-specialty screening program, screening preferences and behaviors among screening-eligible patients in a primary care population appear to be heterogeneous.

Abbreviations
CI: Confidence Interval; CMS: Center for Medicare and Medicaid Services; EHR: Electronic Health Record; LDCT or CT: Low-Dose Computed Tomography or Computed Tomography; NLST: National Lung Screening Trial; US: United States; USPSTF: United States Preventive Services Task Force; VHA: Veterans Health Administration

Acknowledgements
The authors would like to acknowledge Adrian Compean García for his contributions in the field, as well as Carolina Health Assessment and Resource Tool (CHART) and the CHART team for their assistance in delivering the intervention and instruments through CHART's online platform. These findings were previously presented at the Preventing Overdiagnosis 2016 Conference on September 20-22, 2016 and the 38th Annual Meeting of the Society for Medical Decision Making on October 23, 2016.

Funding
This study was supported in part by a grant from NCI (P30-CA16086) to the Lineberger Comprehensive Cancer Center, and the Cancer Prevention and Control Intervention Research, an initiative of the University Cancer Research Fund and the UNC Lineberger Comprehensive Cancer Center, at the University of North Carolina at Chapel Hill (UNC). Other support for this study came from the North Carolina Translational and Clinical Sciences Institute at the University of North Carolina (Grant No. 1UL1TR001111; UNC IRB#s 14–1813 and 14–2012).

Authors' contributions
DR conceived of the study, interpreted the results, and composed the manuscript. LC collected participant data, interpreted results, and contributed substantially to writing the manuscript. AB provide input on study design, analyzed and interpreted data and contributed substantially to writing the manuscript. RH provided input on study design, interpreted results, and contributed to writing the manuscript. BM collected participant data and reviewed the manuscript. MP provided input on study design, interpreted results, and contributed to writing the manuscript. All authors read and approved the final version of the manuscript.

Competing interests
Michael Pignone is a member of the US Preventive Services Task Force. The views presented here are not necessarily those of the Task Force.

Author details
[1]Department of General Medicine and Clinical Epidemiology, University of North Carolina School of Medicine, Cecil G Sheps Center for Health Services Research, University of North Carolina at Chapel Hill, 725 Martin Luther King Jr. Blvd, CB 7590, Chapel Hill, NC 27599, USA. [2]Lineberger Comprehensive Cancer Center, Cecil G Sheps Center for Health Services Research, University of North Carolina at Chapel Hill, 725 Martin Luther King Jr. Blvd, CB 7590, Chapel Hill, NC 27599, USA. [3]Department of General Medicine and Clinical Epidemiology, University of North Carolina, School of Medicine, Ambulatory Care Center, University of North Carolina at Chapel Hill, 101 Mason Farm Road, Chapel Hill, NC 27599-7745, USA. [4]Department of Medicine, Dell Medical School, The University of Texas at Austin, 1912 Speedway, Campus Mail Code D2000, Austin, TX 78712, USA.

References
1. American Cancer Society. Cancer Facts & Figures 2017. Atlanta: American Cancer Society; 2017.
2. National Lung Screening Trial Research Team, Aberle DR, Adams AM, et al. Reduced lung-cancer mortality with low-dose computed tomographic screening. N Engl J Med. 2011;365(5):395–409.
3. Patz EF Jr, Pinsky P, Gatsonis C, et al. Overdiagnosis in low-dose computed tomography screening for lung cancer. JAMA Int Med. 2014;174(2):269–74.
4. Moyer VA. U. S. Preventive Services Task Force. Screening for lung cancer: U. S. Preventive Services Task Force recommendation statement. Ann Intern Med. 2014;160(5):330–8.
5. de Koning HJ, Meza R, Plevritis SK, et al. Benefits and harms of computed tomography lung cancer screening strategies: a comparative modeling study for the U.S. Preventive Services Task Force. Ann Intern Med. 2014; 160(5):311–20.
6. Humphrey L, Deffebach M, Pappas M, et al. Screening for lung cancer: systematic review to update the US Preventive Services Task Force recommendation. MD: Rockville; 2013.
7. Wender R, Fontham ET, Barrera E Jr, et al. American Cancer Society lung cancer screening guidelines. CA Cancer J Clin. 2013;63(2):107–17.
8. Harris RP, Sheridan SL, Lewis CL, et al. The harms of screening: a proposed taxonomy and application to lung cancer screening. JAMA Int Med. 2014; 174(2):281–5.
9. Hoffman RM, Lewis CL, Pignone MP, et al. Decision-making processes for breast, colorectal, and prostate cancer screening: the DECISIONS survey. Med Decis Mak. 2010;30(5 Suppl):53S–64S.
10. Schwartz LM, Woloshin S, Fowler FJ Jr, Welch HG. Enthusiasm for cancer screening in the United States. JAMA. 2004;291(1):71–8.
11. Hoffman RM, Elmore JG, Fairfield KM, Gerstein BS, Levin CA, Pignone MP. Lack of shared decision making in cancer screening discussions: results from a national survey. Am J Prev Med. 2014;47(3):251–9.
12. Hoffman RM, Couper MP, Zikmund-Fisher BJ, et al. Prostate cancer screening decisions: results from the National Survey of medical DECISIONS (DECISIONS study). Arch Intern Med. 2009;169(17):1611–8.
13. Lafata JE, Divine G, Moon C, Williams LK. Patient-physician colorectal cancer screening discussions and screening use. Am J Prev Med. 2006;31(3):202–9.
14. Wunderlich T, Cooper G, Divine G, Flocke S, Oja-Tebbe N, Stange K, Lafata JE. Inconsistencies in patient perceptions and observer ratings of shared decision making: the case of colorectal cancer screening. Patient Educ Couns. 2010; 80(3):358–63.
15. Decision Memo for Screening for Lung Cancer with Low Dose Computed Tomography (LDCT) (CAG-00439N). https://www.cms.gov/medicare-coverage-database/details/nca-decision-memo.aspx?NCAld=274. Accessed 5 Feb 2015.
16. Crothers K, Kross EK, Reisch LM, et al. Patients' attitudes regarding lung cancer screening and decision aids. A survey and focus group study. Ann Am Thorac Soc. 2016;13(11):1992–2001.
17. Brenner A, Howard K, Lewis C, et al. Comparing 3 values clarification methods for colorectal cancer screening decision-making: a randomized trial in the US and Australia. J Gen Intern Med. 2014;29(3):507–13.
18. Volk RJ, Linder SK, Leal VB, et al. Feasibility of a patient decision aid about lung cancer screening with low-dose computed tomography. Prev Med. 2014;62:60–3.
19. Lau YK, Caverly TJ, Cao P, et al. Evaluation of a personalized, web-based decision aid for lung cancer screening. Am J Prev Med. 2015;49(6):e125–9.
20. Mazzone PJ, Tenenbaum A, Seeley M, Petersen H, Lyon C, Han X, Wang XF. Impact of a lung cancer screening counseling and shared-decision-making visit. Chest. 2017;151(3):572–8.
21. Reuland D, Brenner A, Harris R, Cubillos L, Vu MB, Pignone M. Using deliberative methods to guide implementation of lung cancer screening: exploring perceptions and understanding of Overdiagnosis. In: 3rd annual preventive Overdiagnosis conference: September 1-3, 2015; Bethesda, MD; 2015.
22. Elwyn G, O'Connor A, Stacey D, et al. Developing a quality criteria framework for patient decision aids: online international Delphi consensus process. BMJ. 2006;333(7565):417.
23. Screening for Lung Cancer. http://www.prevention.va.gov/docs/ LungCancerScreeningHandout.pdf. Accessed 1 Sept 2014.
24. Patient and Physician NLST Study Guide. https://www.cancer.gov/types/ lung/research/NLSTstudyGuidePatientsPhysicians.pdf. Accessed 1 Sept 2014.
25. Hersch J, Barratt A, Jansen J, et al. Use of a decision aid including information on overdetection to support informed choice about breast cancer screening: a randomised controlled trial. Lancet. 2015;385:1642–52.
26. Brenner AT, Hoffman R, McWilliams A, et al. Colorectal cancer screening in vulnerable patients: promoting informed and shared decisions. Am J Prev Med. 2016;51(4):454–62.

27. Lung-RADS Version 1.0 Assessment Categories. https://www.acr.org/-/media/ACR/Files/RADS/LungRADS/Lung-RADS_AssessmentCategories.pdf. Accessed 23 Aug 2016.
28. O'Connor A, Cranney A. User manual-acceptability. Ottawa: Ottawa Hospital Research Institute; 2002.
29. Kinsinger LS, Anderson C, Kim J, et al. Implementation of lung cancer screening in the veterans health administration. JAMA Intern Med. 2017;177: 399–406.
30. Elwyn G, Frosch D, Thomson R, et al. Shared decision making: a model for clinical practice. J Gen Intern Med. 2012;27(10):1361–7.
31. O'Connor AM, Stacey D, Entwistle V, et al. Decision aids for people facing health treatment or screening decisions. Cochrane Database Syst Rev. 2003; 2:CD001431.
32. Aberle DR, Adams AM, Berg CD, Clapp JD, Clingan KL, Gareen IF, Lynch DA, Marcus PM, Pinsky PF. Baseline Characteristics of Participants in the Randomized National Lung Screening Trial. JNCI J Natl Cancer Inst. 2010; 102(23):1771–1779.
33. Lau YK, Caverly TJ, Cherng ST, Cao P, West M, Arenberg D, Meza R. Development and validation of a personalized, web-based decision aid for lung cancer screening using mixed methods: a study protocol. JMIR Res Protoc. 2014;3(4):e78.

12

A model for predicting utilization of mHealth interventions in low-resource settings: case of maternal and newborn care

Stephen Mburu[*] [iD] and Robert Oboko

Abstract

Background: In low-resource settings, there are numerous socioeconomic challenges such as poverty, inadequate facilities, shortage of skilled health workers, illiteracy and cultural barriers that contribute to high maternal and newborn deaths. To address these challenges, there are several mHealth projects particularly in Sub-Sahara Africa seeking to exploit opportunities provided by over 90% rate of mobile penetration. However, most of these interventions have failed to justify their value proposition to inspire utilization in low-resource settings.

Methods: This study proposes a theoretical model named Technology, Individual, Process-Fit (TIPFit) suitable for user-centred evaluation of intervention designs to predict utilization of mHealth products in low-resource settings. To investigate the predictive power of TIPFit model, we operationalized its latent constructs into variables used to predict utilization of an mHealth prototype called *mamacare*. The study employed single-group repeated measures quasi-experiment in which a random sample of 79 antenatal and postnatal patients were recruited from a rural hospital. During the study conducted between May and October 2014, the treatment involved sending and receiving SMS alerts on vital signs, appointments, safe delivery, danger signs, nutrition, preventive care and adherence to medication.

Results: Measurements taken during the study were cleaned and coded for analysis using statistical models like Partial Least Squares (PLS), Repeated Measures Analysis of Variance (RM-ANOVA), and Bonferroni tests. After analyzing 73 pretest responses, the model predicted 80.2% fit, and 63.9% likelihood of utilization. However, results obtained from initial post-test taken after three months demonstrated 69.1% fit, and utilization of 50.5%. The variation between prediction and the actual outcome necessitated improvement of mamacare based on feedback obtained from users. Three months later, we conducted the second post-test that recorded further drop in fit from 69.1 to 60.3% but utilization marginally improved from 50.5 to 53.7%.

Conclusions: Despite variations between the pretest and post-test outcomes, the study demonstrates that predictive approach to user-centred design offers greater flexibility in aligning design attributes of an mHealth intervention to fulfill user needs and expectations. These findings provide a unique contribution for decision makers because it is possible to prioritize investments among competing digital health projects.

Keywords: Behaviour science, Design science, Fit, mHealth, Predictive modeling, Self-efficacy, Short message service (SMS), Structural equation modeling, Utilization

* Correspondence: smburu@uonbi.ac.ke
School of Computing and Informatics, University of Nairobi, P.O. Box
30197-00100, Nairobi, Kenya

Background

To exploit opportunities provided by mobile penetration in developing countries, there is proliferation of technology innovations aimed at improving healthcare service delivery [1–4]. This is the motivation behind numerous mobile health (mHealth) interventions aimed at overcoming challenges like poor infrastructure, staff shortages, and limited budgets that characterize low-resource settings [5–7]. Despite these initiatives, a global observatory survey conducted by World Health Organization (WHO) and International Telecommunication Union (ITU) revealed that majority of mHealth systems are weak platforms that have failed to transit to actual practice [8]. Prior studies have also attributed failure of mHealth interventions to misalignment to realistic needs and expectations of the target users [9–11]. Since most mHealth initiatives in Sub-Sahara Africa are donor-funded projects, we argue that low utilization of most of these interventions may be due to poor understanding of users, tasks and technology context during design. Several case studies have revealed that design of some of mHealth systems is based on "perceived problems", then "pushed" for adoption and use by consumers who were least involved in designing the intervention [8, 12].

To scale up utilization of mHealth innovations, there is need for user-centred evaluation of design specifications to predict usage behaviour after workplace implementation. Some of the reviewed studies on technology adoption have demonstrated how to predict utilization based on theoretical knowledge of causal connections [13–15]. For example, Davis and Venkatesh [14] used Technology Acceptance Model (TAM) to predict acceptance and use of a new system based on perceived usefulness. The same approach was used by Bhattacherjee and Premkumar [15] to provide empirical evidence on predictive approach to user acceptance testing. This study therefore builds on similar approaches to predicting acceptance and use of mHealth interventions in low-resource settings. Due to gaps identified in the reviewed models and theories [16–22], we derived a structural model for predicting utilization of mHealth interventions. The model called *TIPFit* comprises of predictor variables X_1 to X_9 shown in Fig. 1; hypothesized to influence *fit* and utilization of an mHealth intervention. **TIPFit** is an acronym derived from **individual, process, technology,** and **fit** constructs. Similar to studies by Strong et al. [21] and Davis and Konsynski [22], **fit** is configured as a surrogate measure of user acceptance to determine temporal changes toward usage of mHealth artifacts. Justification and detailed reasoning regarding inclusion of each construct as a predictor variable is provided in the methods section.

To validate the model, we conducted within-subjects repeated measures quasi-experiment. The validation process was done in a practical scenario to investigate how well user's perceptions predicted utilization of *mamacare* prototype. Mamacare is an integrated mobile and web-based application optimized to run on low-cost smartphones because most health facilities in low-resource settings have limited access to computers, power and broadband internet. Furthermore, WHO [10] recommends use of mobile phones to facilitate

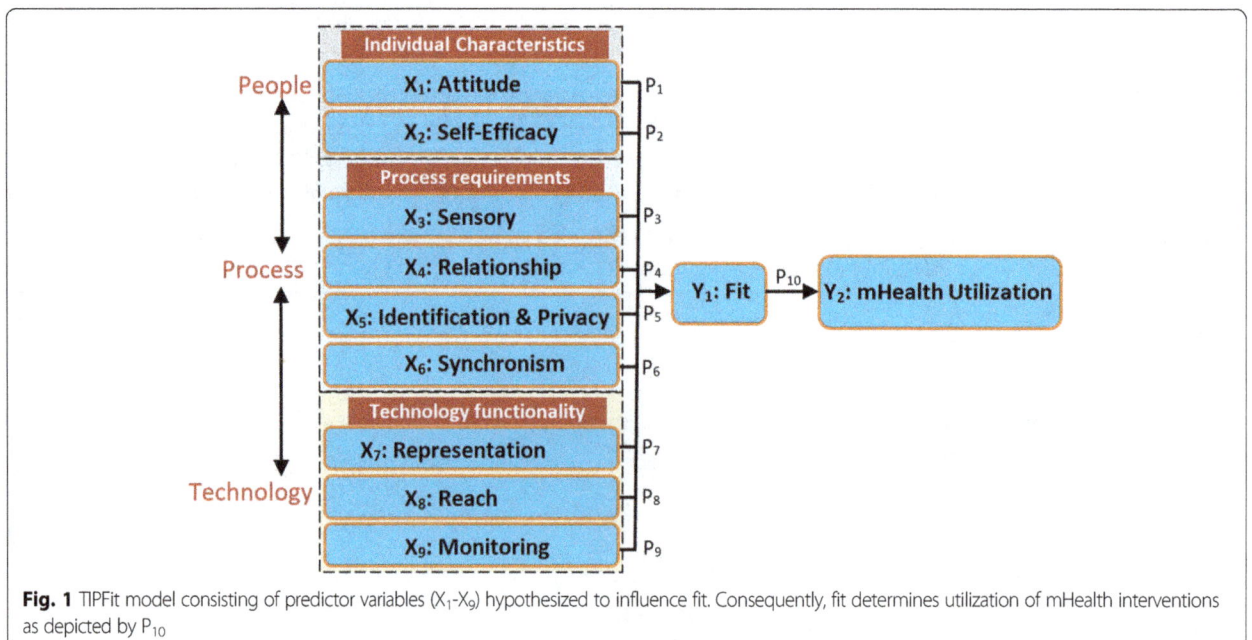

Fig. 1 TIPFit model consisting of predictor variables (X_1-X_9) hypothesized to influence fit. Consequently, fit determines utilization of mHealth interventions as depicted by P_{10}

timely delivery and access to healthcare services. There is no doubt that acceptance and use of mHealth innovations has the potential to achieve Sustainable Development Goals (SDGs) aimed at reversing maternal and newborn deaths by 2030 [23].

Methods

To build a strong case for the predictive method employed in this study, we first justify inclusion of eleven TIPFit variables classified into five constructs: individual, process, technology, fit and utilization of mHealth [14, 15, 23, 24].

Attitude (X₁)

Prior studies in behaviour science have shown that attitude influences one's judgment on certain behaviour, subject or action [25–27]. Therefore, inclusion of attitude as a predictor variable was informed by our pre-study experience, and empirical findings from studies that are based on Theory of Planned Behaviour (TPB) [16, 26, 27]. In TIPFit model, attitude is crucial in measuring patients' and caregivers' perception before and after exposure to an intervention. We hypothesized that attitude changes over time as benefits of an intervention becomes more realistic due to continued use.

Self-efficacy (X₂)

Self-efficacy as a predictor variable was derived from Technology Acceptance Model (TAM) and Computer Self-Efficacy (CSE) [17, 20]. The variable is intended to measure one's ability to use technology to access healthcare services and information. In particular, we used this predictor to measure one's ability to use mobile phones to access maternal care services and information in rural areas.

Sensory requirements (X₃)

Sensory requirements as a predictor variable was derived from Process Virtualization Theory and Impact of IT (PVT-IT) [18, 22]. Overby and Konsynski [22, 28] demonstrated that sensory requirements of touch, smell, sight and taste makes it difficult to virtualize some physical processes. Moreover, Overby [18] argues that if a process requires sensory experience of smell, taste or touch, it would be more difficult to replicate these senses in a virtual (electronic) environment. For example, during routine maternal care visits, clinicians use medical devices to physically take clinical tests such as temperature, blood pressure, blood sugar, and haemoglobin. Although some of these vital signs may be taken remotely using wireless sensors, it may be difficult or costly to deploy such technologies in low-resource settings. This is why sensory requirements variable is crucial in predicting the degree to which mobile phones

and point-of-care devices can be used to fulfil sensory requirements in maternal and newborn care.

Relationship (X₄)

Relationship as a predictor variable was derived from PVT-IT [18, 22] to investigate the degree of interaction between caregivers and patients in remote areas. We observe that in clinical processes, relationship is important because it builds mutual trust between patients and caregivers.

During physical encounter, verbal and non-verbal communications convey vital information resulting to mutual trust and better inter-personal relationships [28]. Although multimedia technology may be used to simulate such interaction, limitations of cost and infrastructure in low-resource settings make multimedia-based interventions unsustainable.

Identification and privacy (X₅)

Identification refers to proof of one's identity while privacy refers to confidentiality of health information. This variable derived from PVT-IT [18, 22] was largely informed by our pre-study experience during focus group discussions. We noted that prove of identity in clinical processes like diagnosis is essential if patients and caregivers are to share sensitive information. For example, a HIV-positive patient may be reluctant to receive reminders on adherence to antiretroviral (ARV) regimen through mobile phones. On the other hand, clinicians may be reluctant to perform diagnosis and prescription electronically to avoid compromising patient's privacy [1, 29].

Synchronism (X₆)

Synchronism as a predictor variable was derived from PVT-IT to measure degree to which time-critical processes are completed with minimal delay [18, 22, 28]. In medical practice, synchronism is crucial in emergency cases like preeclampsia that require urgent clinical attention. Our pre-study experience revealed that delays in detecting complications related to pregnancy and postpartum are some of the major causes of deaths in developing countries [4, 5, 13]. Therefore, synchronization was included as a predictor variable to measure degree to which use of mobile phones and point-of-care devices reduce delays in executing clinical tasks.

Representation (X₇)

This variable was derived from PVT-IT [18, 22] and Task Technology-Fit (TTF) [19, 21, 22] to investigate capabilities of technology to simulate or present information relevant to clinical processes [18, 22]. For example in telemedicine, mobile phones may be integrated with wireless sensors and multimedia tools to provide remote consultation between patients and doctors. However, due to poor connectivity, it becomes difficult to provide such services in low-resource settings [28]. In this study, we used representation as a predictor variable to measure degree to which mHealth artifacts could be used to simulate a clinical process like diagnosis.

Reach (X_8)

Inclusion of reach as a predictor variable was informed by empirical findings relating to PVT-IT [18, 22]. The variable is a measure of technology capability to provide sufficient access to maternal care services at reduced cost and time. In reviewed studies, it is evident that most mHealth interventions fail to provide adequate access to maternal care services and information due to long distances, inadequate health facilities, and cultural barriers [5–7, 28]. Therefore, we used reach to investigate how mobile phones and point-of-care devices could provide sufficient reach by reducing time and cost of accessing maternal care services and information.

Monitoring (X_9)

This variable was adapted from PVT-IT [18] to measure capability of technology to monitor patient's health status. During antenatal and postnatal care, mothers are required to make at least four visits to monitor their progress. However, in remote areas, most patients fail to honour such visits hence resulting to complications like stillbirth and haemorrhage. To provide sufficient patient monitoring in such places, mobile-based interventions that use wireless body sensors may be considered. Nevertheless, such interventions may not be feasible due to limitations relating to poor infrastructure, cost, privacy and cultural beliefs. In this study, we used the variable to predict degree to which mobile devices could be used to provide sufficient patient follow-up in low-resource settings.

Fit (Y_1)

In the context of this study, fit refers to perceived usefulness, suitability or benefits of a planned intervention. Justification of including fit as a mediating variable was informed by studies conducted by Goodhue and Thompson [19], Strong et al. [21], and Overby and Konsynski [22]. Our reasoning is that perception on fit in terms of user, task and technology requirements determine utilization of an mHealth intervention [14, 17–19]. We posit that the higher the perception on fit, the higher the likelihood of utilizing an intervention.

mHealth utilization (Y_2)

In this context, utilization is the behaviour of using technology to accomplish some tasks [19]. Justification of

including utilization as the outcome (dependent) variable was based on the premise that intention to use or usage of an mHealth system or product is influenced by perceived fit [14, 15, 19, 21]. In this study, we used the variable to measure the intention or utilization level of an mHealth intervention [30–32].

TIPFit constructs as predictor variables

The ability to make predictions from a structural model depends on knowledge of causal relationship between predictor variables and the outcome [24]. Therefore, to test the predictive power of TIPFit model, we converted the causal relationships depicted using P_1 to P_{10} into Structural Equation Model (SEM). The structural model comprises of a system of multi-linear regressions represented using the following equation:

$$Y_j = \beta_i X_i + \varepsilon_i$$

In the equation, X_i represents the predictor variables (X_1, X_2...X_9) hypothesized to influence fit [33–35]. The Y_j term denotes two variables, i.e., Y_1 and Y_2 that represents fit and utilization of mHealth respectively. The term β_i (β_1 to β_9) represent path coefficients P_1 to P_9 used to determine the effect of each variable on fit. Path P_{10} on TIPFit is an aggregate coefficient used to measure cumulative effect of fit on mHealth utilization. The error term, i.e., $_i$ represents unexplained variations in each of the predictor variable X_1 to X_9.

To measure the degree to which a variable predicts changes in fit and utilization, we operationalized the model into ten hypotheses. Table 1 lists a set of null hypotheses denoted by H_01 to H_010 used to test the causal relationships represented by paths P_1 to P_{10} on TIPFit model. Inferences from the hypotheses were drawn from path weights (β_i) computed using Partial Least Squares (PLS) algorithm in SmartPLS [36].

Operationalizing TIPFit into structural path model

To test hypothesized cause-and-effect relationships, we operationalized TIPFit into a path model consisting of two parts namely measurement, and structural model. Figure 2 shows how three of the nine variables were operationalized into measurement, and structural models.

The measurement model represents predictor variables (X_1 to X_9) measured using manifest variables represented using initials in the leftmost boxes. The manifest variables shown on the legend of the diagram are scale items in the measurement instruments provided as Additional files 1, 2, 3, 4 and 5. The inner part of the model comprises of path coefficients from β_1 to β_9 hypothesized to influence fit. Consequently, β_{10} is used as a measure of how fit as an intervening variable

Table 1 Hypotheses for predicting fit and utilization of mHealth

Path	Prediction hypotheses
H_01	Attitude has no significant change on fit before, and after use of mHealth intervention
H_02	Self-efficacy in use of mobile devices has no significant change on fit before, and after mHealth intervention
H_03	Sensory requirements have no significant change on fit before, and after use of mHealth intervention
H_04	Relationship requirement has no significant change on fit before, and after use of mHealth intervention
H_05	Identification and privacy requirements have no significant change on fit before, and after use of mHealth intervention
H_06	Synchronism requirement has no significant change on fit before, and after use of mHealth intervention
H_07	Representation capability of technology has no significant effect on fit before, and after use of mHealth intervention
H_08	Reach capability of technology has no significant change on fit before, and after use of mHealth intervention
H_09	Monitoring capability of technology has no significant change on fit before, and after use of mHealth intervention
H_010	Perceived fit has no significant change before, and after use of mHealth intervention

Source: Researchers' TIPFit hypothetical model

functionally determines utilization of an mHealth artifact. It is this graphical model that formed the basis for predicting fit and utilization of an intervention using SmartPLS 2.0.

Study design

The study was conducted for a period of six months starting from 5th May to 31st October 2014. This was after we obtained ethical approval issued by the Kenyatta Hospital/University of Nairobi Ethics Research Committee (KNH/UoN-ERC) on 23rd November 2013. Our study setting was the Maternal and Newborn Healthcare (MNH) section of a rural hospital called *Kimbimbi Sub-county Hospital*. The hospital, located in Kirinyaga County 110 km from Nairobi serves patients; most of whom are farmers from Mwea Rice Irrigation and Settlement Scheme.

Maternal care intervention

To develop mamacare, we employed user-centred design to understand the study environment, user needs, and maternal care process. Figure 3 shows the approach used; a customized model of agile development methodology.

During conceptualization phase, TIPFit was instrumental in measuring perceived fit of mobile-based intervention as a basis for predicting post-deployment utilization [14, 15]. Some of the user-centred techniques employed to understand the target users and clinical tasks in MNH include storyboards, mock-ups, interviews and focus group discussions. Feedback obtained from these interactions was used as the basis for the next phase of designing *mamacare*; a mobile and web-based prototype. Mamacare is an acronym derived from two words, i.e., mama that stands for "mother" across many languages, and care referring to maternal and newborn healthcare.

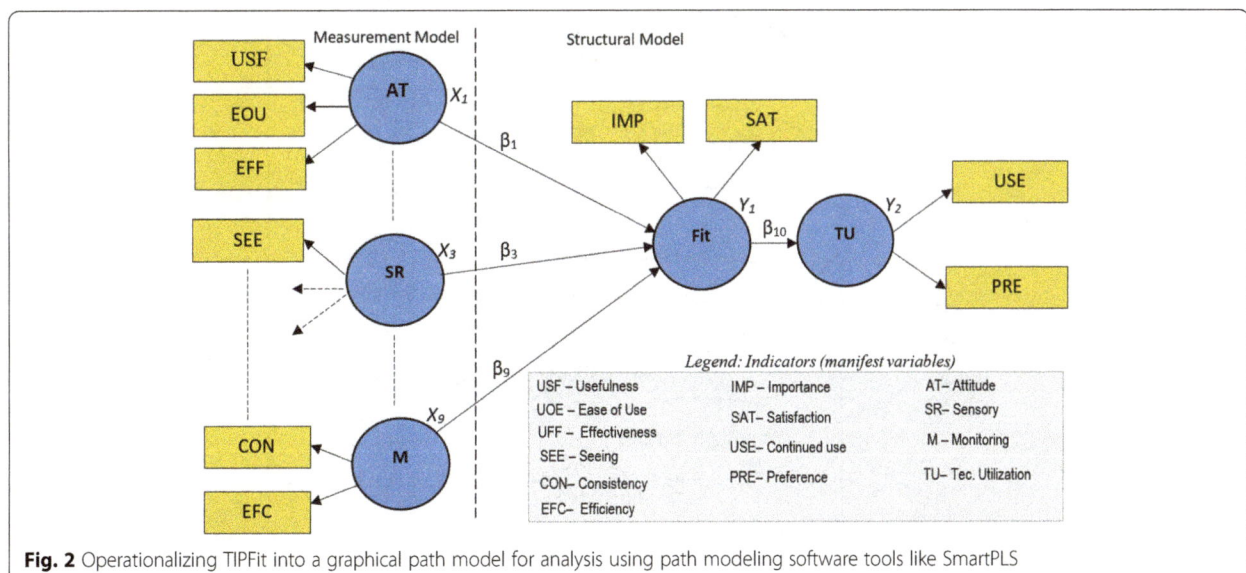

Fig. 2 Operationalizing TIPFit into a graphical path model for analysis using path modeling software tools like SmartPLS

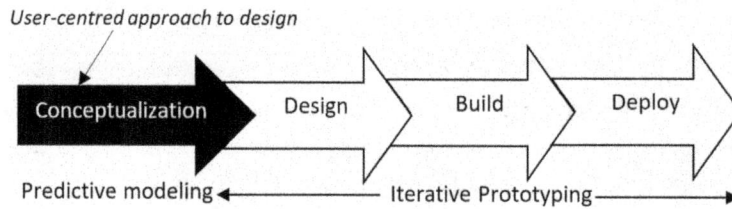

Fig. 3 Approach employed in the development of mamacare prototype that was used to support maternal and newborn care

In design phase, we used unified modeling language (UML) tools to align the planned intervention to user requirements identified during conceptualization. Figure 4 is a sample use case diagram that depicts interaction between mamacare and clinicians (caregivers) that were involved in the study.

To improve access to maternal care services and information through mobile, Fig. 5 shows a sample use case diagram depicting interaction between mamacare and patients.

During the build phase, we used web development tools like HTML5, CSS3 and JavaScript to implement the web portal used by caregivers to process and manage patients' health records. The Short Message Service (SMS) module was implemented using open source SMS Server Tools3 while the back-end was implemented using MySQL, Apache web server and PHP. Figure 6 depicts the architecture used to deploy mamacare in the study setting. The primary database server was installed in the hospital while a backup server was hosted at University of Nairobi for redundancy and security purpose.

To enhance user experience, the web interface was designed to adapt to multiple device profiles depending on the screen size and orientation. Figure 7 shows how the same web portal appears on desktop computer and mobile phone. This responsive behaviour makes mamacare suitable for use in places with limited access to computers.

Before mamacare was deployed, we agreed with the hospital management that the system was complementary to standard procedure for managing antenatal and postnatal patients. The complementary mechanism involved sending SMS messages on appointments, danger signs, safe delivery, nutrition and preventive care to registered patients. Mamacare also receives vital signs for temperature, blood pressure, and blood sugar to enhance monitoring of mothers and their children. Figure 8(a) shows vital signs received via SMS while Fig. 8(b) shows a sample SMS reminder on clinic appointment otherwise referred to as "To Come Again (TCA)" in maternal care context.

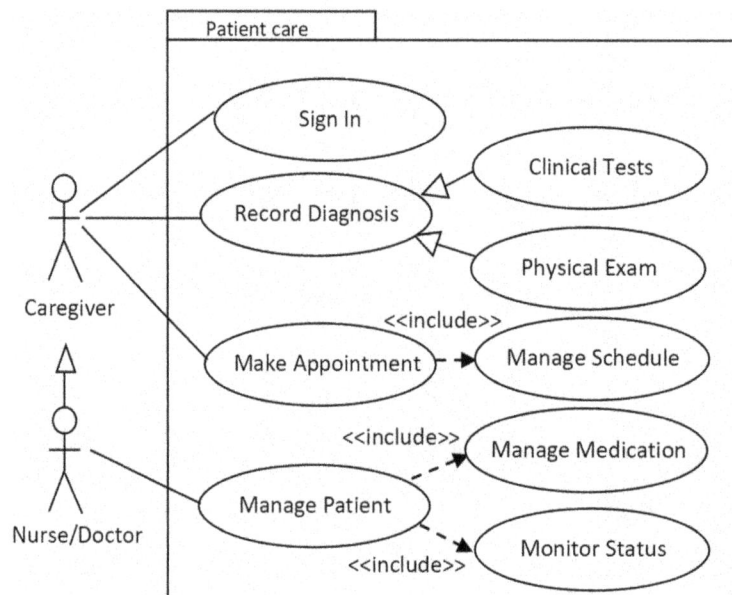

Fig. 4 Use case model depicting the interaction between mamacare system and caregivers

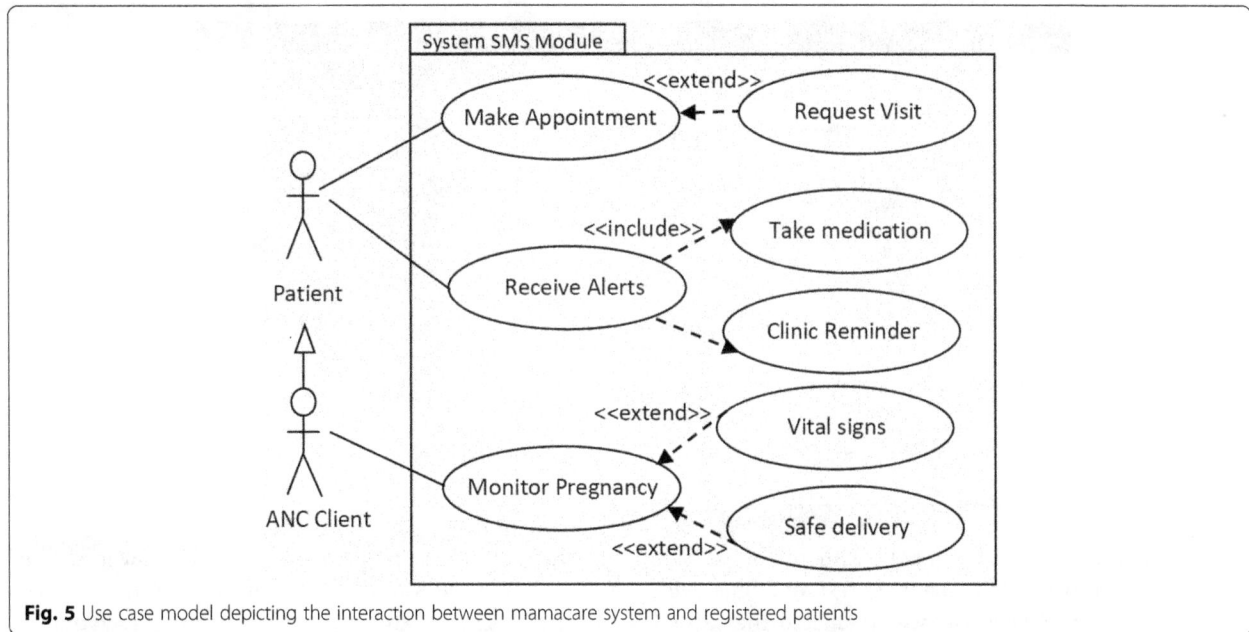

Fig. 5 Use case model depicting the interaction between mamacare system and registered patients

Design of repeated measures quasi-experiment

To measure the predictive power of TIPFit model, we used quasi-experiment to repeatedly measure responses from the same group of respondents before, and after intervention. Despite shortcomings of quasi-experiments in terms of internal and external validity, single-group repeated measures design is desirable in clinical environment where randomization may raise political, ethical or legal issues. In this regard, our study protocol approved by KNH/UoN-ERC required use of study designs that would not deny subjects benefits of the planned intervention. This was the main reason that influenced choice

of single-group (within-subjects) repeated measures design. In this design, each subject served as her own experimental control hence making it possible to detect the effect of predictor variables on fit and utilization of mamacare. Figure 9 shows how the three measures were taken before, and after exposure to mamacare intervention for a period of six months.

Before the intervention, a pretest (T_0) was used to measure perceptions based on benefits of mamacare communicated to participants during health education sessions organized by the hospital. Three months after the subjects were exposed to intervention, we conducted

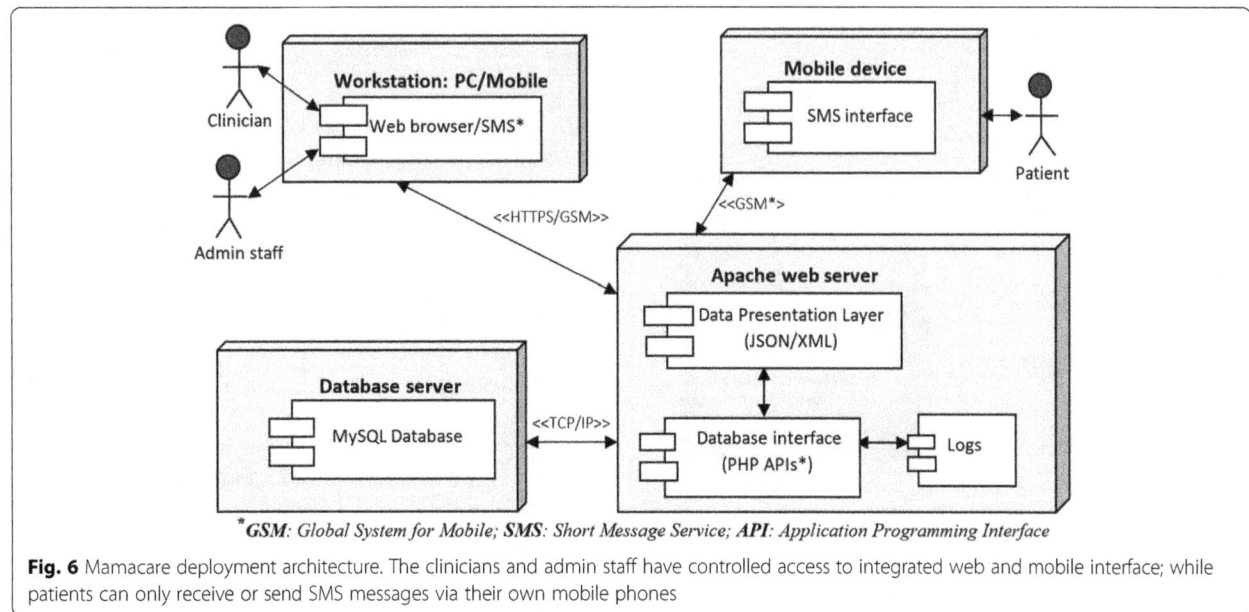

GSM: Global System for Mobile; SMS: Short Message Service; API: Application Programming Interface

Fig. 6 Mamacare deployment architecture. The clinicians and admin staff have controlled access to integrated web and mobile interface; while patients can only receive or send SMS messages via their own mobile phones

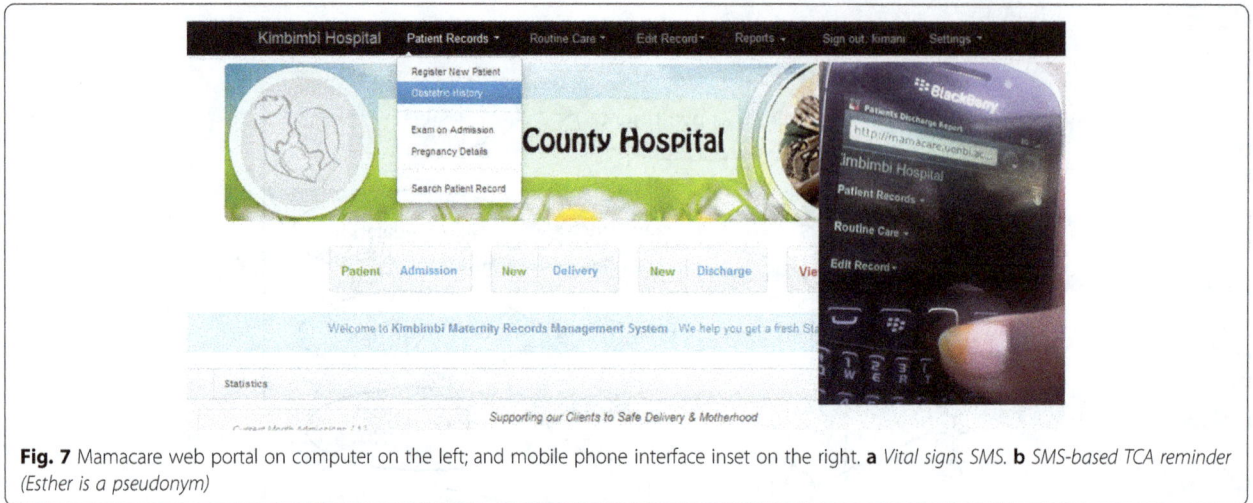

Fig. 7 Mamacare web portal on computer on the left; and mobile phone interface inset on the right. **a** *Vital signs SMS.* **b** *SMS-based TCA reminder (Esther is a pseudonym)*

the first post-test (T_1) to compare with predicted outcome. To compare the initial post-test outcome with reactions after prolonged use, we conducted the second post-test (T_2) using the same tools employed in the initial post-test evaluation.

Sampling and inclusion of study population

During the inception stage of this study, we visited the Maternal and Newborn Healthcare (MNH) section of Kimbimbi Sub-county hospital to review the antenatal and postnatal registers. The reviewed registers had a total of 226 women most of whom were receiving either antenatal or postnatal care services. To get a representative proportion from this population, we used simple random sampling with age, education, gestation, residence, and ownership of mobile phone as inclusion criteria. Empirical findings from related studies have shown that factors like age, environment, and education influence individual's attitude and ability to use technology [16, 17, 26, 27]. The gestation factor was considered because during pregnancy, women tend to change their

attitude and ability to perform tasks. The ownership of mobile phone was also important because the purpose of the present study was to investigate utilization of mobile devices in maternal and newborn care. Therefore, to get an optimal sample from the population of 226 registered patients, we used the following formula to determine the optimal sample size:

$$n = \frac{z^2 \times p \times q \times N}{e^2(N\text{-}1) + z^2 \times p \times q}$$

In the equation, *n* represents the sample size; z = critical value at 5% significance level; p = sample proportion (degree of variability) set as conservative value of 50%; *N* is size of finite population; *e* is the level of precision set at ±5%; and q = 1 − p. By taking $N = 226$; z = ±1.96 based on 5% significance level; p as 50% (0.5); e = 0.05; and q = 0.5 (1−0.5) we obtained our sample size as follows:

$$n = \frac{1.96^2 \times 0.5 \times 0.5 \times 226}{0.05^2(226\text{-}1) + 1.96^2 \times 0.5 \times 0.5} = 143$$

This implies that a sample of at least 143 subjects was required for the study. After contacting these subjects through mobile calls and SMS, only 95 women accepted to attend a formal training session organized through the hospital. During the two-hour training, benefits and limitations of using mobile phones were communicated to the participants. Based on this information, 79 participants were recruited after they agreed to participate in the study by signing consent forms. The other 16 participants refused to participate due to issues relating to financial constraints, attitude and privacy.

Although the number of participants recruited was half of the expected, it was sufficient to get reliable inferences. Goodhue et al. [37] demonstrated that a sample of 40 subjects is sufficient to achieve reliable results in PLS. Furthermore, Overby and Konsynski demonstrated

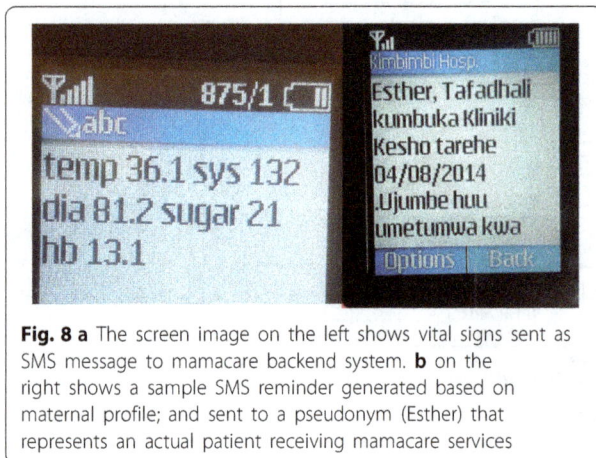

Fig. 8 a The screen image on the left shows vital signs sent as SMS message to mamacare backend system. **b** on the right shows a sample SMS reminder generated based on maternal profile; and sent to a pseudonym (Esther) that represents an actual patient receiving mamacare services

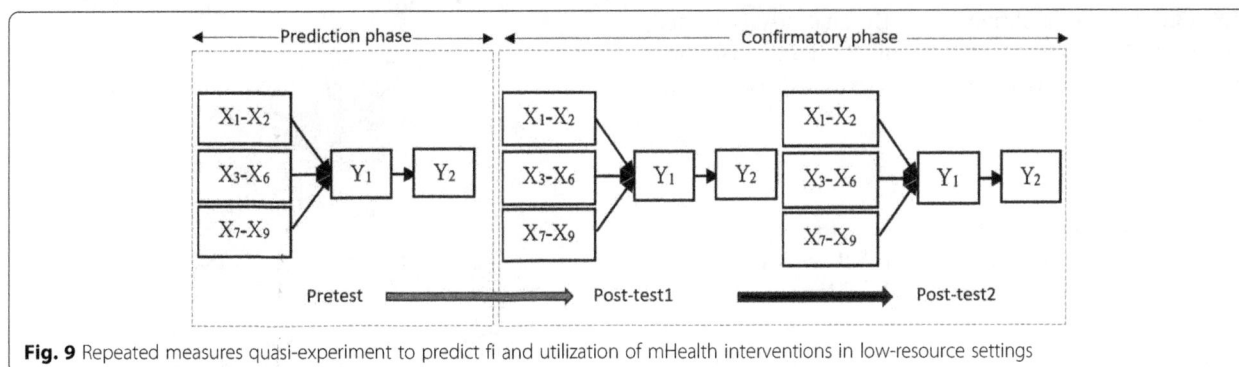

Fig. 9 Repeated measures quasi-experiment to predict fi and utilization of mHealth interventions in low-resource settings

that a sample of 60 subjects is sufficient to detect small and medium effect [22, 38, 39].

Measurements

The study used three measures at different points in time to investigate the predictive power of a hypothetical model. The measurement instruments used before and after intervention were based on indicators derived from TIPFit model.

Before mamacare was deployed, we conducted a pretest as a baseline for predicting post-deployment utilization based on perceived benefits. The measurement instruments included basic demographic scale items such as age, education and gestation assumed to influence attitude and ability to use technology. Since the same subjects were involved in the entire study, the post-test scale items comprised of closed and open-ended Likert-type questions on a scale of 1 to 5. Samples of the pretest and post-test questionnaires used are provided as Additional files 1, 2, 3, 4 and 5.

To take care of participants with low literacy level, two research assistants were recruited from the local community to guide the respondents through the questionnaires in local languages.

To validate the data collection instruments, we used composite reliability, and Cronbach's alpha (α) to test internal consistency. We also analyzed validity of the structural model using convergence and discriminant validity. Given our relatively small sample, we performed these tests using PLS algorithm in SmartPLS [36]. Table 2 gives a summary of composite reliability, and Cronbach's α values generated from the pretest (T_0), and post-test (T_1 and T_2) datasets.

The table shows that composite reliability for all the variables were above the recommended 0.70. However, the four values highlighted in Cronbach's alpha column were slightly less than 0.70. Despite these minor variations, the results indicate good internal consistency of the pretest and post-test scale items.

The results also indicated that Average Variable Extracted (AVE) for all the constructs were above

0.50. According to Chin and Newstead [38], proof of convergent and discriminant validity requires the AVE score for each construct to be above 0.50 (50%). Analysis from the three datasets indicates that each of the eleven constructs has an AVE score above 0.50; hence indicating that TIPFit model has good convergence, and discriminant validity. This confidence in the reliability and validity of the structure of the model was a greenlight to path analysis and hypothesis testing.

Data analysis

To analyze the pretest and post-test datasets collected during the experiment, incomplete and wrongly filled questionnaires were eliminated. The valid responses were coded into numerical values and keyed into Statistical Package for Social Scientists (SPSS) to determine the frequency, percentage, and statistical mean of each demographic item.

Regarding predictive modeling, the responses were entered into Microsoft Excel spreadsheet and exported into SmartPLS workspace for analysis using

Table 2 Reliability test using composite, and Cronbach's alpha

Predictor variable	Composite reliability			Cronbach alpha		
	T_0	T_1	T_2	T_0	T_1	T_2
Attitude	0.85	0.91	0.92	0.73	0.86	0.88
Efficacy	0.84	0.88	0.92	0.77	0.80	0.88
Sensory	0.85	0.89	0.81	0.75	0.81	*0.67*
Relation	0.88	0.85	0.86	0.80	0.73	0.75
Privacy	0.90	0.86	0.86	0.83	0.76	0.76
Synch	0.85	0.84	0.91	*0.66*	*0.62*	0.80
Represent	0.83	0.86	0.89	0.71	0.76	0.82
Reach	0.82	0.88	0.86	*0.68*	0.80	0.75
Monitor	0.92	0.91	0.91	0.82	0.79	0.80
Fit	0.94	0.93	0.93	0.88	0.84	0.85
Utilization	0.88	0.90	0.94	0.74	0.79	0.86

Source: Primary Data. [NB: The italicized values under Cronbach's alpha falls below the recommended threshhold of 0.70]

PLS [36–38]. In addition to path analysis, we used Repeated Measures Analysis of Variance (RM-A-NOVA), and Bonferroni post hoc test to draw reliable conclusions from the study.

Results
Basic demographic characteristics
Most adoption studies have shown that demographic attributes such as gender, age and education influence one's belief, attitude and ability to perform tasks using technology [9, 14, 15, 17, 21, 22]. In this study, we analyzed these attributes to gain insight on characteristics of the subjects that influence acceptance and use of the planned mHealth intervention. From 79 participants who participated in the pretest conducted before the intervention, we obtained 73 valid questionnaires. The six questionnaires that were disregarded were either incomplete or wrongly filled. Analysis of age distribution using SPSS showed that majority of the respondents were aged between 20 and 25. Table 3 shows the age distribution of 73 valid responses; demonstrating that most of the subjects were within the reproductive age between 20 and 35 years.

Analysis on education revealed that 34.2% of the subjects have studied up to primary school level (Grade 8), and 47.9% up to secondary (Grade 12) as shown in Fig. 10. The pie chart also indicates that 15.1% have studied up to college while only 2.7% have studied up to university. This is a clear reflection that majority of the subjects have low literacy skills that could have been a barrier to effective use of mobile and point-of-care technologies [14–16].

Path analysis
To determine the ability of TIPFit in predicting fit and utilization, we used SmartPLS to analyze path weights of the structural model. This is because PLS is variance-based structural equation models that does not impose restrictions on sample size and normality of distribution [37, 38]. Figure 11 shows the structural model generated from the pretest dataset using scale items as reflective indicators of their corresponding predictor variables. The path weights represent

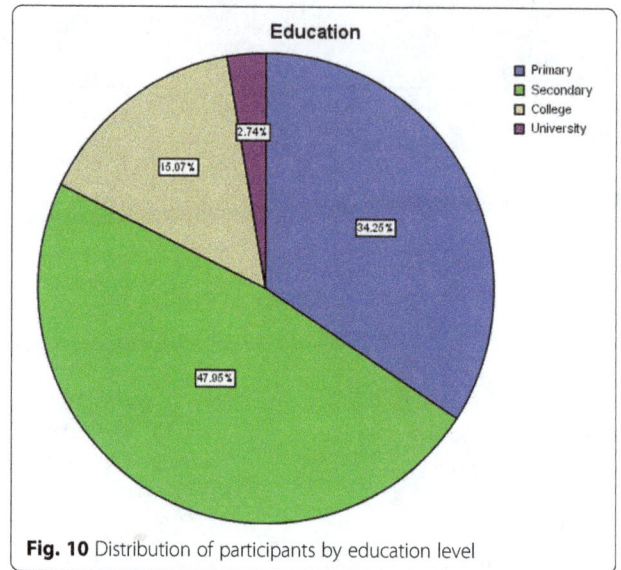

Fig. 10 Distribution of participants by education level

coefficients β_1 to β_{10} in the equation model, and P_1 to P_{10} on TIPFit model.

The coefficient of determination (R^2) values of 0.802 and 0.639 indicate that the pretest model has high predictive power of 80.2% on fit, and 63.9% likelihood of utilization. This assumption is based on Overby and Konsynski [22] assertion that a structural model with $R^2 > 0.25$ is considered to have good predictive power.

After the subjects were exposed to an intervention, dataset collected during the first post-test was cleaned and analyzed using SmartPLS. Figure 12 shows the path weights; R^2 of 69.1% on fit, and 50.5% of actual utilization. The observed variations between the pretest predictions and actual outcome necessitated improvement of mamacare to address issues raised by the users during the first post-test evaluation.

Three months later, we conducted the second post-test as a follow-up measure. However, due to voluntary exit of six subjects, 73 out of 79 initial participants filled the questionnaires. The post-test2 questionnaire was similar to that used in post-test1 but with additional questions for measuring user satisfaction from enhanced mamacare. The enhancements were mostly on the user interface, language used to send messages, and SMS module for receiving vital signs such as blood pressure, temperature, haemoglobin and blood sugar. The vital signs were used by caregivers to monitor health trends using dynamic charts. This made it easier for caregivers in MNH to easily detect pregnancy and postpartum complications that require urgent attention.

Figure 13 shows the model path weights and coefficients of determination after modeling post-test2 dataset

Table 3 Distribution of participants by age categories

Age category		Frequency	Percent (%)	Valid Percent
Valid	15–19	8	11.0	11.0
	20–25	39	53.4	53.4
	26–30	16	21.9	21.9
	30–35	10	13.7	13.7
	Total	73	100.0	100.0

Source: Primary data

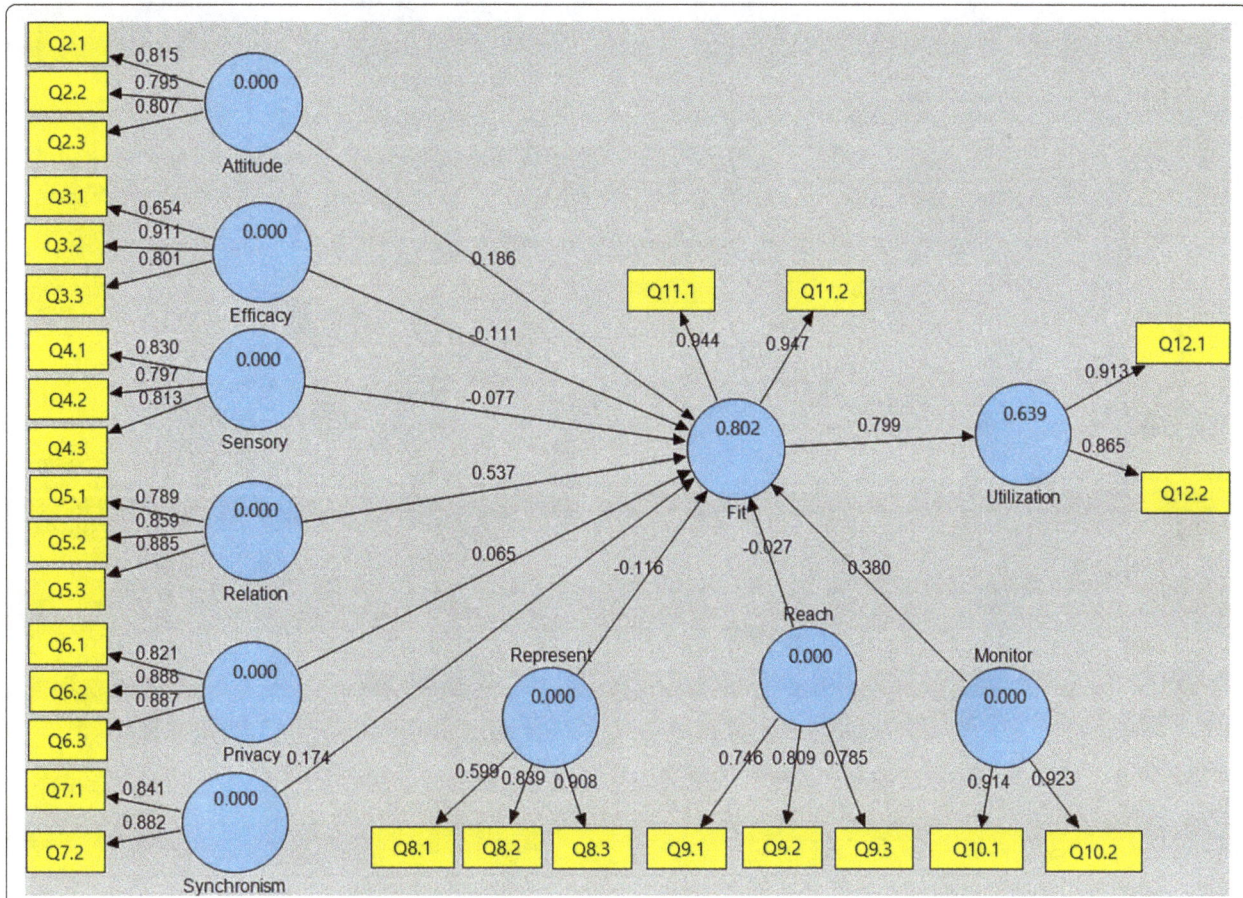

Fig. 11 Pretest (prediction) model generated from pretest dataset showing coefficient of determination (R²) and path weights. The yellow boxes represent reflective indicators (manifest variables)

using SmartPLS. The results indicate marginal drop on fit from 69.1% recorded in the first post-test to 60.3%. Conversely, the results revealed slight improvement on utilization of mamacare from 50.5% recorded in the first post-test to 53.7%.

In summary, Table 4 shows structural model path weights generated from the pretest and two post-test datasets.

The table shows that attitude towards fit was positive before and after intervention. However, Self-efficacy was initially negative but marginally improved after prolonged use of mamacare. We also observe that path weights obtained from sensory requirements were consistently negative before and after the intervention. The cumulative path weights between fit and mHealth utilization shows high positive scores; indicating that fit has strong influence on utilization before, and after intervention.

Comparative analysis

Due to some inconsistencies observed from the structural path models, we used alternative methods in order

to draw reliable conclusions. First, we ran bootstrapping algorithm available in SmartPLS to determine significance of path weights. Table 5 gives a summary of t values after bootstrapping the three path models at 5% significance level.

Physical inspection on each column indicates temporal changes in hypothesized causation. For example, attitude was consistently positive and significant because its t values were greater than the critical value of 1.96 ($t > 1.96$). Sensory requirements variable consistently returned negative outcomes.

These observations may be interpreted to mean that attitude towards mobile use in maternal care was positive but may not sufficiently address sensory requirements. However, due to inconsistences observed in synchronism, representation and monitoring, we opted to use parametric tests as an alternative to structural path modeling.

Bonferroni post hoc test

To analyze changes in usage behaviour before and after intervention, we used Bonferroni post hoc test available

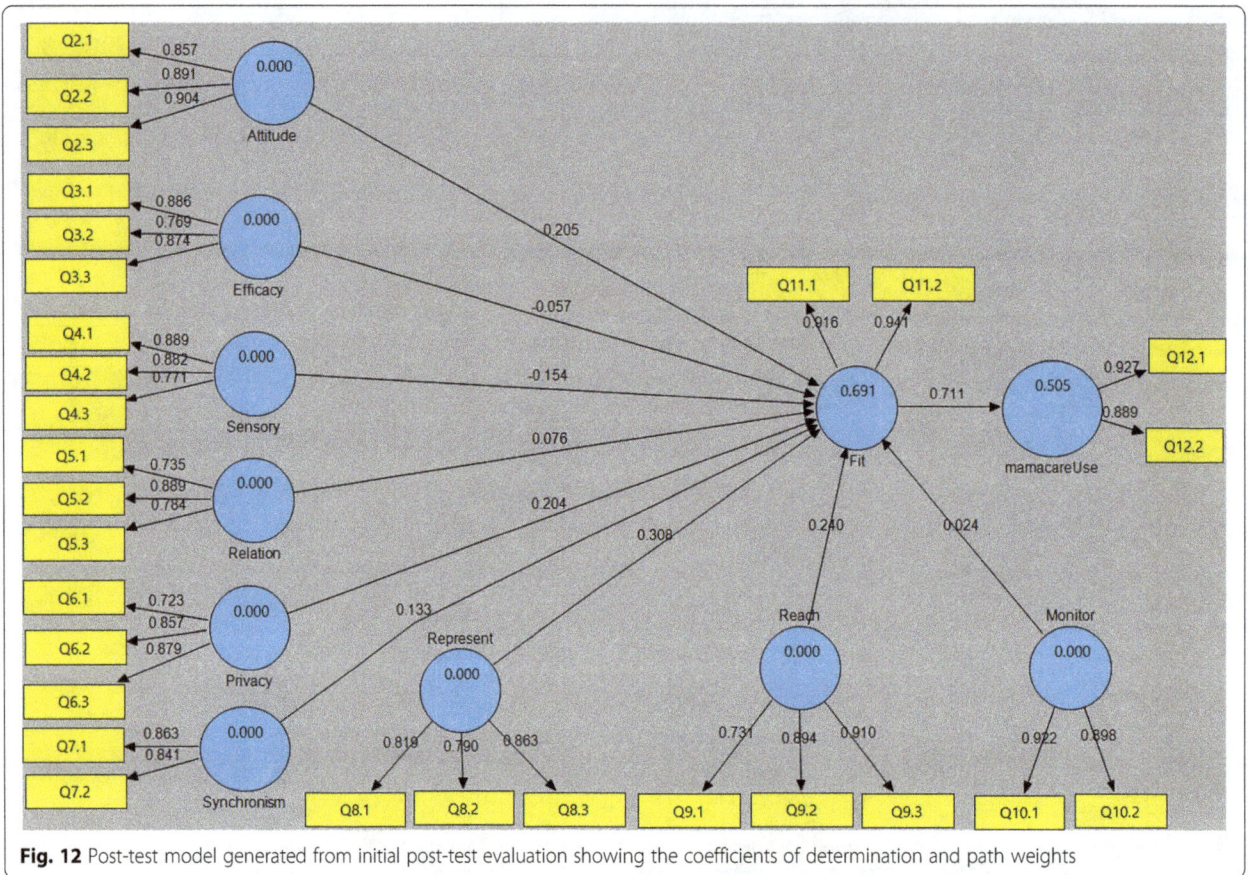

Fig. 12 Post-test model generated from initial post-test evaluation showing the coefficients of determination and path weights

in SPSS. This test is suitable in studies that seek to establish effect of experimental treatment. Table 6 shows summary of pairwise comparison between the pretest and post-test1 (T_0-T_1); post-test1 and post-test2 (T_1-T_2); and pretest and post-test2 (T_0-T_2).

The table shows that there is significant differences between the pretest and post-test1 in sensory requirements, identification and privacy, synchronism, monitoring, fit and utilization of mHealth. However, comparison between T_1 and T_2 shows significant differences in *self-efficacy*, and *monitoring* variables. These findings suggest that reactions before the intervention had better predictions after stable use of mamacare. We therefore assume that after improvement of mamacare, usage behaviour almost matched pretest predictions on utilization of mamacare. To investigate these variations, we further analyzed the three datasets using Repeated Measures ANOVA (RM-ANOVA).

Repeated measures ANOVA

Three essential requirements for using RM-ANOVA are inspection of underlying data for normality of distribution, outliers and sphericity. Although the results from these tests showed the three datasets

satisfied the first two requirements, there were some violations of sphericity. Table 7 shows a summary of RM-ANOVA statistics after correcting violations of sphericity in six variables that have *p* values less than 0.05.

Visual inspection on RM-ANOVA column indicates that there is no significant differences in four variables with p values less than 0.05. These are attitude, sensory requirements, representation, and reach. This inference implies that mamacare intervention did not change participants' perception on these predictor variables. In summary, Table 8 shows conclusions drawn from Repeated Measures ANOVA results to either support or reject hypothesized relationships.

From these inferences, we conclude that *attitude, sensory requirements, representation* and *reach* variables estimated actual outcome observed after exposing the study cohort to mamacare intervention.

By comparing these results with those drawn from structural path models, we observe similarities and some inconsistences. Despite these variations, conclusions drawn from both structural modeling and parametric analyses demonstrate that TIPFit model is capable of predicting utilization of mHealth interventions in the early design stage.

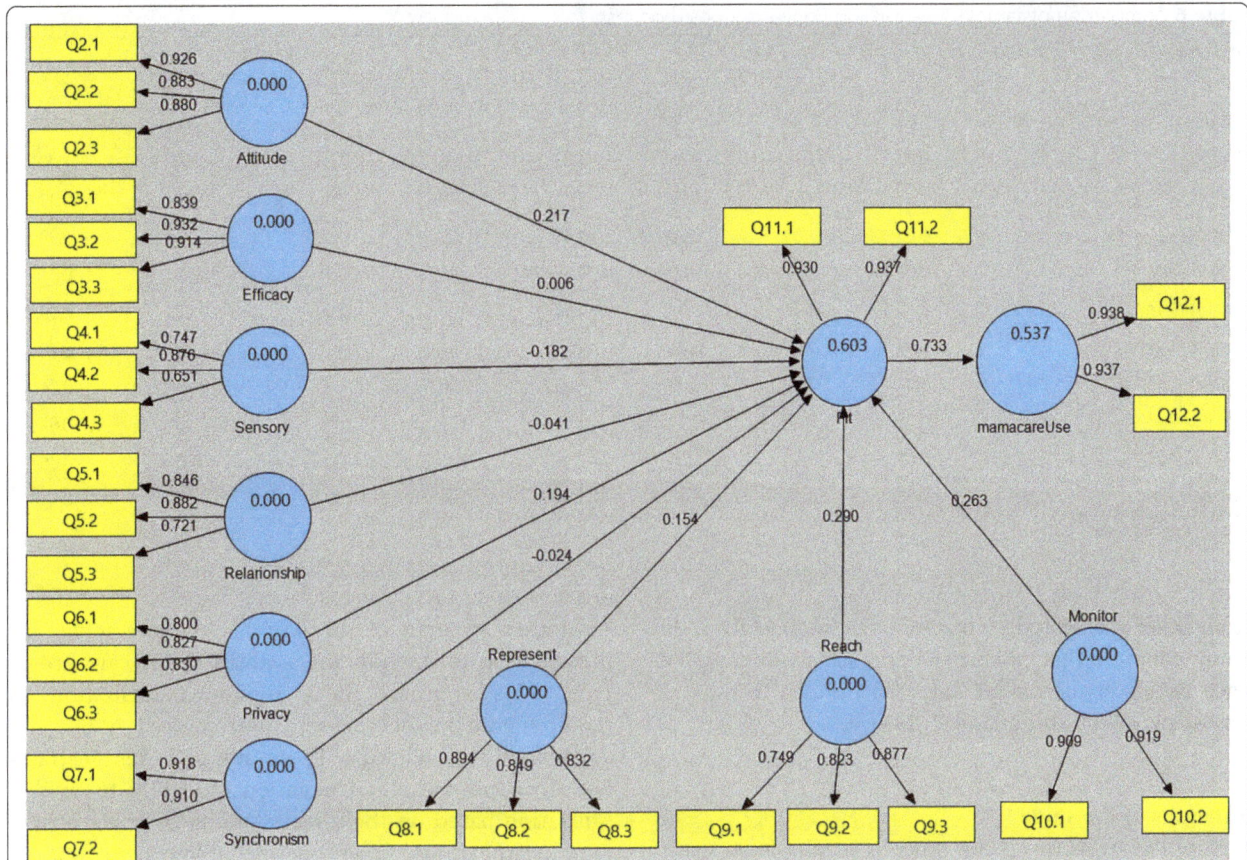

Fig. 13 Post-test model generated from the second post-test showing R² and path weights. The model indicates a marginal improvement on utilization of mamacare

Discussions

This study used repeated measures quasi-experiment on a single group to measure the power of TIPFit model in predicting utilization of mHealth interventions. To validate the model, a pretest was administered on a study cohort of 79 subjects before exposure to mamacare intervention. The intervention involved sending and receiving SMS alerts and reminders on maternal care services through mobile phones.

Predictive power of TIPFit model

The study findings revealed interesting trends before and after exposing the study subjects to mamacare

intervention. Inferences on the pretest and post-test structural path models revealed that user's perception on fit constantly dropped after exposing the subjects to the intervention. Moreover, results from RM-ANOVA revealed the intervention had significant change on seven predictor variables. These are self-efficacy, relationship, identification and privacy, synchronism, monitoring, fit and mamacare utilization.

These results are a confirmation to Davis and Venkatesh assertion that; evaluating user acceptance during design can be used to predict post-implementation acceptance and use of a new system [40]. Furthermore, the study shows some similarities to the findings by Bhattacherjee and Premkumar [15] in their study on predicting usage

Table 4 Summary of path weights from pretest and post-tests models

Test	Atti.	Self	Sense	Rela	Priv	Syn	Rep	Reach	Mo	Fit.
T_0	0.19	−0.11	−0.08	0.54	0.07	0.17	0.12	−0.03	0.38	*0.79*
T_1	0.21	−0.06	−0.15	0.08	0.20	0.13	0.31	0.24	0.02	*0.71*
T_2	0.22	0.01	−0.18	−0.04	0.19	−0.02	0.15	0.29	0.26	*0.73*

Source: Primary Data. [NB. The italicized entries in the Fit column indicates that the values are cummulative path weights from the 9 predictor variables X_1 to X_9]

Table 5 Significance test results for the bootstrapped path weights

Test	Att	Self	Sens	Rel	Prv	Sync	Rep	Reac	Mon	Fit
T_0	2.38	−1.71	−1.79	5.07	0.75	2.28	1.43	−0.37	2.73	20.48
T_1	2.96	−0.83	−3.53	1.09	3.40	1.30	3.91	5.09	0.30	19.52
T_2	3.16	0.08	−3.65	−0.59	2.14	−0.25	1.94	3.64	3.86	20.39

Source: Primary Data

Table 6 Comparison of sample means using Bonferroni post-hoc test

Predictor Variable	Pretest		Post-test1		Post-test2		Mean differences (p-value)		
	$\bar{x}=\mu$	SE	$\bar{x}=\mu$	SE	$\bar{x}=\mu$	SE	$T_0 - T_1$	T_1-T_2	$T_0 -T_2$
Attitude	1.56	0.06	1.39	0.06	1.54	0.06	0.11	0.17	0.99
Efficacy	1.55	0.07	1.35	0.06	1.55	0.06	0.10	0.04	1.00
Sensory	2.23	0.12	1.98	0.12	2.11	0.08	0.05	0.21	0.39
Relation	1.81	0.09	1.53	0.06	1.66	0.06	0.11	0.17	0.99
ID. & Privacy	1.89	0.09	1.51	0.07	1.58	0.06	0.01	0.86	0.01
Synchronism	1.84	0.10	1.43	0.07	1.61	0.06	0.00	0.09	0.09
Representation	1.63	0.07	1.47	0.06	1.52	0.05	0.11	0.83	0.48
Reach	1.74	0.07	1.59	0.08	1.65	0.06	0.47	0.93	0.64
Monitor	1.66	0.08	2.00	0.00	1.60	0.06	0.00	0.00	0.92
Fit	1.77	0.09	1.36	0.06	1.54	0.06	0.00	0.06	0.06
mHealth Use	1.69	0.08	1.43	0.07	1.51	0.06	0.02	0.74	0.18

Source: Primary Data

from belief and attitude. Therefore, the findings from this study confirms that predictive approach to user acceptance testing at the design stage can be used to estimate post-deployment utilization [11, 14, 15].

Strengths of the study

One of the strengths of this study is emphasis on use of open source software to implement mamacare that runs on low-end mobile devices. Mamacare back-end was implemented using Apache web server, MySQL database, PHP, and SMS Tools3 gateway. To make the front-end adaptive to multiple device profiles, we used Twitter bootstrap; a framework that supports HTML5, CSS3 and JavaScript. This makes mamacare a low-cost digital health solution for supporting maternal and newborn care in low-resource settings.

Table 7 Test of overall treatment effect using RM-ANOVA

Predictor	Sphericity		RM-ANOVA:		Effect	Remarks
	χ2	p-value	F ratio	p-value	Eta²	p < 0.05
Attitude	0.534	0.766	2.595	0.078	0.036	Not sign.
Self-Efficacy	3.432	0.180	3.258	0.041	0.045	Significant
Sensory	5.109	0.078	1.233	0.295	0.018	Not sign.
Relationship	22.076	< 0.001	4.038	0.029	0.055	GG: Sign.
ID and Privacy	9.980	0.007	7.462	0.001	0.098	GG: Sign.
Synchronism	13.683	0.001	8.022	0.001	0.104	GG: Sign.
Representation	10.664	0.005	2.373	0.105	0.033	GG: Not Sign
Reach	5.034	0.081	1.117	0.330	0.016	Not sign.
Monitoring	20.082	< 0.001	13.384	< 0.001	0.162	GG: Sign.
Fit	8.516	0.014*	10.144	< 0.001	0.128	GG: Sign.
mHealth use	1.350	0.509	4.152	0.018	0.057	Sign.

Source: Primary Data

Another strength of the study is the predictive approach used to develop and evaluate mamacare prototype. This approach is a unique contribution to requirements engineering and user-centred system development methodology. The study also demonstrates how to apply structural equation modeling to predict utilization based on the understanding of user's behaviour, healthcare processes, and technology contexts.

Study limitations

Theoretical models focusing on **fit** do not give sufficient attention to the fact that system artifacts must be utilized before they deliver performance impacts [19]. Moreover, there is no evidence that quality of an mHealth system leads to increased voluntary utilization. In our pre-study [13], we observed poor systems being utilized extensively in low-income settings due to donor funding, social benefits, ignorance, and availability. For this reason, we argue that increased utilization of mHealth innovations in low-resource settings may not necessarily result to improved quality of health outcomes. This is because there are other socioeconomic and technical factors that influence delivery of healthcare services such as the cost of care, infrastructure, governance, culture, and skilled workforce. Unfortunately, TIPFit model does not consider these factors but only focuses on the three elements of people, process and technology used to evaluate success of information systems.

Another limitation of this study was on the design used to predict utilization. Although single-group repeated measures design used is closer to randomized experiments, the datasets collected from the same subjects may have had likelihood of reporting bias. To

Table 8 Conclusions drawn from RM-ANOVA analysis

Predictor	H_0	Prediction hypotheses	Conclusion drawn (p < 0.05)
Attitude	H_01	Attitude has no significant change on fit before, and after use of mHealth intervention	Nonsignificant - accept
Self-Efficacy	H_02	Self-efficacy has no significant change on fit before, and after use of mHealth intervention	Significant - reject
Sensory	H_03	Sensory requirements have no significant change on fit before, and after use of mHealth intervention.	Nonsignificant - accept
Relationship	H_04	Relationship requirement has no significant change on fit before, and after use of mHealth intervention	Significant - reject
Identification and Privacy	H_05	Identification and privacy has no significant change on fit before, and after use of mHealth intervention	Significant - reject
Synchronism	H_06	Synchronism requirement has no significant change on fit before, and after use of mHealth intervention	Significant - reject
Representation	H_07	Representation capability of technology has no significant effect on fit before, and after use of mHealth intervention	Nonsignificant - accept
Reach	H_08	Reach capability of mHealth technology has no significant change on fit before, and after use of mHealth intervention	Nonsignificant - accept
Monitoring	H_09	Monitoring capability of technology has no significant change on fit before, and after use of mHealth intervention	Significant - reject
Fit for Use	H_010	Perceived fit has no significant change before, and after use of mHealth intervention	Significant - reject

Source: Primary data

maximize on internal and external validity, it is important to observe caution in sample selection, and time difference allowed before taking measurements. This explains the reason why this study lasted for six months. Some of the shortcomings of longitudinal studies are high cost, and decrease in number of subjects due to natural attrition or voluntary withdrawal.

Conclusions

This study concludes that there is a myriad of mHealth projects that have failed to inspire utilization due to poor alignment to user needs, clinical tasks, technology and environmental context. To address this gap, we demonstrated that measuring intended users' perceptions on a planned intervention is crucial to predicting acceptance and use.

In practice, it is crucial for developers of mHealth systems to ensure that user-centred evaluation is performed thoroughly in the early design stage. This is because perceived benefits and user expectations measured during the design stage could provide valuable insights on post-deployment utilization of the intervention [40].

In terms of policy, this study demonstrates that increased utilization of mHealth innovations has the potential to accelerate attainment of Universal Health Coverage (UHC) and Sustainable Development Goals (SDGs) in developing countries. However, success of mHealth interventions depends on how value is driven by aligning the artifacts to health needs and expectations at the design stage.

Additional files

Additional file 1: Pretest questionnaire used prior to implementation of mamacare to measure perception on usefulness mobile and point-of-care devices in maternal care. (DOC 149 kb)

Additional file 2: Post-test questionnaire used after deployment of mamacare prototype to measure user acceptance, satisfaction and actual utilization. (DOC 150 kb)

Additional file 3: Pretest dataset obtained from randomly selected antenatal and post-natal women. The dataset was used as the baseline for predicting post-deployment utilization of mamacare services. (CSV 5 kb)

Additional file 4: Initial post-test dataset obtained from the study cohort after exposing the subjects to mamacare intervention. (CSV 5 kb)

Additional file 5: Second post-test dataset obtained from the cohort after prolonged exposure to enhanced mamacare services. (CSV 4 kb)

Abbreviations
ANOVA: Analysis of Variance; eHealth: electronic health; ICT: Information and Communication Technology; ITU: International Telecommunication Union; PLS: Partial Least Squares; SDGs: Sustainable Development Goals; SMS: Short Message Service; TIPFit: Technology, Individual, Process Fit; WHO: World Health Organization

Acknowledgements
We are grateful to University of Nairobi Deans Committee for funding pre-study fieldwork during this study. We acknowledge immense support from Mr. Onesmus Kamau, Head of eHealth in the Ministry of Health, Kenya. We also highly appreciate valuable guidance from the Late Prof. Okelo-Odongo, and Ms. Dorothy Iseu of University of Nairobi. Thanks to Prof. Alexander Schill, Thomas Springer, and Elke Franz of TU Dresden, Germany for their dedicated academic mentorship and support.

Funding
This research was partly supported by grants from University of Nairobi Deans' Research Committee. However, the funder had no role in the design of the study, data collection, analysis, interpretation of data and writing of this manuscript.

Authors' contributions

SM and RO designed TIPFit model and data collection tools. SM collected data and wrote the manuscript. All the authors proofread, edited and approved the revised manuscript.

Competing interests

The authors declare that they have no competing interests.

References

1. Njoroge M, et al. Assessing the feasibility of eHealth and mHealth: a systematic review and analysis of initiatives implemented in Kenya. Medical Informatics and Decision Making. 2017;10(90):1–11.
2. Omachonu VK, Einspruch NG. Innovation in healthcare delivery systems: a conceptual framework. The Innovation Journal: The Public Sector Innovation Journal. 2010;15(2):1–20.
3. Breen G, Matusitz J. An evolutionary examination of telemedicine: a health and computer-mediated communication. Perspective Soc Work Public Health. 2010;25:59–71.
4. WHO: mHealth New horizons for health through mobile technologies: second global survey on eHealth 2011.
5. Mechael P, et al. Barriers and gaps affecting mHealth in low and middle income countries: Policy White Paper. Columbia: Academic Center for Global Health and economic development earth institute; 2010.
6. Yu P, Wu MX, Yu H, Xiao GQ. The challenges for the adoption of m-health. Shanghai: IEEE Int. Conf. on Service Operations and Logistics and Informatics; 2006. p. 181–6.
7. International Telecommunication Union (ITU): Mobile eHealth for developing countries. ITU-telecommunication development bureau 2010.
8. WHO, ITU. eHealth and innovation in women's and children's health: a baseline review: based on the findings of the 2013 survey of CoIA countries by the WHO global observatory for eHealth. Geneva; 2014.
9. Breen G, Wan TTH, Ortiz J. Information technology adoption in rural health clinics: a theoretical analysis. Journal of Information Technology Impact. 2010;10(1):1–14.
10. Huang, et al. Effects of and satisfaction with short message service reminders for patient medication adherence: a randomized controlled study. BMC Med Inform Decis Mak. 2013;13:127.
11. Mburu S. Application of structural equation modelling to predict acceptance and use of mHealth interventions at the design stage. Journal of Health Informatics in Developing Countries. 2017;11:1–17.
12. Omary Z, Lupiana D, Mtenzi F, Wu B. Analysis of the challenges affecting E-healthcare adoption in developing countries: a case of Tanzania. International Journal of Information Studies. 2010;2:38–50.
13. Mburu S, Franz E, Springer T. A conceptual framework for designing mHealth solutions for developing countries. In: in MobileHealth Proceedings of the 3rd ACM MobiHoc workshop on Pervasive wireless healthcare; 2013. p. 31–6.
14. Davis FD, Venkatesh V. Toward pre-prototype user acceptance testing of new information systems: implications for software Project Management. IEEE Trans on Engineering Management. 2004;51:31–46.
15. Bhattacherjee A, Premkumar G. Understanding changes in belief and attitude toward information technology usage: a theoretical model and longitudinal test. MIS Q. 2004;28(2):229–54.
16. Ajzen I. The theory of planned behavior. Organ Behav Hum Decis Process. 1999;50:179–211.
17. Davis FD. Perceived usefulness, perceived ease of use, and user acceptance of information technology. MIS Q. 1989;13:319–40.
18. Overby EM. Process virtualization theory and the impact of information technology. Organ Sci. 2008;19:277–91.
19. Goodhue DL, Thompson RL. Task-technology fit and individual performance. MIS Q. 1995;19:213–36.
20. Compeau DR, Higgins CR. Computer self-efficacy: development of measure and initial test. MIS Q. 1995;19:189–211.
21. Strong DM, Dishaw MT, Bandy DB. Extending task technology fit with computer self-efficacy. The DATA BASE for Advances in Information Systems. 2006;37(2 & 3):96–107.
22. Overby EM, Konsynski B. Task-technology fit and process virtualization theory: an integrated model and empirical test. Res Pap. 2010:10–96.
23. United Nations. Progress towards the sustainable development goals. Economic and Social Council. 2016:5–7.
24. Gregor S. The nature of theory in IS. MIS Q. 2006;30(3):612–42.
25. Hevner AR, March ST, Park J, Ram S. Design science in information systems research. MIS Q. 2004;28:75–105.
26. Armitage CJ, Conner M. Efficacy of the theory of planned behaviour: a meta-analytic review. Br J Soc Psychol. 2001;40:471–99.
27. Hagger MS, Chatzisarantis NLD, Biddle SJH. A meta-analytic review of theories of reasoned action and planned behavior in physical activity: predictive validity and contribution of additional variables. J Sport Exerc Psychol. 2002;24:3–32.
28. Overby EN, Slaughter SA, Konsynski B. The design, use, and consequences of virtual processes. Information Systems Research, INFORMS. 2010;21:700–10.
29. Oluoch T, Katana A, Ssempijja V, et al. Electronic medical record systems are associated with appropriate placement of HIV patients on antiretroviral therapy in rural health facilities in Kenya: a retrospective pre-post study. J Am Med Inform Assoc. 2014;21:1009–14.
30. Ammenwerth E, Iller C, Mahler C. IT-adoption and the interaction of task, technology and individuals: a fit framework and case study. BMC Med Inform Decis Mak. 2006;6(3):1–13.
31. Yusof MM, Kuljis J, Papazafeiropoulou A, Stergioulas LK. An evaluation framework for health information systems: human, organization and technology fit factors (HOT-fit). Int J Med Inform. 2008;77:386–98.
32. Becker MH, Maiman LA, Kirscht JP, Haefner DP, Drachman RH. The health belief model and prediction of dietary compliance: a field experiment. J Health Soc Behav. 1977;18:348–66.
33. Henseler J, Ringle CM, Sinkovics RR. The use of partial least squares in international marketing. New Challenges to International Marketing, Advances in Int Marketing. 2009;20:277–319.
34. Fornell C, Larcker DF. Evaluating structural equation models with unobservable variables and measurement error. J Mark Res. 1981;18:39–50.
35. Bagozzi RP, Yi Y. On the evaluation of structural equation models. Acad Market Sci J Acad Mark Sci. 1998;16:74–94.
36. Wong KK. Partial least squares structural equation modeling (PLS-SEM) techniques using SmartPLS, Marketing Bulletin. Technical Note. 2013:1.
37. Goodhue DL, et al. PLS, Small Sample Size, and Statistical Power. Proceedings of the 39th Int. Conf. on System Sciences, Hawaii: MIS Research; 2006. p. 1–10.
38. Chin WW, Newsted PR. Structural Equation Modelling analysis with Small Samples using Partial Least Squares, Statistical Strategies for Small Sample Research, Sage Publications; 1999. p. 307–41.
39. Cohen J. Quantitative methods in psychology: a power primer. American Psychological Association Bulletin. 1992;112:155–9.
40. DeLone WH, McLean ER. The DeLone and Mclean model of information system success: a ten-year update. J Manag Inf Syst. 2003;19(4):9–30.

13

The relationship between hospital and ehr vendor market dynamics on health information organization presence and participation

Sunny C. Lin[1][*] [iD] and Julia Adler-Milstein[2]

Abstract

Background: Health Information Organizations (HIOs) are third party organizations that facilitate electronic health information exchange (HIE) between providers in a geographic area. Despite benefits from HIE, HIOs have struggled to form and subsequently gain broad provider participation. We sought to assess whether market-level hospital and EHR vendor dynamics are associated with presence and level of hospital participation in HIOs.

Methods: 2014 data on 4523 hospitals and their EHR vendors were aggregated to the market level. We used multivariate OLS regression to analyze the relationship between hospital and vendor dynamics and (1) probability of HIO presence and (2) percent of hospitals participating in an HIO.

Results: 298 of 469 markets (64%) had HIO presence, and in those markets, 47% of hospitals participated in an HIO on average. In multivariate analysis, four characteristics were associated with HIO presence. Markets with more hospitals, markets with more EHR vendors, and markets with an EHR vendor-led HIE approach were *more likely* to have an HIO. Compared to markets with low hospital competition, markets with high hospital competition had a 25 percentage point *lower probability* of HIO presence. Two characteristics were associated with level of hospital HIO participation. Markets with more hospitals as well as markets with high vendor competition (compared to low competition) had lower participation.

Conclusion: Both hospital and EHR vendor dynamics are associated with whether a market has an HIO as well as the level of hospital participation in HIOs.

Keywords: Health information exchange, Electronic health records, Systems integration

Background

Fragmented healthcare delivery has resulted in silos of health information and the challenge of ensuring that patient information is shared between providers. Information sharing is vital to care coordination, and when done electronically, can be more comprehensive, accurate, and timely, leading to a reduction in redundant testing, improved patient safety, and better quality of care [1, 2]. Health Information Organizations (HIOs) are third party organizations that provide the governance and technical infrastructure to enable electronic health information exchange (HIE) between providers in a geographic area. As opposed to other HIE approaches that place restrictions on who can participate in sharing data, such as Enterprise Health Information Exchanges or EHR Vendor Exchanges, HIOs promote community-wide HIE participation [3] and are a community approach to HIE that may be less likely to lead to information blocking (the intentional and unreasonable interference with electronic exchange of health information) [4].

Although HIOs represent an important option for community-level connectivity, HIOs have struggled to identify sustainable business models, which may be driving the observed decline in the number of HIOs [5] and

* Correspondence: sunnylin@umich.edu
[1]Department of Health Management and Policy, School of Public Health, University of Michigan, Ann Arbor, MI, USA
Full list of author information is available at the end of the article

leads to uncertainty about their viability. Critical to HIO sustainability is whether hospitals perceive participation as valuable, which is influenced both by hospital dynamics and by how EHR vendors work with HIOs. Hospitals have expressed concern about the potential loss of patients and revenue that could result from sharing data with competitors through HIOs, particularly if participation costs are high. Anecdotal reports of EHR vendors charging prohibitive fees or withdrawing support for connectivity have raised concerns about the influence of EHR vendors on the sustainability of HIOs, especially as EHR vendors are increasingly offering their own HIE networks [6].

While prior studies on HIOs have examined what predicts whether or not hospitals participate in an HIO [7], it is not yet known whether market conditions, particularly those related to dynamics of hospitals and EHR vendors, are associated with HIO presence and the level of hospital participation. This question has important implications for understanding the future of HIOs and the effectiveness of policies designed to promote their sustainability. In particular, many HITECH policies seeking to increase HIE have targeted individual organizations. To the extent that market characteristics predict HIO presence and level of hospital participation, it may be more effective to pursue policies at the market level.

In this study, we sought to understand how hospital and EHR vendor market dynamics are related to HIO presence and level of hospital participation in HIOs. Market dynamics may hinder **HIO presence** if an HIO is unable to negotiate tensions between competing hospitals or vendors. Even in markets that have successfully established an HIO, these same market dynamics may limit**the level of hospital participation in HIOs**. We answer the following questions: (1) Do market-level hospital and EHR vendor characteristics differ in markets with and without an HIO? (2) In markets with an HIO, are market-level characteristics associated with the level of hospital participation in HIOs?

Methods

Data

Data on US hospitals (excluding mental, children's, and federal government hospitals) from the 2014 AHA Survey and 2014 AHA IT Supplement were aggregated to the Health Service Area (HSA) and merged with data from the 2012 Dartmouth Atlas and the 2014 Area Health Resource File. When 2014 AHA data was missing, we used the most recently available data from the 2008–2013 American Hospital Association (AHA) Surveys and 2012–2013 AHA IT Supplements. Because many HSAs contain a single hospital, areas bound by HSAs may not adequately capture interactions between hospitals. We therefore combined HSAs within Health

Referral Regions (HRRs, larger geographic areas created by aggregating HSAs based on patient referrals for tertiary medical care) based on whether or not there was at least one HIO in the HSA. This effectively split HRRs into two areas, one that contains all HSAs in the HRR that have HIO presence, and one that contains all HSAs in the HRR that do not have HIO presence. Each of these areas was considered an individual market.

Markets were dropped if there were not enough hospitals in the market that responded to the AHA IT Supplement. If there were at least 7 hospitals in the market, at least one-third of the hospitals in the market had to have responded to the IT supplement to remain in the data set. If there were fewer than 7 hospitals in the market, at least 3 of the hospitals had to have responded to remain in the data set. Additional markets were dropped if no hospitals had data available for the following revenue-related measures: percent of inpatient days from Medicare, percent of inpatient days from Medicaid, and percent of revenue from shared risk or capitated payment sources. A total of 72 markets were dropped (63 missing IT data and 9 missing hospital revenue-related data) resulting in a final analytic data set of 469 markets, representing 2648 HSAs and 4523 hospitals (Table 1).

Dependent variables

HIO presence in a market was measured using responses to a question from the AHA IT Supplement that asked about HIOs in a hospital's area. An HSA was considered as having an HIO if at least one hospital in the HSA indicated that there was an HIO in their area, even if they did not participate. Level of hospital participation in HIOs was calculated using the percent of hospitals in the market that reported *actively participating* in an HIO on the AHA IT Supplement. Because HIO participation can, by definition, only occur in markets with an HIO, analysis of HIO participation was limited to markets with HIO presence.

Independent variables

We selected six independent variables—three related to hospital dynamics and three related to vendor dynamics—that we hypothesized would be related to both the likelihood of HIO presence and the level of hospital HIO participation in markets with HIOs (Please see Additional file 1: Conceptual Model). We chose these variables based on those included in previous hospital-level studies that sought to predict which hospitals engage in HIE and adopt other types of health information technologies [8, 9].

Hospital market size

A greater number of hospitals may be associated with higher probability of HIO presence and a higher level of

Table 1 Characteristics of markets by HIO presence and level of hospital participation

Variables	All Areas	No HIO Presence	HIO Presence	P-value	Hospital Participation	P-value
Number of Markets	469	171	298		298	
Categorical Variables	*n(%)*	*n(%)*	*n(%)*	*P-value*	Mean (SD)	*P-value*
Number of Hospitals				< 0.001		< 0.001
Low (1–4)	175 (37%)	106 (62%)	69 (23%)		58% (32)	
Moderate (5–8)	128 (27%)	36 (21%)	92 (31%)		41% (24)	
High (9+)	166 (35%)	29 (17%)	137 (46%)		47% (25)	
Total	469	171	198			
Hospital Competition (HHI)				< 0.001		0.33
Non-Competitive (0.46–1.00)	127 (27%)	67 (39%)	60 (20%)		59% (32)	
Moderately Competitive (0.25–0.45)	166 (35%)	62 (36%)	104 (35%)		45% (26)	
Highly Competitive (0.00–0.24)	176 (37%)	42 (25%)	134 (45%)		43% (20)	
Total	469	171	298			
For-Profit Hospital Marketshare				0.003		< 0.001
Low For-Profit Marketshare (0–57%)	357 (76%)	117 (68%)	240 (81%)		34% (34)	
High For-Profit Marketshare (> 57%)	112 (24%)	54 (32%)	58 (19%)		18% (18)	
Total	469	171	298			
No. of EHR Vendors				< 0.001		< 0.001
Low (1–2)	141 (30%)	21 (12%)	120 (40%)		55% (32)	
Moderate (3–4)	146 (31%)	45 (26%)	101 (34%)		44% (25)	
High (5+)	182 (39%)	105 (61%)	77 (26%)		44% (19)	
Total	469	171	298			
Vendor Competition (HHI)				< 0.001		0.35
Non-Competitive (0.63–1.00)	144 (31%)	76 (44%)	68 (23%)		57% (31)	
Moderately Competitive (0.38–0.62)	162 (35%)	57 (33%)	105 (35%)		46% (25)	
Highly Competitive (0.00–0.37)	163 (35%)	38 (22%)	125 (42%)		42% (20)	
Total	469	171	298			
Alternative HIE Approach (%)				< 0.001		< 0.001
No (0–49% of hospitals on Epic)	256 (55%)	135 (79%)	121 (41%)		44% (27)	
Yes (50–100% of hospitals on Epic)	213 (45%)	36 (21%)	177 (59%)		49% (24)	
Total	469	171	298			
Continuous Variables	*Mean (SD)*	*Mean (SD)*	*Mean (SD)*	*P-value*	Coefficient (SE)	*P-value*
Number of HSAs	6 (6)	5 (4)	6 (6)	0.018	0.16 (0.23)	0.46
% HIO Participation	30 (30)	0 (0)	47 (25)	< 0.001		
% Hospital Participation in Patient Centered Medical Home and/or Accountable Care Organizations	27 (27)	17 (26)	33 (25)	< 0.001	0.003 (0.001)	< 0.001
% Revenue Shared Risk Programs	1 (4)	1 (3)	2 (4)	0.062	0.12 (0.33)	0.72
% Inpatient Days Medicare	52 (21)	53 (15)	51 (9)	0.088	0.18 (0.16)	0.25
% Inpatient Days Medicaid	19 (9)	18 (10)	19 (8)	0.066	0.32 (0.19)	0.10
Hospital Beds per 1000 residents	24 (31)	15 (16)	29 (36)	< 0.001	−0.09 (0.04)	0.03
FTE Hospital Staff per 1000 residents	164 (197)	98 (91)	202 (229)	< 0.001	−0.01 (0.01)	0.12
Percentage of Hospitals in Urban Settings	62 (35)	46 (39)	72 (29)	< 0.001	−0.04 (0.05)	0.50
Number of Physicians (Weighted County Average)	409 (769)	260 (737)	495 (775)	0.001	0.00 (0.00)	0.65

HIO Health Information Organization,*HHI* Herfindahl-Hirschman Index, *EHR* Electronic Health Record, *HSA* Health Service Area, *FTE* Full Time Equivalent, *SD* Standard Deviation, *SE* Standard Error

Note: Percentages may not add up to 100% due to rounding; *p*-values based on ANOVA for categorical variables and linear regression for continuous variables

hospital HIO participation, because markets with more hospitals have more fragmented care and therefore see a greater need to establish an HIO and share information. Markets were categorized as having a low, moderate, or high number of hospitals using tertiles, which are cutoffs that split the sample into three equal parts and resulted in the following categories: low = 1–5 hospitals, moderate = 6–10, high = 11 + .

Hospital market competition

Hospital competition may be associated with lower probability of HIO presence and lower hospital participation because hospitals that are highly competitive may prefer more selective ways to exchange information, such as through Enterprise HIE or direct connections [3, 8, 10, 11]. We categorized markets as non-competitive, moderately competitive, and highly competitive using the Herfindahl-Hirschman index (HHI). The HHI is calculated using the sum of the squared market share of each hospital in the market. Market share was determined using the number of hospital beds in a hospital system. After calculating the HHI for the market, markets were categorized as non-competitive, moderately competitive, or highly competitive based on whether they were in top, middle, or bottom third of the distribution for HHI, respectively (HHI of 0.447–1 = noncompetitive, 0.239–0.439 = moderately competitive, 0–0.238 = highly competitive).

Hospital market ownership

For-profit hospitals may see HIO participation as a risky way to exchange information, since HIO participation makes valuable patient data more accessible and could reduce barriers for patients to receive care at competitors. Markets with a large for-profit market share may have lower probability of HIO presence and lower hospital participation. For-profit market share was calculated using the percent of beds owned by for-profit hospitals. Markets were considered as having high for-profit marketshare if they were in the top quartile of for-profit marketshare (> 57%).

EHR vendor market size

A higher number of EHR vendors that are used by hospitals in the market might increase the technical complexity and associated costs of connecting multiple EHR systems from different vendors [12–14]. This could improve the attractiveness of an HIO because each hospital would only need to establish a single connection to the HIO, increasing both the probability of HIO presence and the level of hospital participation. Alternatively, having more EHR vendors could increase the cost of HIO formation and hospital participation, decreasing the probability of HIO presence and reducing participation. The number of EHR vendors was calculated by counting the number of unique inpatient EHR vendors used by hospitals in the market. Markets were categorized as having a low, moderate, or high number of vendors using tertiles (low = 1–2 vendors, moderate = 3–4, high = 5+).

EHR vendor market competition

In competitive vendor markets, competing EHR vendors may be reluctant to support hospital participation in HIOs in an effort to maintain vendor lock-in [13, 15–17]. As a result, markets with competitive EHR vendors may have lower probability of HIO presence and lower hospital participation. Similar to hospital competition, vendor competition was determined using the Herfindahl-Hirschman Index of vendors in the market. Vendor market share was based on the number of hospital beds in hospitals that use the vendor's inpatient EHR product. Markets were categorized as non-competitive, moderately competitive, and highly competitive based on whether they were in the top, middle, or bottom third of the distribution for vendor HHI (HHI of 0.592–1.000 = noncompetitive, 0.357–0.592 = moderately competitive, and 0–0.356 = highly competitive).

Market penetration of alternative (vendor-led) HIE approach

One specific EHR vendor - Epic - has a mature intra-Epic HIE in which the vast majority of Epic clients participate. Therefore, markets dominated by Epic have an alternative to HIOs and there may be a sufficient number of hospitals that prefer to exchange data through Epic's HIE platform instead of an HIO, resulting in both a lower probability of HIO presence and lower hospital participation. Market penetration of an alternative (vendor-led) HIE approach was measured by calculating Epic marketshare using the percent of beds owned by hospitals whose primary inpatient vendor was Epic. A market was considered to have an alternative HIE approach if the Epic marketshare was greater than 50%.

We included seven market-level controls: percent of hospitals that participate in a Patient Centered Medical Home and/or Accountable Care Organization, average percent of revenue from alternative payment models (e. g. shared risk programs and capitated payments), average percent of inpatient days from Medicare/Medicaid, number of hospital beds per 1000 residents, number of full time hospital employees per 1000 residents, number of physicians per 1000 residents, and percent of hospitals in urban settings. These control variables were chosen because they may confound the relationship between hospital and EHR vendor market dynamics and HIO presence and hospital participation in HIOs. In markets where a higher percentage of hospital revenue is from shared risk programs, hospitals may be more likely to participate in an HIO effort to improve care coordination [12]. In markets where hospitals have a greater percentage of inpatient days paid for by Medicare and Medicaid, hospitals may be more inclined to participate in an HIO in order to meet Meaningful Use criteria [18]. Markets with a higher density of hospital beds, hospital staff, and physicians, as well as greater urbanicity, may have greater need for HIE to facilitate care coordination.

Analysis

To answer our first research question about how hospital and vendor market characteristics differ for markets with and without an HIO, we conducted bivariate analyses on market characteristics and HIO presence, and then ran a multivariate linear probability model with state fixed effects. A linear probability model was chosen over the logistic model for ease of interpretation, such that coefficients can be interpreted as a change in the predicted probability of HIO presence given a unit change in the independent variable. However, as a robustness test, we ran a logistic regression model and the resulting odds ratios were compared with the linear probability model (Additional file 2: Logistic Regression Model for HIO Presence in Marekts with different Hospital and Vendor Characteristics).

To address our second research question about how characteristics of markets are associated with hospital participation, we conducted bivariate analyses on hospital participation and market characteristics using one-way ANOVAs for categorical variables and linear regression for continuous variables. We then ran a multivariate linear regression model with state fixed effects using hospital participation as the dependent variable for all markets with HIO presence.

In our dataset, the number of hospitals and number of vendors in the market were highly correlated (correlation coefficient = 0.83), while the number of hospitals and hospital competition, the number of vendors and vendor competition, and hospital and vendor competition were moderately correlated (correlation coefficients = 0.50, 0.74, 0.74 respectively). High multicollinearity may lead to two problems: (1) invalid interpretations of model coefficients as "the expected change in an outcome *holding all other variables constant*", since, as a result of collinearity, a change in one variable necessitates a change in the collinear variable, and (2) high standard errors for collinear variables leading to insignificance. We addressed multicollinearity in three ways. First, in our primary models, we use tertiles of number of hospitals and vendors, and hospital and vendor competition instead of continuous variables. Second, as a robustness test, we ran our models using continuous variables, to ensure that the directionality of the estimated effect was

consistent with our primary models. Finally, we ran our models and systematically excluded each of the collinear variables, and then compared standard errors and statistical significance to our primary models.

Results

HIO presence

In bivariate analyses, markets with and without an HIO differed significantly for all independent variables, but not always in the predicted direction: markets with an HIO had more hospitals ($p < 0.001$), had higher hospital competition ($p < 0.001$), were less likely to have high for-profit hospital marketshare ($p = 0.003$), had more EHR vendors ($p < 0.001$), had more competitive EHR vendors ($p < 0.001$) and were more likely to have an alternative HIE approach (i.e., be Epic dominant; $p < 0.001$, Table 1).

In the multivariate probability regression, most of these variables continued to be significantly related to HIO presence. Compared to markets with a low number of hospitals, markets with a moderate number of hospitals had a 19 percentage-point higher probability of HIO presence ($p = 0.032$) and markets with a high number of hospitals had a 19 percentage-point higher probability of HIO presence ($p = 0.006$, Table 2). Compared to non-competitive hospital markets, highly-competitive hospital markets had 25 percentage-point lower probability of HIO presence ($p = 0.003$, Table 2). Moderately-competitive hospital markets had a 12 percentage-point lower probability of HIO presence, though this effect was not statistically significant ($p = 0.058$, Table 2). Markets in the top quartile of for-profit hospital marketshare had a 7 percentage-point lower probability of HIO presence, though this effect was also not statistically significant ($p = 0.163$, Table 2).

Markets with more EHR vendors were more likely to have HIO presence. Compared to markets with a low number of vendors, markets with a moderate number of vendors had a 21 percentage-point higher probability of HIO presence ($p = 0.002$) while markets with a high number of vendors had a 32 percentage-point higher probability of HIO presence ($p = 0.001$, Table 2). Vendor competition did not have a statistically significant relationship with probability of HIO presence. Finally, having an alternative HIE approach was associated with a 14 percentage-point higher probability of HIO presence ($p = 0.001$, Table 2).

Hospital participation in HIO

Bivariate analyses comparing hospital participation by market characteristics in the 298 markets with HIO presence revealed that markets with a higher level of HIO participation were more likely to have: (1) a low number of hospitals ($p < 0.001$), (2) low for-profit hospital marketshare ($p < 0.001$), (3) a low number of EHR

Table 2 HIO Presence and Hospital Participation in Markets with different Hospital and Vendor Characteristics

Variables	Linear Probability Model Coefficients for HIO Presence		Linear Regression Coefficients for Hospital Participation	
Constant	−0.232	(0.158)	54.8**	(17.4)
Hospital Dynamics				
Number of Hospitals (Ref: Low 1–4)				
Moderate (5–8)	0.185*	(0.079)	−5.2	(5.8)
High (9+)	0.190**	(0.068)	−10.9*	(4.7)
Hospital Competition (Ref: Non-competitive, HHI= 0.46–1.00)				
Moderately Competitive (0.25–0.45)	−0.118	(0.063)	−8.4	(4.7)
Highly Competitive (0.00–0.24)	−0.252**	(0.078)	−10.2	(6.0)
For-Profit Hospital Market Share (Ref: Low 0–57%)				
High For-Profit Hospital Market Share (> 57%)	−0.067	(0.053)	−5.6	(3.9)
EHR Vendor Dynamics				
Number of EHR Vendors (Ref: Low 1–2)				
Moderate (3–4)	0.208**	(0.070)	5.4	(5.0)
High (5+)	0.318***	(0.095)	7.0	(6.6)
Vendor Competition (Ref: Non-competitive, HHI= 0.63–1.00)				
Moderately Competitive (0.38–0.62)	0.033	(0.059)	−6.9	(4.5)
Highly Competitive (0.00–0.37)	−0.039	(0.072)	−11.2*	(5.6)
Alternative HIE Approach (Ref: No)				
Yes (50–100% of hospitals on Epic)	0.144**	(0.046)	1.2	(3.1)
Community Controls				
% Hospital Participation in Patient Centered Medical Home and/or Accountable Care Organizations	0.004***	(0.001)	0.1	(0.21)
Avg. % Revenue from Shared Risk Programs	0.004	(0.005)	0.1	(0.3)
% Inpatient Days Medicare	0.002	(0.002)	0.1	(0.2)
% Inpatient Days Medicaid	0.007	(0.004)	0.1	(0.3)
Hospital Beds per 1000 residents	−0.001	(0.002)	0.1	(0.2)
FTE Hospital Staff per 1000 residents	0.000	(0.000)	0.0	(0.0)
Percentage of Hospitals in Urban Settings	0.005***	(0.001)	0.0	(0.1)
Number of Physicians (Weighted County Average)	−0.000*	(0.000)	0.0	(0.0)
State Fixed Effects	Included		Included	
n	469		298	
R^2	0.44		0.16	

Note: * $p<0.05$, ** $p<0.01$, *** $p<0.001$. All models include state fixed effects. Robust standard error in parentheses

vendors ($p < 0.001$), and (4) have an alternative HIE approach ($p < 0.001$, Table 1).

In multivariate regression analysis, two independent variables were significantly associated with hospital participation in HIOs. Compared to markets with a low number of hospitals, markets with a high number of hospitals had on average 11 percentage-points lower hospital participation ($p = 0.023$, Table 2). Though not statistically significant, markets with a moderate number of hospitals had on average 5 percentage-points lower hospital participation ($p = 0.350$, Table 2). Compared to markets with low vendor competition, markets with high vendor competition had on average 11 percentage-points lower hospital participation ($p = 0.043$, Table 2). Though not statistically significant, markets with moderate vendor competition had 7 percentage-points lower hospital participation ($p = 0.151$, Table 2).

Robustness tests

Odds ratio estimates from the logistic regression model were similar to estimates from the linear probability model in both relative magnitude and significance (Additional file 2: Logistic Regression Model for HIO PResence in Markets with Different Hospital and Vendor

Characteristics). The result of the robustness tests for multicollinearity showed that using continuous variables resulted in coefficients in the same direction as in the primary models (Additional file 3: Continuous Variable Models for HIO Presence and Level of Participation in HIOs). Excluding collinear variables did not substantially change standard errors (Additional file 4 and Additional file 5: Robustness Tests for Multicolinearity). While statistical significance did change in some cases, these changes suggest that the collinear variables are picking up the effect of the excluded variables, resulting in either significance if the excluded variable had an effect in the same direction of the collinear variable, or insignificance if the excluded variable had an effect in the opposite direction. These results suggest that the overall conclusions still hold.

Discussion

This study examined the relationship between hospital and EHR vendor market dynamics, and HIO presence and hospital participation. We found that both hospital and EHR vendor dynamics (number of hospitals, hospital competition, number of vendors, and having an alternative HIE approach) are associated with HIO presence, while a greater number of hospitals and high vendor competition predicts lower hospital participation. These results supported some of our hypothesized relationships and contradicted others.

Consistent with what we predicted, markets with more hospitals and vendors were more likely to have an HIO. This suggests that markets with many hospitals or vendors may perceive a greater need for an HIO, leading to a greater likelihood of HIO presence. However, also as we predicted, competitive dynamics among hospitals appear to work against HIO presence. More competitive hospital markets were less likely to have an HIO. Contrary to what we predicted, vendor dynamics did not additionally limit HIO presence. Markets with an alternative, EHR vendor-led approach to HIE were more likely to have an HIO (and vendor competition was unrelated). While this finding contradicts our hypothesis that hospitals in markets with an alternative approach may be less inclined to support an HIO because the majority of hospitals can use Epic's Care Everywhere platform to engage in HIE, a possible explanation is that this measure is serving as a proxy measure for health IT market maturity, which we would expect to increase the likelihood of having an HIO.

Our results on the level of hospital participation in markets with HIOs similarly pointed to the influence of hospital dynamics. Markets with more hospitals had lower HIO participation, which was surprising given our expectation that more hospitals would lead to greater HIO participation. It may be that hospital perception of

HIO value is a function of the percent of hospitals in the market participating in the HIO. That is, HIOs in larger markets may have a harder time recruiting hospitals to participate since it takes many more participating hospitals to achieve the same value. Greater vendor competition was also associated with lower HIO participation, which was consistent with our prediction and suggests that competitive dynamics among vendors may impact how easy they make it for hospitals to connect to an HIO. Both findings point to the ongoing challenges facing HIO viability.

Our study contributes to the growing literature on HIO development and sustainability. While studies have found that hospital participation in health information exchange is growing [19], they do not identify how market dynamics may be influencing the *types* of exchanges that are developing. The types of health information exchange efforts in a market have important consequences for whether information exchange serves to enhance patient care or strengthen strategic relationships between providers [20]. Our study is consistent with prior work that has found that hospitals in highly competitive markets are less likely to participate in HIOs [7, 8, 16, 19]. However, by examining EHR vendor dynamics as well as market-level hospital dynamics as potential inhibitors of HIO presence, we meaningfully extend these findings by revealing that hospital competition is a potential inhibitor of HIO *presence* in a market, while EHR vendor competition may subsequently inhibit hospital participation in HIOs. An investigation of the effect of EHR vendor dynamics on HIOs is important to our understanding of HIO development and sustainability as EHR vendors are key stakeholders in HIE efforts and have the potential to make or break efforts to achieve community-level information exchange.

Our work has important policy implications. Through the CMS Meaningful Use Program and HITECH funding for HIOs, policymakers have tried to create conditions under which HIOs can become established and achieve broad provider participation. Recent concerns about their viability have primarily stemmed from vendor dynamics – including information blocking [6] and proprietary HIE networks [21]. In this context, we find that both hospital dynamics and vendor dynamics appear to be inhibiting HIO viability. It could be that competition between hospitals inhibits the formation of HIOs, while in areas with HIO presence, vendor competition gives rise to information blocking behaviors that create barriers to high hospital participation.

In the interim, our results suggest that efforts to-date have not created sufficient demand for geographically-based HIE. Policymakers may therefore be best off targeting market dynamics in their efforts to promote

HIOs. For example, our results suggest that payment reform efforts (e.g. PCMH and ACO models) that incentivize hospitals to take on greater risk for the cost and quality of care that occurs in the market at large may introduce needed incentives for hospitals to participate in HIOs. Under these models, hospital participation in HIOs may improve the quality of care transitions, reducing readmission rates and subsequent penalties. It will be important to study these mechanisms directly as well as more broadly monitor changes in HIO activity as these policies progress and mature.

Limitations

Our study has several limitations. First, missing data from the AHA IT supplement and AHA survey resulted in dropping 72 markets. These markets had fewer HSAs, lower hospital participation in PCMH and/or ACO models, fewer hospital beds, fewer employees, fewer physicians, fewer hospitals, were less urban, were more likely to be non-competitive hospital markets, and have a higher for-profit marketshare than the markets that were not dropped (Additional file 6: Descriptive Statistics for Areas in Sample and those Dropped from the Sample), which could limit generalizability of our results. Second, we were unable to determine whether hospitals in a given market participated in the same or different HIOs. Without this information, our analysis is unable to examine the possible confounding effect of HIO competition on HIO presence and HIO participation. Lastly, the analyses are associative and should not be used to draw conclusions about causality. Relatedly, we are unable to say whether our key independent variables contribute to HIO *formation*, or whether our key independent variables prevent HIO *closures*. There could also be *interactions* between hospital and vendor market dynamics that our measures failed to capture. Future research should examine these as well as the impact of ambulatory provider dynamics on HIO activity [22], since a major function of HIE is to facilitate information exchange with ambulatory providers.

Conclusions

Market dynamics related to hospital competition appear to be the key factor impeding HIO presence while vendor competition may be a key factor limiting hospital participation in HIOs. Taken together these results suggest that efforts to improve HIO sustainability may need to address possible information blocking behaviors stemming from competitive vendor dynamics and make HIO participation more appealing to hospitals in competitive, larger markets, which may be best facilitated by expanding payment reform efforts and strengthening market-level incentives for valuable activities that HIOs enable.

Additional files

Additional file 1: Conceptual Model. Conceptual model illustrating relationship between hospital and EHR vendor market dynamics, costs and benefits of HIO, perceived value of HIO, HIO presence, and level of participation in HIO. (DOCX 71 kb)

Additional file 2: Logistic Regression Model for HIO Presence in Markets with different Hospital and Vendor Characteristics. Sensitivity Analysis Results from Logistic Regression Model. (DOCX 172 kb)

Additional file 3: Continuous Variable Models for HIO Presence and Level of Participation in HIOs. Sensitivity Analysis Results from Continuous Variable Models (DOCX 93 kb)

Additional file 4: Robustness Test for Multicollinearity, Linear Probability Model. Sensitivity Analysis Results from Probability Models testing for Multicollinearity. (DOCX 109 kb)

Additional file 5: Robustness Test for Multicollinearity, Coefficients for Linear Regression Model. Sensitivity Analysis Results from Linear Regression Models testing for Multicollinearity. (DOCX 104 kb)

Additional file 6: Descriptive Statistics for Areas in Sample and those Dropped from the Sample. Descriptive Statistics for In and Out of Sample Observations. (DOCX 76 kb)

Abbreviations

ACO: Accountable Care Organization; AHA: American Hospital Association; ANOVA: Analysis of Variance; CMS: Centers for Medicare & Medicaid Services; EHR: Electronic Health Record; HHI: Herfindahl-Hirschman Index; HIE: Health Information Exchange; HIO: Health Information Organization; HITECH: The Health Information Technology for Economic and Clinical Health (HITECH) Act; HRR: Health Referral Region; HSA: Health Service Area; OLS: Ordinary Least Squares; PCMH: Patient Centered Medical Home

Acknowledgements

The authors would like to thank Jordan Everson for his assistance with refining the methods used in this study.

Authors' contributions

SCL conceived the research question, designed the study, analyzed the data, and drafted the manuscript. JAM helped designed the study, interpret the results, and draft the manuscript. Both authors read and approved the final manuscript.

Competing interests

The authors declare that they have no competing interests.

Author details

[1]Department of Health Management and Policy, School of Public Health, University of Michigan, Ann Arbor, MI, USA. [2]Department of Medicine, Center for Clinical Informatics and Improvement Research, University of California, San Francisco, CA, USA.

References

1.   Ferlie EB, Shortell SM. Improving the quality of health care in the United Kingdom and the United States: a framework for change. Milbank Q. 2001; 79(2):281–315.
2.   Kaelber DC, Bates DW. Health information exchange and patient safety. J Biomed Inform. 2007;40(6, Supplement):S40–5.
3.   Vest JR, Campion TR, Kaushal R. Challenges, alternatives, and paths to sustainability for health information exchange efforts. J Med Syst. 2013;37(6):9987.
4.   Vest JR, Greenberger MF, Garnatz A. Diverging views on health information exchange organizations. Learning Health Systems. 2017;1(3).
5.   Adler-Milstein J, Lin SC, Jha AK. The number of health information exchange efforts is declining, leaving the viability of broad clinical data exchange uncertain. Health Aff. 2016;35(7):1278–85.

6. Office of the National Coordinator for Health IT. Report to Congress: Report on Health Information Blocking. Washington, D.C.: Department of Health and Human Services; 2015.

7. Adler-Milstein J, Jha AK. Health information exchange among U.S. hospitals: who's in, who's out, and why? Healthcare. 2014;2(1):26–32.

8. Vest JR. More than just a question of technology: factors related to hospitals' adoption and implementation of health information exchange. Int J Med Inform. 2010;79(12):797–806.

9. Burke DE, Wang BBL, Wan TTH, Diana ML. Exploring Hospitals' adoption of information technology. J Med Syst. 2002;26(4):349–55.

10. Terry K. The rocky road to RHIOs. Med Econ. 2006;83(4):TCP8–TCP12.

11. Adler-Milstein J, DesRoches CM, Jha AK. Health information exchange among US hospitals. Am J Manag Care. 2011;17(11):761–8.

12. Vest JR, Gamm LD. Health information exchange: persistent challenges and new strategies. J Am Med Inform Assoc. 2010;17(3):288–94.

13. Carr K, Bangalore D, Benin A, Holmboe ES. Leveraging the benefits of health information technology to support healthcare delivery model redesign. J Healthc Inf Manag. 2006;20(1):31.

14. Miller RH, Miller BS. The Santa Barbara County care data exchange: what happened? Health Aff. 2007;26(5):w568–80.

15. Allen A. Doctors say data fees are blocking health reform. In: Politico. 2015. http://www.politico.com/story/2015/02/data-fees-health-care-reform-115402.html. Accessed 6 Nov 2017.

16. Miller AR, Tucker C. Health information exchange, system size and information silos. J Health Econ. 2014;33:28–42.

17. Yaraghi N. A sustainable business model for health information exchange platforms: the solution to interoperability in healthcare IT. Washington, D.C.: The Brookings Institution; 2015.

18. Williams C, Mostashari F, Mertz K, Hogin E, Atwal P. From the office of the National Coordinator: the strategy for advancing the exchange of health information. Health Aff. 2012;31(3):527–36.

19. Furukawa MF, Patel V, Charles D, Swain M, Mostashari F. Hospital electronic health information exchange grew substantially in 2008–12. Health Aff. 2013;32(8):1346–54.

20. Everson J. The implications and impact of 3 approaches to health information exchange: community, enterprise, and vendor-mediated health information exchange. Learning Health Systems. 2017;1(2).

21. Everson J, Adler-Milstein J. Engagement in hospital health information exchange is associated with vendor marketplace dominance. Health Aff. 2016;35(7):1286–93.

22. Grossman JM, Bodenheimer TS, McKenzie K. Hospital-physician portals: the role of competition in driving clinical data exchange. Health Aff. 2006;25(6):1629–36.

Effective behavioral intervention strategies using mobile health applications for chronic disease management

Jung-Ah Lee[1], Mona Choi[2*] (iD), Sang A Lee[3] and Natalie Jiang[4]

Abstract

Background: Mobile health (mHealth) has continuously been used as a method in behavioral research to improve self-management in patients with chronic diseases. However, the evidence of its effectiveness in chronic disease management in the adult population is still lacking. We conducted a systematic review to examine the effectiveness of mHealth interventions on process measures as well as health outcomes in randomized controlled trials (RCTs) to improve chronic disease management.

Methods: Relevant randomized controlled studies that were published between January 2005 and March 2016 were searched in six databases: PubMed, CINAHL, EMBASE, the Cochrane Library, PsycINFO, and Web of Science. The inclusion criteria were RCTs that conducted an intervention using mobile devices such as smartphones or tablets for adult patients with chronic diseases to examine disease management or health promotion.

Results: Of the 12 RCTs reviewed, 10 of the mHealth interventions demonstrated statistically significant improvement in some health outcomes. The most common features of mHealth systems used in the reviewed RCTs were real-time or regular basis symptom assessments, pre-programed reminders, or feedbacks tailored specifically to the data provided by participants via mHealth devices. Most studies developed their own mHealth systems including mobile apps. Training of mHealth systems was provided to participants in person or through paper-based instructions. None of the studies reported the relationship between health outcomes and patient engagement levels on the mHealth system.

Conclusions: Findings from mHealth intervention studies for chronic disease management have shown promising aspects, particularly in improving self-management and some health outcomes.

Keywords: Mobile applications, Disease management, Mobile health, Chronic disease management, Self-management

Background

The prevalence of chronic diseases, such as cancer, cardiovascular diseases, chronic pain, diabetes, and respiratory diseases is continuously increasing with regard to an aging society worldwide. According to the World Health Organization, chronic diseases are the leading cause of mortality in the world, accounting for more than 60% of all deaths [1]. Chronic disease is, therefore, a global burden. For example, according to the report by the Centers for Disease Control and Prevention (CDC) in the United States (US), about half of all American adults, approximately 117 million people, have one or more chronic disease conditions including heart disease, stroke, cancer, type 2 diabetes, obesity, or arthritis [2]. One in four adults in the US had two or more chronic diseases in 2012 [2]. Chronic diseases are the main cause of death among Americans, with 48% dying from cancer or heart diseases in 2010 [3]. In 2010, about 86% of Americans' health care expenditure was for chronic disease treatment [4]. Therefore, chronic disease management is now a major public health issue in the US. Likewise, managing chronic diseases is also a challenge

* Correspondence: monachoi@yuhs.ac
[2]College of Nursing, Mo-Im Kim Nursing Research Institute, Yonsei University, 50 Yonsei-ro, Seodaemun-gu, Seoul, Republic of Korea03722
Full list of author information is available at the end of the article

in other countries [5, 6]. For instance, over 40% of the population aged 15 years or older had a chronic disease condition in the European Union countries [5] and chronic diseases accounted for a substantial proportion of deaths throughout Southeast Asia [6].

With advances in mobile technologies, approaches based on mobile health (mHealth)—defined as "an area of electronic health (eHealth) with the provision of health services and information via mobile technologies such as mobile phones and Personal Digital Assistants (PDAs)" [7]—have been very popular in health care and public health [8–11]. Current evidence shows that the advantages of using mHealth devices are not only for the improvement of diagnosis and treatment but also the social connection with people [12]. Behavioral interventions using mobile applications (apps) on smartphones or tablet computers in enhancing self-management for patients with chronic diseases, such as heart failure [13] or diabetes [14], have been studied [9, 12]. For instance, a food intake diary, physical activity monitoring, and home blood sugar monitoring via mHealth systems are commonly used for diabetes management [14–16] while monitoring of weight, symptoms, and physical activity are common features of heart failure interventions [13, 17].

However, the evidence from current literature using the mHealth approach on improving health outcomes is inconsistent; some studies have shown that mHealth-based behavioral interventions are potentially effective in chronic disease management, whereas other studies did not obtain supportive results [9]. Previously, the evaluation of mHealth-based research focused on feasibility and acceptability of mHealth tools.

Rather than relying on feasibility research, which often does not utilize randomization in their intervention and/ or a control group, and often lacks an effective size, a number of systematic or integrated reviews examined randomized controlled trials (RCTs) in diabetes management. These studies have demonstrated positive physiological and behavioral outcomes as well as incentive driven outcomes with mHealth systems [14–17]. However, there is limited literature showing that mHealth approaches can be useful for the self-management in patients with other chronic diseases. Therefore, an in-depth evaluation of RCTs on interventions that employ mHealth technologies and participants' adherence to the interventions, training methods, intervention dosage, and length of follow-ups as outcomes of interest should be performed to provide recommendations on what factors make mHealth interventions effective for chronic disease management.

Thus, the purpose of this study was to perform a systematic review of RCTs using mHealth interventions for chronic disease management in adult populations to examine the effectiveness of mHealth interventions on health outcomes and process measures.

Methods

The Preferred Reporting Items for Systematic Review and Meta-Analysis (PRISMA) guidelines [18] were used in this systematic review. The PICOS (participants, interventions, comparisons, outcomes, and study design) approach was used to develop a research question to guide the search strategies and review: that is, do interventions using mobile health applications improve health outcomes and process measures for adults with chronic diseases in RCTs?

Search strategies

Searches were performed to retrieve studies that were published in peer-reviewed journals from January 2005 to March 2016, and written in English; the following databases were used: PubMed, CINAHL, EMBASE, the Cochrane Library, PsycINFO, and Web of Science. We used combinations of the key words and indexing terms such as MeSH or Emtree linked to the search domains. An example of a PubMed search strategy is as follows: for mobile interventions, *"Mobile Applications"[Mesh] OR "Cell Phones"[Mesh] OR "Computers, Handheld"[-Mesh] OR "mobile health" OR "m-health" OR mhealth OR "mobile-health" OR smartphone* OR "smart-phone*" OR "mobile phone*" OR "mobile-phone*" OR "cellular phone*" OR "cellular-phone*" OR "smart device*" OR "smart-device*" OR "tablet* PC*" OR "tablet-based" OR "tablet* device*"*; for chronic disease outcomes, *"Disease Management"[Mesh] OR "Chronic Disease/prevention and control"[Mesh] OR "Chronic Disease/therapy"[Mesh] OR "disease* manag*" OR "disease* monitor*" OR monitor* OR "health promot*" OR Promot**, and for method, *"Randomized Controlled Trial" [Publication Type] OR "Randomized Controlled Trials as Topic"[Mesh] OR "Controlled Clinical Trial"[Publication Type] OR randomized[Title/Abstract] OR randomised[Title/Abstract] OR randomly[Title/Abstract] OR "random* assign*"[Title/Abstract] OR trial*[Title/Abstract]*. Then, those three groups of search results were combined with "AND" (see Additional file 1 for search strategy for each database).

Study selection

The inclusion criteria were as follows: adult patients with chronic diseases (except diabetes) as the target population, an intervention that involved using a mobile application for smartphones or tablets, and assessing the health outcomes and process measures. The exclusion criteria were as follows: studies that focused on a healthy population, pregnant women, non-adults (i.e., adolescents and children), or healthcare providers (e.g., apps for physicians' or nurses' use only); studies that used only qualitative methods (e.g., focus groups or group/individual interviews) or simple usability tests; and studies that measured psychological outcomes only (Table 1). Two reviewers (MC and SAL) independently screened titles, abstracts, and full-text articles to decide whether an article was relevant to the review. In case of disagreement, a third person was consulted (JL). We excluded studies of diabetes management because several systematic reviews and integrated reviews have already been published to report the effectiveness of mHealth-based interventions [14–17]. Only studies published in peer-reviewed journals were included.

Data extraction
Data were extracted from the selected articles and entered into an electronic data sheet. The contents of the data sheet included year of publication, research question or purpose, study design, types of disease, types of outcome and measurement, and the main results. In instances of disagreement, each case was discussed by the authors.

Assessment of risk of bias
Selection bias (random sequence generation and allocation concealment), performance bias (blinding of participants and personnel), detection bias (blinding of outcome assessment), attrition bias (incomplete outcome data), reporting bias (selective reporting), and other biases (determined according to sample size calculation method, inclusion/exclusion criteria for patients' recruitment, comparability of baseline data, funding sources, and any other potential methodological flaw that might have influenced the overall assessment) were assessed with the tool for risk of bias given in the Cochrane Handbook for Systematic Reviews of Intervention [19]. For each risk of bias item, the studies were classified as "unclear," "low," or "high" risk of bias respectively. Two reviewers (MC and SAL) assessed the

Table 1 Inclusion and exclusion criteria

Inclusion criteria	• studies that included adult patients with chronic diseases (except diabetes) as the target population • studies that involved using a mobile application • studies that focused on disease management or health promotion
Exclusion criteria	• studies that included healthy people, pregnant women, non-adults (i.e., adolescents and children), and healthcare providers • studies that used only qualitative methods or simple usability tests • studies that measured psychological outcomes only

trials independently and disagreements between two authors were resolved via discussion.

Operational definitions of the terms used in this review
Studies on feasibility assess whether or not an intervention is appropriate for further testing, whereas studies on acceptability (which is a component of feasibility) determine how recipients react to that intervention [20]. Effectiveness is defined as an intervention study that shows statistical differences of one or more outcomes of interest measured between intervention and control groups. Health outcomes included physiological outcomes (e.g., gait and balance in patients with Parkinson's disease or fatigue in patients with cancer) and psychological outcomes (e.g., quality of life, depressive symptoms, anxiety). Process measures [21] included participants' adherence to, satisfaction with, and/or the level of engagement with mHealth systems. These process measures could be assessed via quantitative tools such as surveys or qualitative methods such as open-ended questions or a focus group interviews with intervention participants.

Results
Figure 1 shows the PRISMA flow diagram indicating the search process to select the final studies that met the inclusion criteria and thus were included in this systematic review. A study conducted by Kristjánsdóttir et al. was published as part 1 [22] and part 2 [23], which corresponded to short-term and long-term follow-ups, respectively. The results of both follow-ups were reviewed. Accordingly, the results of this systematic review are based on 12 studies from 13 published articles with quantitative evaluations.

Table 2 presents the summary of 12 RCT studies reviewed in this paper. The variety of chronic diseases managed using mobile apps included allergic rhinitis and asthma, cancer, cardiovascular diseases, chronic pain, chronic kidney disease, lung transplantation, Parkinson's disease (PD), and spinal bifida. Diabetes management using mHealth apps has been evaluated in other literature and thus was not included. Among the 12 studies reviewed, 10 studies showed statistically significant mHealth app intervention effects on some variables that were examined in each study, while two of the 12 studies reviewed showed no statistically significant mHealth intervention effects on outcomes of interest when comparing between treatment and control groups. Two studies in this review were feasibility studies aimed at testing mHealth interventions for chronic disease management [24, 25] and one study was a pilot study evaluating a smartphone-based symptom management system for chemotherapy management [26]. These studies were also listed as RCTs.

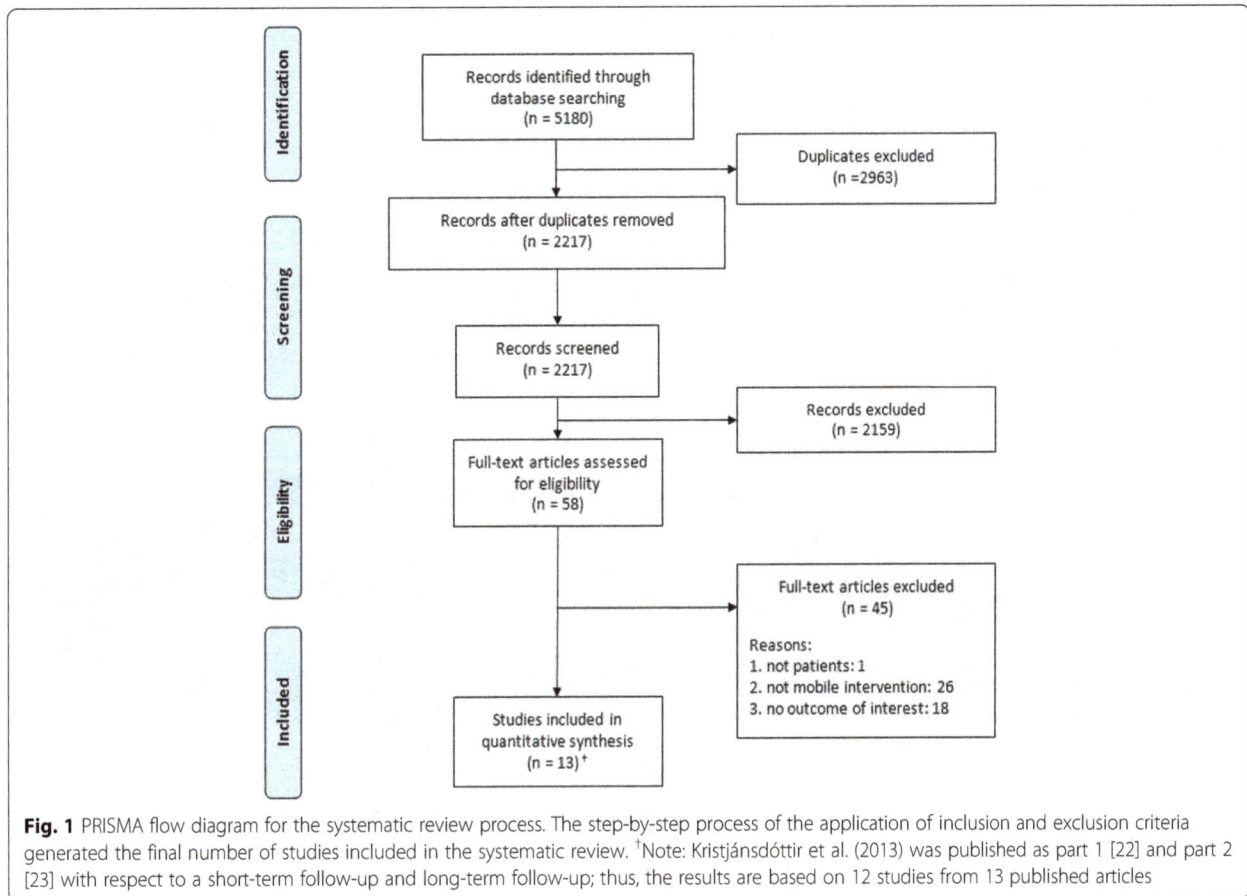

Fig. 1 PRISMA flow diagram for the systematic review process. The step-by-step process of the application of inclusion and exclusion criteria generated the final number of studies included in the systematic review. [†]Note: Kristjánsdóttir et al. (2013) was published as part 1 [22] and part 2 [23] with respect to a short-term follow-up and long-term follow-up; thus, the results are based on 12 studies from 13 published articles

Studies reporting significant effects on outcomes

The majority of mHealth RCT-studies in this systematic review (10 out of 12 studies, 83.3%) showed statistically significant effects on health outcomes by incorporating mobile applications in managing chronic diseases. Those studies demonstrated improved physical functioning, adherence to prescribed medications, and/or ease of symptom evaluation and reports to care providers, as well as process measures including patient satisfaction with mHealth management and feasibility of smart-phone-based self-management interventions.

Kearney et al. [26] in the United Kingdom reported significant improvement in fatigue (odds ratio, OR = 2.29; 95% CI, 1.04–5.05; $P = 0.040$) and hand-foot syndrome (OR control/intervention $= 0.39$; 95% CI, 0.17–0.92; $P = 0.031$) in patients with lung, breast, and colorectal cancer using a mobile phone-based remote monitoring of chemotherapy-related symptoms in comparison to the usual care group. In Norway, Kristjánsdóttir et al. [22, 23] showed a favorable effect on pain management in a 4-week follow-up (catastrophizing score lower for *Intervention, M* = 9.20, SD = 5.85, compared to *Control, M* = 15.71, SD = 9.22, $P < 0.01$, with a large effect size, Cohen's $d = 0.87$) but not in the 5-month and 11-month follow-ups (outcome variables

including catastrophizing, acceptance, functioning, and symptom level, all $P > 0.1$). In Spain, Garcia-Palacios et al. [27] developed an ecological momentary assessment (EMA) for chronic pain in fibromyalgia patients and found that patients with less familiarity with technology using a mobile EMA system via their smartphones showed higher levels of compliance than patients with a paper-based diary (complete record $t = -4.446$, $d = 1.02$, reference Cohen's $d > = 0.8$, large effect). In Turkey, Cingi et al. [28] reported that patients with allergic rhinitis or asthma displayed better quality of life or well-controlled asthma scores by using the mHealth intervention compared to the control group (all $P < 0.05$). Dicianno et al. [24] demonstrated the feasibility of a mHealth intervention for patients with spina bifida to improve self-management skills and high usage of the mobile system was associated with positive changes in the self-management skills. In Sweden, Hägglund et al. [29] tested a tablet-based intervention in patients with heart failure (HF) and found improved self-care and health-related quality of life (HRQoL) and a reduction in HF-related hospital days (risk ratio, RR = 0.38; 95% CI, 0.31–0.46; $P < 0.05$). In Israel, Ginis et al. [25] conducted home-based smartphone-delivery automated feedback training for gait in people with PD, and found significant

Table 2 Summary of studies reviewed

Year/Author/Country	Purpose of Study	Sample	Types of Disease	Types of Outcomes and Measurements	Main Results
2009 Kearney et al. United Kingdom	To evaluate the impact of a mobile phone-based remote monitoring, advanced symptom management system (ASyMS©) on the incidence, severity and distress of six chemotherapy-related symptoms in patients with lung, breast, or colorectal cancer.	*n* = 112 (56 in each intervention or control group) patients from 7 clinical sites throughout the UK. Inclusion criteria: commencing a new course of chemotherapy treatment, receiving outpatient chemotherapy, age ≥ 18, written informed consent given, able to read and write English, and deemed by members of the clinical team as being physically and psychologically fit to participate in the study.	Chemotherapy related toxicity in patients with lung, breast, or colorectal cancer	• Severity and distress of the six symptoms including vomiting, nausea, diarrhea, hand-foot syndrome, sore mouth/throat, and fatigue. • Incidence – (did symptom occur? Y/N), Severity and distress (scores 0–3) of the six individual symptoms. • ASyMS has integrated the Common Toxicity Criteria Adverse Events (CTCAE) grading system and the Chemotherapy Symptom Assessment Scale. • Paper version of the electronic symptom questionnaire was administrated at baseline, chemotherapy cycles 2, 3, 4, and 5 in both groups.	• Two of the six symptoms measured (fatigue and hand-foot syndrome) showed statistical significance between the control and intervention groups (respectively, $p = 0.040$, $p = 0.031$). • Patients reported improved communication with health professionals, improvements in the management of their symptoms, and feeling reassured their symptoms were being monitored while at home when using ASyMS.
2013 Kristjánsdóttir et al. Norway	To study the long term effects of a 4-week smartphone intervention with diaries and therapist feedback following an inpatient chronic pain rehabilitation program (11-month follow up of 2013 Kristjánsdóttir et al. study)	*n* = 135 (intervention group: 69/control group: 66) Inclusion criteria: female, age ≥ 18, participating in the inpatient multidimensional rehabilitation program for chronic widespread pain, having chronic widespread pain > 6 months (with or without diagnosis of fibromyalgia), not participating in another research project at the rehab center, being able to use a smartphone, and not being diagnosed with a profound psychiatric disorder.	Chronic widespread pain or Fibromyalgia	• Catastrophizing [Pain catastrophizing scale (PCS)] • Acceptance [Chronic pain acceptance questionnaire (CPAQ)] • Emotional distress [modified General Health Questionnaire (GHQ)] • Importance and success in living according to one's own values in 6 domains (family, intimate relationships, friendship, work, health, and personal growth) [Chronic Pain Values Inventory (CPVI)] • Pain, fatigue, sleep disturbance [Visual analog scales (VAS)] • Impact of Fibromyalgia on functioning and symptom levels the past week [Fibromyalgia Impact Questionnaire (FIQ)] • Functioning [Short-Form Health Survey (SF-8)] • Use of noninteractive website [self-report at T3 (4 weeks after discharge)]	Short-term follow-up results: • Intervention group reported less catastrophizing ($p < 0.001$). • Results from the per-protocol analysis indicate intervention with diaries and written personalized feedback reduced catastrophizing and increased acceptance and effects persisted 5 months after the intervention. • Increased improvement in values-based living in the intervention group • Control group showed an increased level of fatigue and a tendency toward an increase in sleep disturbance at the 5-month follow-up. Long-term 11-month follow-up results: • The between-group differences on catastrophizing, acceptance, functioning, and symptom level

Table 2 Summary of studies reviewed (Continued)

Year/Author/Country	Purpose of Study	Sample	Types of Disease	Types of Outcomes and Measurements	Main Results
				· Feasibility of the smartphone intervention (single question for post-intervention)	were no longer evident (p > 0.10). · More improvement in catastrophizing scores during the follow-up period (T2-T5) in the intervention group (p = 0.045) · Positive effect on acceptance was found within the intervention group (p < 0.001). · Small to large negative effects were found within the control group on functioning and symptom levels, emotional distress, and fatigue (p = 0.05). · Reduction in disease impact (measured by FIQ) found for intervention group (p = 0.03). · Long-term results are ambiguous.
2013 Garcia-Palacios et al. Spain	To compare compliance with paper diary vs. smartphone diary, aggregated ecological momentary assessment (EMA) data vs. retrospective data, and assess acceptability of EMA procedures.	n = 40 (intervention group:20/control group:20) Inclusion criteria: met criteria for FMS, defined by the American College of Rheumatology and were diagnosed by a rheumatologist.	Fibromyalgia syndrome (FMS)	· EMA pain and fatigue (0–10 Numerical Rating Scales) · Mood (face-based pictorial 7-point scale) · Weekly retrospective rating of pain and fatigue [Brief Pain Inventory (BPI) and Brief Fatigue Inventory (BFI)] · Acceptability and preferences (self-report)	· Smartphone condition (smartphone diary) showed higher levels of compliance than paper condition (paper diary) (p < 0.01). · Retrospective assessment produces overestimation of events (pain and fatigue, p < 0.01). · Smartphone condition preferred and accepted over paper diary, even in participants with low familiarity with technology.
2014 Vuorinen et al. Finland	To study whether multidisciplinary care with telemonitoring leads to decreased HF-related hospitalization	n = 94 (intervention group: 47/ control group: 47) Inclusion criteria: diagnosis of systolic heart failure, age 18–90 years, NYHA (New Work Heart	Heart failure (HF)	· Number of HF-related hospital days (data from hospital electronic health record system) · Clinical effectiveness [death from any cause, heart transplant operation or listing for transplant operation, left ventricular ejection fraction (LVEF,%)	· No difference found in the number of HF-related hospital days (p = 0.351). · Intervention group used more health care resources. · No statistically significant differences in patients' clinical health status or self-care behavior.

Table 2 Summary of studies reviewed (Continued)

Year/Author/Country	Purpose of Study	Sample	Types of Disease	Types of Outcomes and Measurements	Main Results
		Association) functional class ≥2, left ventricular ejection fraction ≤35%, need for a regular check-up visit, and time from the last visit of less than 6 months.		measured by echocardiography, plasma concentration of N-terminal of the prohormone brain natriuretic peptide (NT-proBNP, ng/1), creatinine, sodium, and potassium] • Self-care behavior (European Heart Failure Self-Care Behavior Scale) • Use of health care resources (analyzed outpatient visits)	
2015 Cingi et al. Turkey	To investigate the impact of a mobile patient engagement application on health outcomes and quality of life	$n = 2282$ interventions (physician on call patient engagement trial, POPET for patients with allergic rhinitis or asthma) POPET-AR (intervention group: 88/control group: 51) POPET-Asthma (intervention group: 60/ control group:29)	Allergic rhinitis (AR) and asthma patients	• Health outcomes and quality of life [AR groups: Rhinitis Quality of Life Questionnaire (RQLQ), asthma groups: Asthma Control Test (ACT)]	• POPET-AR group showed better clinical improvement than the control group in terms of overall RQLQ score as well as measures of general problems, activity, symptoms other than nose/eye, and emotion domains ($p < 0.05$). • More patients in the POPET-Asthma group achieved a well-controlled asthma score compared to the control group ($p < 0.05$).
2015 Dicianno et al. United States	To determine feasibility of the interactive mobile health and rehabilitation (iMHere) system and its effects on psychosocial and medical outcomes	$n = 23$ (intervention group:13/ control group:10) Inclusion criteria: age 18–40, primary diagnosis of myelomeningocele with hydrocephalus, ability to use smartphone, and living within 100 miles of testing site to allow for technical support.	Spina bifida (SB)	• Usage (the number of participant responses to reminders, use of secure messaging, or photo uploads) • Physical independence (Craig Handicap Assessment and Reporting Technique Short Form, Physical independence domain) • Self management skill (Adolescent Self-Management and Independence Scale II) • Depressive symptoms (The Beck Depression Inventory-II) • Perception of patient-centered care	• Smartphone system was found to be feasible and associated with short-term self-reported improvements in self-management skills.

Table 2 Summary of studies reviewed (Continued)

Year/Author/Country	Purpose of Study	Sample	Types of Disease	Types of Outcomes and Measurements	Main Results
				(Patient Assessment of Chronic Illness Care) • Quality of Life (World Health Organization Quality of Life Brief Instrument) • Number of UTIs (diagnosed UTIs) • Number of wounds (unique skin breakdown episodes that were at least stage II) • Number of emergency department (ED) visits (ED visits for any reason) • Number of ED visits due to UTI or wound • Number of planned and unplanned hospitalizations • Number of hospitalizations due to UTI or wound	
2015 Hägglund et al. Sweden	To evaluate whether a home intervention system (HIS) using a tablet had an effect on self-care behavior.	n = 82 (intervention group: 42/control group:40) Inclusion criteria: hospitalized and diagnosed for HF with reduced ejection fraction (HFrEF) and/or preserved EF (HFpEF), treatment with diuretics, and referred straight to primary care.	Heart failure (HF)	• Disease-specific self-care (European Heart Failure Self-Care Behavior Scale) • Health-related quality of life (HRQoL) (Kansas City Cardiomyopathy Questionnaire) • Adherence (frequency of HIS use) • Knowledge (Dutch Heart Failure Knowledge Scale) • HF-related hospital days (patients' case books)	• Intervention group showed improvement in self-care and HRQoL, reduction in HF-related hospital days.
2015 Martin et al. United States	To investigate whether a fully automated mHealth intervention with tracking and texting components increases physical activity.	n = 48 [unblinded = 32 (smart texts = 16, no texts = 16), blinded = 16] Unblinded participants were randomized to smart texts or no texts in phase II (weeks 4–5). Inclusion criteria: ages 18–69, using a Fitbug compatible smartphone (iPhone≥4S, Galaxy≥S3).	Cardiovascular disease (CVD)	• Mean change in accelerometer-measured daily step count (measured by Fitbug Orb) • Attainment of prescribed 10,000 steps/day goal (measured by Fitbug Orb) • Changes in total daily activity and aerobic time (measured by Fitbug Orb)	• Intervention with texting component increased physical activity (p < 0.001).
2015 Piette et al. United States	To compare the effects of systematic feedback to HF patients' caregivers and HF patients receiving standard mHealth.	n = 372 (intervention group:189/ control group: 183) Inclusion criteria: HF diagnosis, ejection fraction < 40%, able to name eligible CarePartner	Heart failure (HF)	• HF-related quality of life (Minnesota Living with Heart Failure Questionnaire) • Patient-CP communication (quantitative telephone surveys) • Medication adherence and self-care (Revised Heart Failure Self-Care Behavior Scale)	• mHealth + CP (intervention) group showed improvement in medication adherence and caregiver communication. • mHealth + CP may improve qualify of life in patients with greater depressive symptoms and also decrease patients'

Table 2 Summary of studies reviewed (Continued)

Year/Author/Country	Purpose of Study	Sample	Types of Disease	Types of Outcomes and Measurements	Main Results
		(CP) that is a relative or friend living outside their home.			risk of shortness of breath and sudden weight gains.
2016 Cubo et al. Spain	To evaluate the cost-effectiveness of home-based motor monitoring (HBMM) with in-office visits versus in-office visits alone in patients with advanced Parkinson's disease	n = 40 (intervention group: 20/control group: 20) Inclusion criteria: non-demented outpatients from a tertiary regional movement disorders clinic, Mini-Mental Scale score > 24, and di agnosed with i diopathic, advanced PD.	Parkinson's disease (PD)	• Motor (Unified Parkinson's Disease Rating Scale and Hoehn and Yahr staging Scale) and non-motor (Non-Motor Symptoms Questionnaire Scale) symptom severities • Cost-effectiveness (incremental cost-effectiveness ratio) • Direct costs (standardized questionnaire) • Quality of life (EuroQoL) • Neuropsychiatric symptoms (Hospital Anxiety Depression Scale, Parkinson Psychiatric Rating Scale) • Comorbidities (Cumulative Illness Rating scale-Geriatric)	• HBMM was found to be cost-effective in improvement of functional status, motor severity, and motor complications.
2016 DeVito Dabbs et al. United States	To compare the efficacy of an mHealth intervention in promoting self-management behaviors and self-care agency, rehospitalization, and mortality at home during the first year after lung transplantation.	n = 201 (intervention group: 99/control group: 102) Inclusion criteria: age > 18, received transplantation at the University of Pittsburgh Medical Center, and could read and speak English.	Lung transplant recipients (LTRs)	• Self-monitoring (percentage of days that LTRs performed self-monitoring) • Adherence to regimen (Health Habits Survey) • Critical health (percentage of critical indicators) • Self-care agency (Perception of Self-Care Agency) • Health outcomes (medical records)	• The intervention group performed self-monitoring ($p < 0.001$), adhered to medical regimen. ($p = 0.046$), and reported abnormal health indicators ($p < 0.001$) more frequently. Than the usual care group. • Both groups did not differ in re-hospitalization ($p = 0.51$) or mortality ($p = 0.25$).
2016 Ginis et al. Israel and Belgium	To determine the feasibility and effectiveness of the gait training CuPiD-system for people with Parkinson's disease in the home environment.	n = 40 (intervention group: 22/control group: 18) Inclusion criteria: ability to walk 0 min continuously, score of ≥24 on Montreal Cognitive Assessment, Hoehn and Yahr Stage II to III in ON-state, and on stable PD medication.	Parkinson's disease (PD)	• Single and dual task gait (gait speed) • Balance (mini-Balance Evaluation Systems Test, Four Square Step Test, Falls Efficacy Scale-International) • Endurance and physical capacity (2 Minute Walk Test,	The CuPiD-system was feasible and effective, as the intervention group improved significantly more on balance and maintained quality of life compared to the control group.

Table 2 Summary of studies reviewed *(Continued)*

Year/Author/Country	Purpose of Study	Sample	Types of Disease	Types of Outcomes and Measurements	Main Results
				Physical Activity Scale for the Elderly) • Disease severity (Movement Disorders Unified Parkinson's Disease Rating Scale – motor examination) • Freezing of gait (New FOG Questionnaire, Ziegler protocol) • Cognition (Color Trail Test A & B, sitting & walking verbal fluency) Quality of life (Short Form 36 Health Survey)	

improvement in balance $(F_{(2,108)} = 3.73, P = 0.04)$ from baseline to post-test.

Martin et al. [30] in the US found that an automated text message system increased physical activity to prevent cardiovascular diseases in phase 1 (weeks 2 to 3) and phase 2 (weeks 4 to 5), all $P < 0.001$. Piette et al. [31] in the US reported that the intervention group involving "CarePartners" connecting to a relative or friend living outside their home showed improvement in medication adherence and caregiver communication (all $P < 0.05$). DeVito Dabbs et al. [32] in the US conducted an RCT for patients with lung transplantation and reported improvement in self-monitoring (OR = 5.11; 95% CI, 2.95–8.87; $P < 0.001$), adherence to medical regimen (OR =1.64; 95% CI, 1.01–2.66, $P = 0.046$), and reported abnormal health indicators more frequently (OR = 8.9; 95% CI, 3.60–21.99; $P < 0.001$).

Studies reporting similar or no effects on outcomes

Two of the twelve studies reviewed (16.7%) showed similar or no effects of mHealth-based interventions on main outcomes of interest compared to control groups. In Finland, Vuorinen et al. [33] found no difference in the number of HF-related hospital days (incidence rate ratio, IRR = 0.812, $P = 0.351$). However, patients in the telemonitoring intervention group used more healthcare resources; increased number of visits to the nurse (IRR = 1.73; 95% CI, 1.38–2.15; $P < 0.001$), more time spent with nurses (mean difference = 48.7 min, $P < 0.001$), and increased number of telephone contacts initiated by nurses (IRR = 5.6; 95% CI, 3.41–7.63; $P < 0.001$). In Spain, Cubo et al. [34] reported a trend of lower PD functional status (the Unified Parkinson's Disease Rating Scale, UPDRS I) in patients on home-based monitoring compared to patients in standard in-office visits ($P = 0.06$), while other outcomes (measured by UPDRS II, III, IV subscales) and HRQoL in PD did not show statistically significant differences between the intervention and control groups. Cubo et al. [34], however, explained that the approach of using home-based motor monitoring via mHealth applications compared to standard office visits in the 1-year follow up was cost-effective (incremental cost-effectiveness ratio, ICER, per unit of UPDRS subscales ranging from €126.72 to € 701.31).

mHealth interventions

Table 3 presents the details of mHealth interventions including duration, mobile app type, app content, and training methods. A quarter of the studies (3 out of 12) reported the feasibility of the mHealth intervention as a pilot study to assess the potential for successful implementation of the mHealth intervention to patients/participants [24–26]. The majority of studies used smartphones as a mobile device, two studies

[29, 34] used tablets for mHealth interventions, and two studies used telemonitoring wireless devices including weight scales for patients with HF [29] or gait detectors for patients with PD [25]. The length of interventions ranged from two weeks to twelve months; half of the studies (6/12, 50%) had more than six-month intervention periods and follow-ups. Most common components of mHealth interventions included remote symptom monitoring and self-assessment as well as tailored automated messages or self-care education to coach patients with chronic disease conditions that needed active disease management. One particular study by Kearney et al. was more inclusive in that it provided real-time feedback and tailored such feedback for symptom management depending on the severity, offering pharmacological, nutritional, or behavioral advice when needed [26].

The sample size of the studies reviewed was between 28 (patients with spina bifida) and 372 (patients with heart failure). In terms of subjects, studies included patients who were 18 years and above, with some studies limited to a particular age range such as 18–40 [24] or up to 69 years [30]. The mean age of participants in the mHealth intervention studies ranged from 30-year-old patients with spina bifida [24] to 75-year-old patients with HF [29]; the approximate average age group in this 12-study review was in the 50s. None of the studies reported effectiveness of mHealth intervention by age categories. These 12 studies also did not report participants' prior experience with mobile devices such as smartphones or educational background, which may have affected the ability to use mHealth apps via mobile devices. Outcomes of interventions were measured either by mHealth systems directly or by paper-based questionnaires.

In terms of mHealth intervention training, either face-to-face information sessions at baseline or paper-based instructions were used in most studies. Kearney et al. [26] found that symptoms were reported differently on a paper-based questionnaire and mobile phone. Participants in the mobile group reported lower levels of fatigue compared to those in the paper-based group (OR $_{non-mobile/mobile}$ = 2.29, 95% CI 1.04–5.05, $P = 0.04$) [26]. Reporting cancer toxicity symptoms (e.g., hand-foot syndrome and mucositis) in real time might allow for more accurate measurement [26].

None of the studies reported process measures, including adherence, level of engagement, and/or satisfaction with the mHealth systems. Potentially, there was limited information on such measures in the published articles with the authors possibly publishing the process measures elsewhere.

Table 3 Details of mobile application intervention for chronic disease management

Study	Length of Intervention	Name of Mobile Application and Platform	Program of Intervention	Delivery of Intervention (Training of mHealth)
2009 Kearney et al. United Kingdom	Five time pointes (baseline, chemotherapy cycle 2, 3, 4, and; each cycle has up to 14 days).	Advanced symptom management system (ASyMS©)	• A mobile phone-based remote monitoring and reporting of chemotherapy-related toxicity. • Participants completed the electronic symptom questionnaire on their mobile phone, took their temperature using an electronic thermometer and entered the value into the application twice a day for 2 weeks after their first 4 cycles of chemotherapy • Patients received tailored self-care advice on their mobile phone based on the severity of symptoms reported	Patients were trained on how to use the system by nurses working in their local clinic who had received training by the study team on how to use the system.
2013 Kristjánsdóttir et al. Norway	4 weeks	Application: Diaries and Daily Situational Feedback Smartphone: HTC TyTN (touchscreen and keyboard)	• The intervention consisted of 4 components: face-to-face session – 1 h individual session with nurse, web-based diaries – 3 diary entries/ day using the smartphone, written situational feedback – daily written feedback from therapist on information provided in diary, and audio files – 4 mindfulness exercises guided by the authors • All participants received access to a non-interactive website with information on self-management strategies for people with chronic pain • Self-reported assessments on paper were gathered before (T1) and after (T2) the inpatient program, immediately after the smartphone intervention which was 4 weeks after discharge (T3), and 5 (T4) and 11 months (T5) after the smartphone intervention	Patients attended an informational group meeting. Participants were lent smartphones and received information about their therapist for the intervention during the face-to-face session.
2013 Garcia-Palacios et al. Spain	2 weeks	Software application: F-EMA (ecological momentary assessment) Smartphone: HTC Diamond 1 (TOUCH Diamond 1, HTC Corporation, New Taipei City, Taiwan) Software: Windows Mobile 6.1	• Session 1 (7 days): participants were randomly assigned a self-record condition and recorded their pain, fatigue, and mood 3 times/day • Session 2 (7 days): acceptability questionnaire and Brief Pain Inventory (BPI) and Brief Fatigue inventory (BFI) were administered regarding the first condition, and participants received the other self-record condition • Session 3: acceptability questionnaire, BPI and BFI, and preference questionnaire were administered regarding the second condition	Participants attended an individual information session during the first week. They were given verbal instructions on the self-record method, explanations of the scales, and practiced rating the scales with the researcher. An information sheet with definitions of each scale and instructions for the self-recording were given to each patient.

Table 3 Details of mobile application intervention for chronic disease management *(Continued)*

Study	Length of Intervention	Name of Mobile Application and Platform	Program of Intervention	Delivery of Intervention (Training of mHealth)
2014 Vuorinen et al. Finland	6 months	Application name not available. Application enabled recording of all necessary measurements and symptoms.	• Patient made measurements (blood pressure, pulse, and body weight), assessed symptoms (dizziness, dyspnea, palpitation, weakness, and edema), and evaluated overall condition (deteriorated, improved, or remained unchanged) once a week • Patient received automatic machine-based feedback of whether parameter was within personal targets set by nurse • Nurse contacted patient each time measurement was beyond target levels	Patients given a home-care package: weight scale, blood pressure meter, mobile phone, and self-care instructions.
2015 Cingi et al. Turkey	1 month (patients with allergic rhinitis(AR)), 3 months (asthma patients)	Application: physician on call patient engagement trial (POPET-AR; POPET-Asthma)	• The application allowed patients to communicate with their physician, record their health status and medication compliance • Provided motivational and educational content • Reminded patients to take prescribed medications	Patients were educated on the recommended use of prescribed medications and informed about the Rhinitis Quality of Life Questionnaire and the Asthma Control Test. Trial information, application training, and technical support was available online.
2015 Dicianno et al. United States	12 months	Application: iMHere Smartphone: Android Provided participants with a phone plan that included unlimited texting and data.	• Intervention consisted of 6 modules, a web-based clinician portal, and a 2-way communication system • Modules served as reminders to perform various self-care tasks, record wounds, manage medications, complete mood surveys, and for secure messaging • Patient problems were triaged on a web-based dashboard for physicians	Participants were instructed to use the modules based on their own prescribed protocols.
2015 Hagglund et al. Sweden	3 months	Application: HIS: OPTILOGG Tablet wirelessly connected to weight scale.	• HIS monitored weight and symptoms, titrated diuretics, and provided information about HF and lifestyle advice	Intervention group received a basal information sheet. The HIS was installed in their home.
2015 Martin et al. United States	5 weeks	Smartphone application: Fitbug Digital physical activity tracker: Fitbug Orb Smartphone texting system: Reify	• Automated mHealth intervention with tracking and texting components • Unblinded participants could view their daily step count, activity time, and aerobic activity time through smartphone and web interfaces;	No training mentioned.

Table 3 Details of mobile application intervention for chronic disease management *(Continued)*

Study	Length of Intervention	Name of Mobile Application and Platform	Program of Intervention	Delivery of Intervention (Training of mHealth)
			blinded participants were unable to view this information • Smart texts delivered coaching 3 times/day aimed at individual encouragement and fostering feedback loops by an automated, physician written, theory-based algorithm with a goal of 10,00 steps/day	
2015 Piette et al. United States	12 months	mHealth application was not mentioned. Intervention used interactive voice response (IVR) telephone calls.	• Standard mHealth group received weekly interactive voice response (IVR) calls with tailored self-management advice • mHealth + CarePartner (CP) group received the same intervention but with automated emails sent to their CP after each IVR call with feedback about the heart failure (HF) patient's status and suggestions to support disease care • CP called their patient-partner weekly to review reports and address identified problems	Both groups were mailed information about HF self-care. CPs received guidelines about how to communicate in a positive motivating way, avoid conflict by respecting boundaries, include in-home caregivers, and respect confidentiality.
2016 Cubo et al. Spain	12 months	System: Kinesia, included tablet software app, wireless finger-worn motion sensor unit, and auto-mated web-based symptom reporting.	• All patients with Parkinson's disease (PD) completed structured questionnaires and were assessed under the beneficial effect of the antiparkinsonian drugs in the clinic every 4 months following the same protocol • PD motor symptoms were monitored at home 1 day/month with 3–6 motor assessments and a structured questionnaire in the HBMM group	Assistant brought Kinesia device and provided training in each participant's home.
2016 DeVito Dabbs et al. United States	12 months	Program: Pocket Personal Assistant for Tracking Health (Pocket PATH)	• Participants recorded daily health indicators, viewed graphical displays of trends, and received automatic feedback messages when reaching critical threshold values using the Pocket PATH system	Patients received scripted discharge instructions from an interventionist and an instruction binder emphasizing the importance of performing daily self-management behaviors at home in 60 min training sessions.
2016 Ginis et al. Israel and Belgium	6 weeks	CuPiD-system: smartphone (Galaxy S3-mini, Samsung, South Korea), docking station, 2 inertial measurement units (EXLs3, EXEL srl., Italy), and 2 applications (the audio-bio feedback, ABF-gait app, the instrumented cueing for freezing of gait, FOG-cue app)	• The CuPiD-system measured gait in real-time, provided positive and corrective auditory biofeedback (ABF) on gait parameters, and rhythmical auditory cueing to prevent or overcome freezing of gait (FOG) episodes	Researchers provided gait training to CuPiD participants for 30 min, 3 times/week for 6 weeks. Participants with FOG were taught ways to avoid FOG and practiced for an additional 30 min, 3 times/week using the FOG-cue app. Pictures and personalized instructions were also given to participants. Telephone consultation was available for system support.

Risk of bias assessment

The risk of bias in the reviewed studies is summarized in Fig. 2 and shown for individual studies in Fig. 3. The intervention studies generally performed well in their risk of bias for random sequence generation (62% low risk), allocation concealment (23% low risk), blinding of participants and personnel (8% low risk), blinding of outcome assessors (15% low risk), incomplete outcome data (69% low risk), and selective reporting (92% low risk) (Fig. 2).

Considering the method of randomization, 5 trials did not present details of randomization [25, 27, 29, 30, 33]. Only 2 studies reported use of an adequate allocation concealment method [22, 32]. Although due to the nature of the mHealth intervention, it is almost impossible to blind participants and healthcare providers, one study described the blinding of participants by providing the same mobile phone application to both experimental and control groups with different functionalities. The experimental group was given communication, health status, or medication usage tracking, and a survey questionnaire, whereas the control group received only the survey questionnaire [28]. Only two trials were identified as blinding the outcome assessors. Four trials failed to provide a full description of participants and losses to follow-up during their trials [24, 28, 29, 31]. All studies had a low risk for reporting bias. Devito et al. had low risk for all items except blinding of participants and personnel [32]. Hägglund et al. had low risk only for reporting bias [29] (Fig. 3).

Discussion

This systematic review has found a potential favorable effect of mHealth interventions on health outcomes and process measures in patients with chronic diseases including asthma, cancer, cardiovascular diseases, chronic pain, spina bifida, or Parkinson's disease. The results from the reviewed RCTs showed improvement in some health outcomes in patients in managing their chronic disease.

There were some commonalities and differences in using mHealth in the reviewed studies. One of the common features useful in mHealth interventions is pre-set and tailored feedback on reported symptoms. The mobile application systems used in the reviewed studies were developed by the study team and validated and refined in the previous studies that were conducted before the RCTs. None of the commercial health apps were used in the reviewed studies. Most studies utilized research staff to provide training in mHealth systems for the participants via face-to-face or information group sessions, or through information materials, while one study [26] used local nurses to train patients. None of the reviewed studies addressed whether their mHealth systems were incorporated into daily medical practice in either clinic settings or acute care hospitals, meaning that there were no signs of their implementation in real health care systems. Challenges in real-life settings may relate to lack of financial incentives for providers in using mHealth tools or uncertainty regarding privacy and security of information transferred via mHealth systems [35].

Interventions to promote self-management in patients with chronic diseases started from web-based and/or telephone-based interventions to mHealth-based interventions. Unlike those previous behavioral interventions limited to places where patients with chronic diseases had access to the treatment advice, mHealth interventions have advanced features such as real-time symptom monitoring and feedback [25, 34, 36]. For example, patients with PD receive real-time feedback on their selected gait parameters during their walks via the preset gait app developed from evidence-based exercise guidelines [25]. This is an example of how using well-designed and validated mHealth apps in daily life can benefit health outcomes.

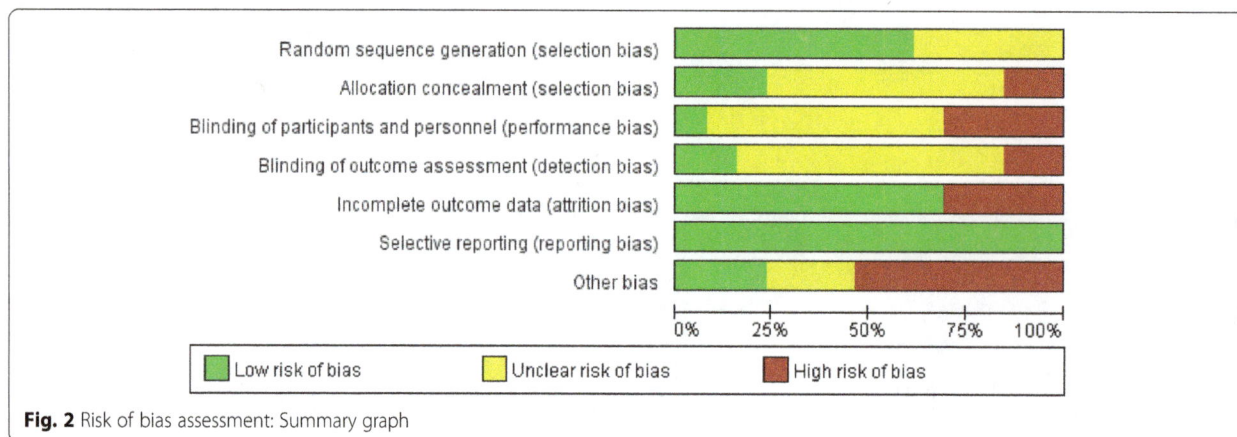

Fig. 2 Risk of bias assessment: Summary graph

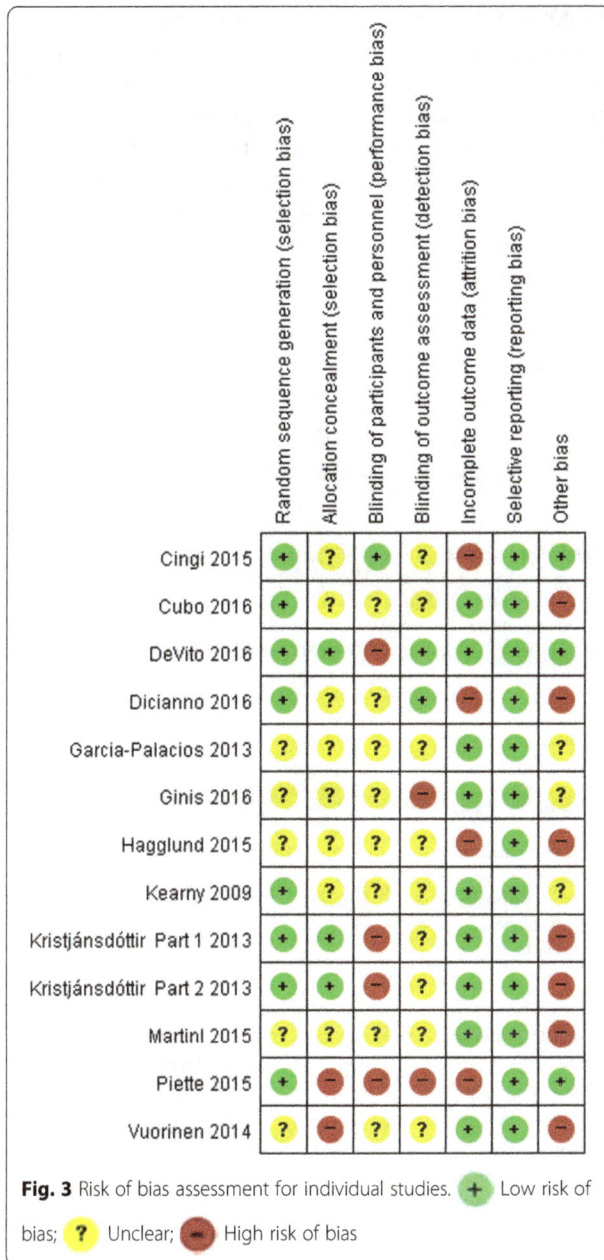

Fig. 3 Risk of bias assessment for individual studies. ⊕ Low risk of bias; ? Unclear; ⊝ High risk of bias

disease management. Piette et al. [31] studied the comparative effectiveness of mHealth interventions supporting HF patients and their family caregivers and showed improvement for medication adherence and caregiver communication. The impact of including caregivers as a part of mHealth users—one of the care supporting groups—on actual patients' health outcomes should continue to be studied in the context of an increasing aging society.

Moreover, long-term follow-ups of responses from patients and caregivers who have used mHealth need to be evaluated. Areas that need to be studied include the optimum length of time and frequency of the mHealth delivery system as well as type of technology and training. For example, effective frequencies of automated reminders or coaching messages, when additional reminders should be sent, and when people become tired or irritated by automated messages need to be studied. Users of mHealth might experience fatigue from automated reminders and eventually mHealth interventions could become ineffective. Other systematic reviews on chronic disease management showed that the frequency of input into mHealth systems was a burden on participants and affected the attrition rate [17]. In this review, the length of the intervention in the 12 studies varied from 2 weeks to 12 months; 5 of 12 studies (about 42%) had less than 2-month interventions while 4 studies (about 33%) had 1 year of intervention. The positive health outcomes of the various studies were not directly related to the length of the intervention or training methods of mHealth in the reviewed studies.

One aspect of mHealth approaches that also needs to be considered is effective clinical communication between patients and healthcare professionals who need to respond to patients' questions via mHealth systems. Cingi et al. [28] reported healthcare providers (i.e., residents) expressed an improvement in communication with patients via mHealth; however, they found that using mHealth tools as the primary method of communication was strongly opposed by the healthcare providers. Vuorinen et al. [33] also reported a significant increase in the communication (i.e., telephone contacts) between nurses and patients which in turn increased the nurses' workload during the trial. One recommendation for reducing health care providers' workload in mHealth interventions is using advanced technology to respond to patients' questions regarding symptoms assessed and reported via the mHealth systems.

While considering positive health outcomes (e.g., reduction of hospital readmission for HF-related conditions or medication adherence) of patients with chronic diseases, burden of healthcare professionals should be measured as an outcome of mHealth interventions. An adequate triage system can decrease healthcare

The number of smartphone users has shown great increases; in the US [37] it is estimated to reach 224.3 million in 2017, up from 171 million in 2014; worldwide it was [38] 2.32 billion in 2017, up from 1.57 billion in 2014. Approximately 77% of people in the US owned smartphones in 2016 [39]. Using mobile devices for mHealth is essential nowadays and approaches of mHealth vary from sending text messaging for medical appointment reminders to monitoring and assessing symptoms in real-time, virtually at any location via wireless networks. Interventions using mHealth have also eased medical coaching for caregivers as care partners with healthcare professionals for effective chronic

professionals' response time for emergency needs reported by mHealth users [28].

Common recommendations discussed in the studies of this systematic review to improve mHealth interventions include a simple and user-friendly-designed mHealth system, data confidentiality, lay language use for structured and automated feedback or advice, positive motivation and improving engagement [28], and inclusion of patient's social supporters, such as family members, friends, and/or peers [31].

There are several limitations in this systematic review. First, we only selected randomized controlled trials for this review and most of them were funded studies. Therefore, the mHealth systems or smartphone apps used in the studies were validated and relatively reliable compared to health apps commercially available on the market. Literature from studies on smartphone-based interventions for chronic disease management that were small scale with or without control group and/or had a short-term follow-up has shown ambivalent results. Thus, we intended to choose robust studies that used randomization, control groups, and relevant follow-ups for outcomes. We looked at the outcome changes at different follow-up points.

Second, we did not include mHealth intervention studies for diabetes management since there is ample literature on diabetes management using mobile technology approaches [14–17]. Third, we excluded studies wherein health apps were used only by health professionals such as physicians or specialized clinical nurses. We focused on patient-centered health apps as a part of mHealth interventions in the review. Lastly, most of the reviewed studies provided smartphones or tablets to participating patients and thus, the results from this review cannot yet be generalized among those who have financial concerns regarding purchasing mHealth tools. Although the availability of wireless networks is increasing, potential mHealth users such as patients with chronic diseases or their caregivers may have limited data services for their mobile devices due to financial concerns. This might be an important issue during an emergency when patients may have no access to evidence-based medical advice via mHealth devices.

Conclusion

The findings from the majority of reviewed studies that used mHealth interventions showed some health outcome improvement in patients with chronic disease conditions. Favorable factors in mHealth approaches are automated text reminders, frequent and accurate symptom monitoring (often in real time), and improved communication between patients and healthcare providers resulting in enhanced self-management in patients with chronic conditions. Thus, the future of mHealth is presumably optimistic. The relationship between engagement of users on mHealth tools and outcome improvement should be further studied. The studies reviewed in this paper showed disease-specific mHealth interventions that might be different from commercial mobile health apps available to the public. Rigorously tested mHealth apps developed through research should be further considered to be made available to the general population.

Abbreviations
CDC: The US Centers for Disease Control and Prevention; EMA: Ecological momentary assessment; HF: Heart failure; mHealth: Mobile health; PD: Parkinson's disease; RCTs: Randomized controlled trials; UPDRS: Unified Parkinson's Disease Rating Scale; US: The United States of America

Acknowledgements
The authors thank Yoori Yang, MSN, College of Nursing, Yonsei University and Laura Narvaez, BS, Sue and Bill Gross School of Nursing at University of California Irvine for their assistance in literature search and abstract reviews. We also thank Dr. Priscilla Kehoe for her thorough editorial support.

Funding
Not applicable.

Authors' contributions
Design of the study protocol: JL, MC; Data collection and analysis: MC, SAL, NJ; Data interpretation: JL, MC, SAL; Drafting the manuscript: JL, MC, SAL, NJ. All authors revised the article critically, gave feedback and approved the final manuscript.

Competing interests
The authors declare that they have no competing interests.

Author details
¹Sue and Bill Gross School of Nursing, University of California Irvine, Irvine, CA, USA. ²College of Nursing, Mo-Im Kim Nursing Research Institute, Yonsei University, 50 Yonsei-ro, Seodaemun-gu, Seoul, Republic of Korea03722. ³College of Nursing and Health Sciences, University of Massachusetts, Boston, MA, USA. ⁴Program in Public Health, University of California Irvine, Irvine, CA, USA.

References
1. World Health Organization. Noncommunicable diseases country profiles 2014. 2014. http://apps.who.int/iris/bitstream/10665/128038/1/9789241507509_eng. pdf. Accessed 22 Dec 2017.
2. Ward BW, Schiller JS, Goodman RA. Multiple chronic conditions among US adults: a 2012 update. Prev Chronic Dis. 2014;11:E62. https://doi.org/10. 5888/pcd11.130389.
3. US Centers for Disease Control and Prevention. Death and Mortality: NCHS FastStats Web Site. 2013. https://www.cdc.gov/nchs/fastats/deaths.htm. Accessed 22 Dec 2017.
4. US Agency for Healthcare Research and Quality. Multiple Chronic Conditions Chartbook: 2010 Medical expenditure panel survey data. AHRQ Publication No Q14–0038. 2014. https://www.ahrq.gov/sites/default/files/ wysiwyg/professionals/prevention-chronic-care/decision/mcc/mccchartbook. pdf. Accessed 22 Dec 2017.

5. Nolte E, Knai C, McKee M. Managing chronic conditions: experience in eight countries. 2008. http://www.euro.who.int/__data/assets/pdf_file/0008/98414/E92058.pdf?ua=1. Accessed 22 Dec 2017.

6. Sharma J. Chronic disease managment in the South-East Asia Region: a need to do more. WHO South East Asia J Public Health. 2013;2(2):79–82. https://doi.org/10.4103/2224-3151.122935.

7. Healthcare Information and Management Systems Society. Definitions of mHealth. 2012. http://www.himss.org/definitions-mhealth. Accessed 22 Dec 2017.

8. Bitsaki M, Koutras G, Heep H, Koutras C. Cost-Effective Mobile-Based Healthcare System for Managing Total Joint Arthroplasty Follow-Up. Healthc Inform Res. 2017;23(1):67–73. https://doi.org/10.4258/hir.2017.23.1.67.

9. Hamine S, Gerth-Guyette E, Faulx D, Green BB, Ginsburg AS. Impact of mHealth chronic disease management on treatment adherence and patient outcomes: a systematic review. J Med Internet Res. 2015;17(2):e52. https://doi.org/10.2196/jmir.3951.

10. Park YT. Emerging New Era of Mobile Health Technologies. Healthc Inform Res. 2016;22(4):253–4. https://doi.org/10.4258/hir.2016.22.4.253.

11. Free C, Phillips G, Felix L, Galli L, Patel V, Edwards P. The effectiveness of M-health technologies for improving health and health services: a systematic review protocol. BMC Res Notes. 2010;3:250. https://doi.org/10.1186/1756-0500-3-250.

12. Fiordelli M, Diviani N, Schulz PJ. Mapping mHealth research: a decade of evolution. J Med Internet Res. 2013;15(5):e95. https://doi.org/10.2196/jmir.2430.

13. Widmer RJ, Collins NM, Collins CS, West CP, Lerman LO, Lerman A. Digital health interventions for the prevention of cardiovascular disease: a systematic review and meta-analysis. Mayo Clin Proc. 2015;90(4):469–80. https://doi.org/10.1016/j.mayocp.2014.12.026.

14. de Ridder M, Kim J, Jing Y, Khadra M, Nanan R. A systematic review on incentive-driven mobile health technology: as used in diabetes management. J Telemed Telecare. 2017;23(1):26–35. https://doi.org/10.1177/1357633X15625539.

15. Cui M, Wu X, Mao J, Wang X, Nie M. T2DM self-management via smartphone applications: a systematic review and meta-analysis. PLoS One. 2016;11(11):e0166718. https://doi.org/10.1371/journal.pone.0166718.

16. Sieverdes JC, Treiber F, Jenkins C. Improving diabetes management with mobile health technology. Am J Med Sci. 2013;345(4):289–95. https://doi.org/10.1097/MAJ.0b013e3182896cee.

17. Whitehead L, Seaton P. The effectiveness of self-management mobile phone and tablet apps in long-term condition management: a systematic review. J Med Internet Res. 2016;18(5):e97. https://doi.org/10.2196/jmir.4883.

18. Liberati A, Altman DG, Tetzlaff J, Mulrow C, Gøtzsche PC, Ioannidis JP, et al. The PRISMA statement for reporting systematic reviews and meta-analyses of studies that evaluate health care interventions: explanation and elaboration. PLoS Med. 2009;6(7):e1000100. https://doi.org/10.1371/journal.pmed.1000100.

19. Higgins JPT, Altman DG, Sterne JAC. Chapter 8: Assessing risk of bias in included studies. In: Higgins JPT, Green S, editors. Cochrane Handbook for Systematic Reviews of Interventions. 2011. http://handbook-5-1.cochrane.org/chapter_8/8_assessing_risk_of_bias_in_included_studies.htm. Accessed 22 Dec 2017.

20. Bowen DJ, Kreuter M, Spring B, Cofta-Woerpel L, Linnan L, Weiner D, et al. How we design feasibility studies. Am J Prev Med. 2009;36(5):452–7. https://doi.org/10.1016/j.amepre.2009.02.002.

21. Hebert M. Telehealth success: evaluation framework development. Stud Health Technol Inform. 2001;84(Pt 2):1145–9.

22. Kristjansdottir OB, Fors EA, Eide E, Finset A, Stensrud TL, van Dulmen S, et al. A smartphone-based intervention with diaries and therapist-feedback to reduce catastrophizing and increase functioning in women with chronic widespread pain: randomized controlled trial. J Med Internet Res. 2013;15(1):e5. https://doi.org/10.2196/jmir.2249.

23. Kristjansdottir OB, Fors EA, Eide E, Finset A, Stensrud TL, van Dulmen S, et al. A smartphone-based intervention with diaries and therapist feedback to reduce catastrophizing and increase functioning in women with chronic widespread pain. part 2: 11-month follow-up results of a randomized trial. J Med Internet Res. 2013;15(3):e72. https://doi.org/10.2196/jmir.2442.

24. Dicianno BE, Fairman AD, McCue M, Parmanto B, Yih E, McCoy A, et al. Feasibility of using mobile health to promote self-management in spina bifida. Am J Phys Med Rehabil. 2016;95(6):425–37. https://doi.org/10.1097/phm.0000000000000400.

25. Ginis P, Nieuwboer A, Dorfman M, Ferrari A, Gazit E, Canning CG, et al. Feasibility and effects of home-based smartphone-delivered automated feedback training for gait in people with Parkinson's disease: a pilot randomized controlled trial. Parkinsonism Relat Disord. 2016;22:28–34. https://doi.org/10.1016/j.parkreldis.2015.11.004.

26. Kearney N, McCann L, Norrie J, Taylor L, Gray P, McGee-Lennon M, et al. Evaluation of a mobile phone-based, advanced symptom management system (ASyMS) in the management of chemotherapy-related toxicity. Support Care Cancer. 2009;17(4):437–44. https://doi.org/10.1007/s00520-008-0515-0.

27. Garcia-Palacios A, Herrero R, Belmonte MA, Castilla D, Guixeres J, Molinari G, et al. Ecological momentary assessment for chronic pain in fibromyalgia using a smartphone: a randomized crossover study. Eur J Pain. 2014;18(6):862–72.

28. Cingi C, Yorgancioglu A, Cingi CC, Oguzulgen K, Muluk NB, Ulusoy S, et al. The "physician on call patient engagement trial" (POPET): measuring the impact of a mobile patient engagement application on health outcomes and quality of life in allergic rhinitis and asthma patients. Int Forum Allergy Rhinol. 2015;5(6):487–97. https://doi.org/10.1002/alr.21468.

29. Hägglund E, Lynga P, Frie F, Ullman B, Persson H, Melin M, et al. Patient-centred home-based management of heart failure. Findings from a randomised clinical trial evaluating a tablet computer for self-care, quality of life and effects on knowledge. Scand Cardiovasc J. 2015;49(4):193–9. https://doi.org/10.3109/14017431.2015.1035319.

30. Martin SS, Feldman DI, Blumenthal RS, Jones SR, Post WS, McKibben RA, et al. mActive: a randomized clinical trial of an automated mHealth intervention for physical activity promotion. J Am Heart Assoc. 2015;4(11).

31. Piette JD, Striplin D, Marinec N, Chen J, Trivedi RB, Aron DC, et al. A mobile health intervention supporting heart failure patients and their informal caregivers: a randomized comparative effectiveness trial. J Med Internet Res. 2015;17(6):e142. https://doi.org/10.2196/jmir.4550.

32. DeVito Dabbs A, Song MK, Myers BA, Li R, Hawkins RP, Pilewski JM, et al. A randomized controlled trial of a mobile health intervention to promote self-management after lung transplantation. Am J Transplant. 2016;16(7):2172–80. https://doi.org/10.1111/ajt.13701.

33. Vuorinen AL, Leppanen J, Kaijanranta H, Kulju M, Helio T, van Gils M, et al. Use of home telemonitoring to support multidisciplinary care of heart failure patients in Finland: randomized controlled trial. J Med Internet Res. 2014;16(12):e282. https://doi.org/10.2196/jmir.3651.

34. Cubo E, Mariscal N, Solano B, Becerra V, Armesto D, Calvo S, Arribas J, Seco J, Martinez A, Zorrilla L, et al. Prospective study on cost-effectiveness of home-based motor assessment in Parkinson's disease. J Telemed Telecare. 2016;23(2):328–38. https://doi.org/10.1177/1357633X16638971.

35. Lee JA, Evangelista LS, Moore AA, Juth V, Guo Y, Gago-Masague S, et al. Feasibility study of a mobile health intervention for older adults on oral anticoagulation therapy. Gerontol Geriatr Med 2016;2:2333721416672970. doi: https://doi.org/10.1177/2333721416672970.

36. Mera TO, Heldman DA, Espay AJ, Payne M, Giuffrida JP. Feasibility of home-based automated Parkinson's disease motor assessment. J Neurosci Methods. 2012;203(1):152–6. https://doi.org/10.1016/j.jneumeth.2011.09.019.

37. Statista. Number of smartphone users in the United States from 2010 to 2022 (in millions). 2017. https://www.statista.com/statistics/201182/forecast-of-smartphone-users-in-the-us. Accessed 22 Dec 2017.

38. Statista. Number of smartphone users worldwide from 2014 to 2020 (in billions). 2017. https://www.statista.com/statistics/330695/number-of-smartphone-users-worldwide. Accessed 22 Dec 2017.

39. Pew Research Center. Record shares of Americans now own smartphones, have home broadband. 2017. http://www.pewresearch.org/fact-tank/2017/01/12/evolution-of-technology. Accessed 22 Dec 2017.

15

Using natural language processing methods to classify use status of dietary supplements in clinical notes

Yadan Fan[1] and Rui Zhang[1,2]*

Abstract

Background: Despite widespread use, the safety of dietary supplements is open to doubt due to the fact that they can interact with prescribed medications, leading to dangerous clinical outcomes. Electronic health records (EHRs) provide a potential way for active pharmacovigilance on dietary supplements since a fair amount of dietary supplement information, especially those on use status, can be found in clinical notes. Extracting such information is extremely significant for subsequent supplement safety research.

Methods: In this study, we collected 2500 sentences for 25 commonly used dietary supplements and annotated into four classes: Continuing (C), Discontinued (D), Started (S) and Unclassified (U). Both rule-based and machine learning-based classifiers were developed on the same training set and evaluated using the hold-out test set. The performances of the two classifiers were also compared.

Results: The rule-based classifier achieved F-measure of 0.90, 0.85, 0.90, and 0.86 in C, D, S, and U status, respectively. The optimal machine learning-based classifier (Maximum Entropy) achieved F-measure of 0.90, 0.92, 0.91 and 0.88 in C, D, S, and U status, respectively. The comparison result shows that the machine learning-based classifier has a better performance, which is more efficient and scalable especially when the sample size doubles.

Conclusions: Machine learning-based classifier outperforms rule-based classifier in categorization of the use status of dietary supplements in clinical notes. Future work includes applying deep learning methods and developing a hybrid system to approach use status classification task.

Keywords: Natural language processing, Rule-based method, Machine learning-based classification, Dietary supplements, Use status, Clinical notes

Background

The consumption of dietary supplements continues to grow worldwide. According to the most recent marketing data, Americans spent nearly $38.8 billion on dietary supplements in 2015 [1]. Due to the Dietary Supplement Health and Education Act (DSHEA) in 1994 [2], dietary supplements in the US markets are sold and regulated as a special category of food without safety testing before

marketing. While dietary supplements are widely believed to be safe, they can cause adverse events, such as bleeding. A study conducted by Centers for Disease Control and Prevention (CDC) and Food and Drug Administration (FDA) estimated that 23,005 emergency department visits per year were attributed to the adverse events caused by dietary supplements [3]. Another major safety concern regarding the use of supplements is that prescribed drugs can interact with dietary supplements. The risk associated with drug-supplement interactions (DSIs) has gained increasing attention due to the widespread prevalence of dietary supplements in recent

* Correspondence: zhan1386@umn.edu
[1]Institute for Health Informatics, University of Minnesota, Minneapolis, MN, USA
[2]Department of Pharmaceutical Care & Health Systems, College of Pharmacy, University of Minnesota, Minneapolis, MN, USA

years, especially among the elderly, who are at greater risk for DSIs. Medications commonly prescribed among this population, such as anticoagulants and nonsteroidal anti-inflammatory drugs (NSAIDs), often tend to have serious interactions with dietary supplements, leading to dangerous clinical outcomes [4]. The bleeding induced by the interaction between warfarin and ginkgo is one example of DSIs [5].

The source information on supplement adverse events and DSIs mainly relies on voluntary reporting through post-marketing surveillance. Starting in 2006, dietary supplements companies were required by Dietary Supplements and Nonprescription Drug Consumer Protection Act to file reports of adverse events associated with dietary supplements to FDA [6]. However, the reporting is often inadequate and underestimated since such reporting is limited to severe adverse events, such as those leading to death, disability, and hospitalization. Moreover, there were very few clinical trials conducted to detect DSIs in the human population. Due to the inherent limitations of clinical trials such as sample size and limited study time, it's often difficult to detect rare events. The lack of such information has posed a great risk to the health of the general population. To improve patient safety, it is imperative to increase our knowledge based on DSIs.

The data in the electronic health records (EHR), especially the clinical notes, serve as a great source for active pharmacovigilance on dietary supplements, as it captures longitudinal real word patient information on almost every aspect of clinical care, particularly those related to patient safety, including medication, laboratory results, signs and symptoms, etc. Similar to the medication information, clinical notes contain rich and valuable information on dietary supplements, especially the use status information. For example, there are mentions such as "She has started ginkgo for memory issue," "Stop taking ginger before surgery," and "The patient has discontinued taking ginseng two months ago." Unlocking such information is critical for subsequent investigation on supplement safety research.

In the clinical domain, a number of studies have investigated the recognition of medication use status in clinical narratives through various methods including machine learning-based and rule-based methods. Pakhomov et al. [7] built a Maximum Entropy classifier along with a variety of different feature sets to categorize medication use status into four categories. Sohn et al. [8] used rule-based method and support vector machine (SVM) only with indication features to detect medication status change (e.g., no change, stop, start) in free text. Meystre et al. [9] performed prescription status classification on heart failure medications using SVM, reaching an accuracy score of 95.49% in the evaluation. Liu et al. [10]

developed an SVM classifier using three types of features (i.e., contextual, semantic, discourse) to detect warfarin use status (ON or OFF) from clinical notes. Clinical notes have been extensively investigated to detect and recognize the medication use status. As for dietary supplements, we have previously investigated the detection of use status from clinical notes using both rule-based [11] and machine learning-based methods [12], and we also compared the performance of both classifiers based on a corpus with a smaller sample size of 1300 sentences [13].

In this study, we doubled the size of the corpus (2500 sentences) compared to our previous studies [13] and compared the performances. We tested more feature sets (e.g., bigrams, TF-IDF) with the supervised machine learning classification algorithms. We focused on 25 commonly used dietary supplements.

Methods

Data collection and annotation

The 25 commonly used dietary supplements were selected based on online consumer survey results [14], peer reviewed publications [15–17] and their availability in our patient cohort, which included alfalfa, biotin, black cohosh, Coenzyme Q10, cranberry, dandelion, Echinacea, fish oil, flax seed, folic acid, garlic, ginger, ginkgo, ginseng, glucosamine, glutamine, kava kava, lecithin, melatonin, milk thistle, saw palmetto, St John's Wort, turmeric, valerian, and Vitamin E. Clinical notes mentioning the 25 supplements listed above were retrieved from clinical data repository (CDR) at the University of Minnesota. Institutional Review Board (IRB) approval was obtained to access the notes. A list of supplement names and their corresponding lexical variants generated by a pharmacist was used in the process of retrieving notes. For example, ginkgo and its lexical variants including ginko, gingko, and ginkoba were used. For each of the 25 dietary supplements, 100 sentences were randomly selected. A total of 2500 sentences were annotated following the annotation guideline in our previous study [11]. The use status of supplement in each sentence was given one of the four classes: Continuing (e.g., "Increase fish oil to 200 mg per day for high triglycerides"; "He was also continued on glutamine and Peridex to protect against mouth sores"), Discontinued (e.g., "The *Ginkgo biloba* was discontinued on admission"; "Pt did stop ginseng Oct 2013"), Started (e.g., "Continued joint pain, has added glucosamine and started exercise regimen last week"; "Patient is to start taking melatonin tonight to help her sleep"), and Unclassified (e.g., "She was advised to take NSAID's PRN and Vitamin E daily"; "Recommend over the counter biotin 3 mg once daily"; "Pt inquiring about milk thistle"; "Avoid grapefruit, ginseng, and St. John's wort"). Ten percent of the corpus was independently annotated by two raters with pharmaceutical background. Inter-annotator agreement was evaluated by Cohen's kappa score (0.83) and percentage agreement (95%).

Data preprocessing and splitting

The data was preprocessed as input to the classifiers. Preprocessing involved lowercasing as well as removing stop words, punctuations, and digits. Because of the time-constrained nature of the clinical setting, abbreviations are abundant in clinical documentation. Physicians often write abbreviations to improve efficiency and save time. For example, they often write "cont" to denote "continue", "info" to denote "information", "discontinue" has several forms of abbreviation, such as "dc", "D/C", "d/ced". These abbreviations were replaced with their standard word form before normalization. All the sentences were then normalized using Lexical Variation Generation (LVG) [18]. The corpus was further split at the supplement level to generate the training and test datasets. Specifically, for each supplement, 100 sentences were randomly divided into two parts: 70 sentences (70%) for training and 30 sentences (30%) for test. In total, 1750 (70%) sentences out of 2500 served as the training data, and the remaining 750 (30%) sentences were used as test data.

Development and evaluation of rule-based classifier

The rule-based classifier was developed on the training data and further tested using the test data. Two of our previous studies [12, 13] have shown that indicator words are extremely important in recognition and detection use status of dietary supplements. Based on the training data, a set of rules were generated using a variety of status indicators, which were compiled from reviewing the clinical notes and incorporated from other works identifying the use status of medications. Such indicator words included "start", "restart", "initiate", "begin", "add", "resume", "try", "increase", "decrease", "continue", "discontinue", "stop", "hold", "off", "recommend", "advise", "avoid", etc. Some negated words were also included, like "no", "not", "never", "decline", "deny". The indicator words were searched for within a window of the supplement mentions. We experimented with different window sizes starting from 0 to 11 tokens on both sides of the target words (supplement mentions). The best window size was selected based on the F-measure on the training data. The rules that were built from the training data were evaluated on the test data. Precision, recall, and F-measure were used as evaluation metrics.

Development and evaluation of machine learning-based classifier

Compared with the previous study [13], more feature sets were trained when building the machine learning-based classifier, such as bigrams, the combination of unigrams, bigrams, and trigrams. Totally, five classification algorithms were trained along with nine types of feature sets on the training data. Five classification algorithms included decision tree, random forest, Naïve Bayes, Maximum Entropy and support vector machine (SVM). Nine types of feature sets were shown as follows: Type 1: raw unigrams without normalization; Type 2: unigrams (normalized); Type 3: TF-IDF (term frequency – inversed document frequency) for unigrams; Type 4: bigrams; Type 5: unigrams + bigrams; Type 6: unigrams + bigrams + trigrams; Type 7: indicator words only; Type 8: unigrams + bigrams + indicator words with distance (window size); Type 9: unigrams + bigrams + trigrams + indicator words with distance. We used 10-fold cross-validation to select the optimal parameters in the training data. All the trained models with optimal parameters were further evaluated on the test data. Precision, recall, and F-measure were used as evaluation metrics.

Performance comparison

The performances of the rule-based and machine learning-based classifiers in terms of four use statuses in the test data were compared. Error analysis was conducted on the rule-based classifier to manually review the sentences that were falsely classified and identify the source of error. The precision, recall, and F-measure of the classifier with the best performance were further compared on each individual dietary supplement to evaluate the generalizability of the classifier across various dietary supplements.

Results
Dataset

In total, there were 604 sentences for C, 323 sentences for D, 425 sentences for S, 398 sentences for U in the training dataset. In the test dataset, there were 233 sentences for C, 166 sentences for D, 178 sentences for S, and 173 sentences for U.

Performance of the rule-based classifier

A total of 68 rules were generated. For each use status, the three most commonly used regular expressions and corresponding examples are shown in Table 1. The F-measure of the rule-based classifier with different window sizes in the training data are shown in Fig. 1. From the figure, we can see that F-measure increased sharply with the increasing distance and reached a stable state when the window size is 6 tokens. After 6 tokens, the performance went up very slowly with the enlarging distance. We arbitrarily set the window size to 7 in order to avoid over-fitting. The precision, recall, and F-measure for the four use statuses of the rule-based classifier on

Table 1 Selected rules and examples

Use status class	Frequently used regular expressions	Selected examples
Continuing (C)	continue(\s + \S+){0,7}\s + sup	Continue fish oil to reduce inflammation.
	increase(\s + \S+){0,7}\s + sup	She has increased her alfalfa tabs and this has eliminated her symptoms and chest tightness.
	take(\s + \S+){0,7}\s + sup	She is also taking a Vitamin E supplement and Tylenol as needed for pain.
Discontinued (D)	Stop(\s + \S+){0,7}\s + sup	Stop Vitamin E supplement.
	discontinue(\s + \S+){0,7}\s + sup	She is to discontinue her St. John's Wort.
	hold(\s + \S+){0,7}\s + sup	You are already holding the fish oil and aspirin.
Started (S)	Start(\s + \S+){0,7} + sup	Started echinacea 1 week ago for cold.
	Add(\s + \S+){0,7} + sup	Add supplements with ginger.
	Begin(\s + \S+){0,7}\s + sup	I have asked him to begin using fish oil 3 capsules a per day, and he is agreeable to this.
Unclassified (U)	Recommend(\s + \S+){0,7}\s + sup	I did recommend taking over-the-counter fish oil, either 500 or 1000 mg per day.
	Avoid(\s + \S+){0,7}\s + sup	Avoid use of st. john's wort on methadone as it can affect systemic level.
	Suggest(\s + \S+){0,7}\s + sup	Also suggested that she could consider trying otc Ginkgo biloba.

the test dataset are shown in Table 2. It shows that the F-measure for the four categories are all above 0.85, among which F-measures for continuing (C) and started (S) status are both 0.90.

Performance of the machine learning-based classifier

The performance of five machine learning-based algorithms with nine types of feature sets in the test data is shown in Table 3. As for the Type 8 and 9 feature sets, we experimented with different window sizes and selected the optimal window size as 6. The results showed that Maximum Entropy with type 8 or type 9 feature achieved the best performance. The precision, recall, and F-measure in terms of four use status of the optimal

model are shown in Table 4. From the results we can see that the machine learning-based classifier achieved a satisfactory performance in terms of the four use statuses, particularly in C, D, and S, which have F-measures over 0.9.

Error analysis of the rule-based classifier

We performed an error analysis for the rule-based classifier by manually reviewing the sentences that were incorrectly classified. In total, there were 89 sentences incorrectly classified by the rule-based classifier. As shown in Table 5, the source of error mainly consists of three parts: missing pattern issue, indicator words issue, and distance issue.

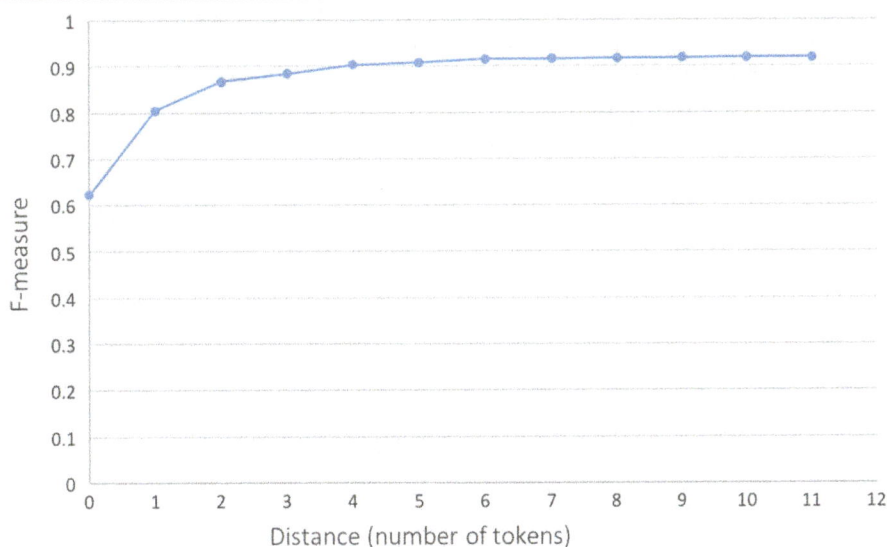

Fig. 1 F-measures of the rule-based classifier with different window sizes on the training data

Table 2 Performance of the rule-based classifier (window size: 7) in the test data

Status	Number of sentences	Precision	Recall	F-measure
Continuing	233	0.90	0.91	0.90
Discontinued	166	0.92	0.80	0.85
Started	178	0.97	0.84	0.90
Unclassified	173	0.78	0.97	0.86
Total (weighted)	750	0.89	0.88	0.88

Performance of machine learning-based classifier on dietary supplement level

The performance of the machine learning-based classifier on the individual dietary supplement in the test data is shown in Table 6. From the results in Table 6 we can see that for most dietary supplements, the F-measure is 0.9. For Vitamin E, the F-measure reached 1. However, the classifier has a poor performance on Coenzyme Q10 and milk thistle, the F-measures for which are below 0.8. Overall, our results demonstrated a good generalizability of the machine learning-based classifier for the majority of the dietary supplements.

Comparing the rule-based and machine learning-based classifiers

Comparing the performance of the two classifiers on the test data, the machine learning-based classifier achieved a better result with respect to the four use statuses, especially in the D status, whose F-measure improved from 0.85 to 0.92. For the C, S, and U status, the performance of the rule-based classifier is close to that of the machine learning-based classifier. Additionally, we also compared both classifiers in terms of the number of sentences which they both correctly classified, they both falsely classified, and only one of them correctly classified. From the detailed comparison results in Table 7, it indicates that the true positive rate in

terms of C, D, and S status of the machine learning-based classifier exceeds that of the rule-based classifier. However, the rule-based classifier is more accurate in recall regarding U status.

Discussion

For all classification algorithms, normalized unigrams have a better performance compared with raw unigrams, indicating that normalization effectively reduces the feature space, thus improving the classification results. For some classification algorithms, such as decision tree and SVM, the TF-IDF features are more informative than unigrams, while for other algorithms, the performance degraded compared with unigrams. Bigrams are the least informative among the features sets, reflected by their poorest performance. Compared with only unigrams, the addition of bigrams and trigrams didn't necessarily contribute to the improvement of the performance. For instance, for the random forest, the performance of Type 2 feature (unigrams) is better than that for Type 5 (unigrams + bigrams) and Type 6 (unigrams + bigrams + trigrams) feature sets. From the results of Type 7 (indicators only), we can see that indicator words hold significant information in use status. For example, for Naïve Bayes, the Type 7 feature set has the best performance compared with other feature sets. For decision tree, the Type 5 feature set (unigrams + bigrams) has the best performance. For random forest, the Type 2 feature set (unigrams) achieved the best result. For SVM, the Type 8 and Type 9 feature sets performed best. Among all the classification algorithms, Maximum Entropy with Type 8 or Type 9 feature sets achieved the same best performance (F-measure: 0.902).

Like the previous study [13], the sources of errors were mainly made up of three parts. First, there are new patterns we failed to generate from the training set. For example, "we reviewed her medications and cut out hyocyamine, biotin and scheduled the bentyl bid," "Was

Table 3 Performances of five classification algorithms with different feature sets in the test data

Type	Features	Decision tree			Random forest			Naïve Bayes			SVM			Maximum Entropy		
		P	R	F	P	R	F	P	R	F	P	R	F	P	R	F
Type 1	raw uni[a]	0.819	0.817	0.816	0.858	0.853	0.853	0.770	0.757	0.755	0.818	0.816	0.815	0.850	0.849	0.849
Type 2	uni	0.846	0.845	0.844	0.878	0.876	0.876	0.793	0.784	0.783	0.837	0.835	0.834	0.874	0.873	0.873
Type 3	tf-idf	0.862	0.857	0.857	0.862	0.857	0.857	0.763	0.704	0.701	0.844	0.839	0.839	0.840	0.831	0.831
Type 4	bi[a]	0.760	0.720	0.716	0.760	0.720	0.716	0.715	0.707	0.702	0.735	0.719	0.720	0.749	0.739	0.739
Type 5	uni + bi	0.872	0.864	0.863	0.872	0.864	0.863	0.815	0.808	0.807	0.881	0.877	0.876	0.890	0.888	0.887
Type 6	uni + bi+tri[a]	0.863	0.852	0.850	0.863	0.852	0.850	0.815	0.808	0.808	0.880	0.876	0.875	0.887	0.883	0.882
Type 7	indi[a] only	0.848	0.847	0.846	0.861	0.860	0.860	0.860	0.849	0.848	0.851	0.849	0.849	0.862	0.859	0.859
Type 8	uni + bi+indi	0.860	0.860	0.860	0.875	0.865	0.864	0.813	0.803	0.801	0.899	0.897	0.897	0.895	0.903	**0.902**
Type 9	uni + bi+tri + indi	0.860	0.857	0.857	0.872	0.861	0.860	0.813	0.803	0.801	0.899	0.897	0.897	0.905	0.903	**0.902**

[a]uni: unigrams; bi: bigrams; tri: trigrams; indi: indicators
Bolded data represent the largest value

Table 4 The performance of Maximum Entropy with Type 8 feature set (unigrams + bigrams + indicators with window size of 6) in the test data

Status	Number	Precision	Recall	F-measure
Continuing	233	0.86	0.95	0.90
Discontinued	166	0.94	0.89	0.92
Started	178	0.92	0.91	0.91
Unclassified	173	0.92	0.84	0.88
Total (weighted)	750	0.91	0.90	0.90

taking milk thistle when he was living at home, but is no longer doing so," "He denies taking any other GNC supplementation other than the ginseng and protein." Second is the indicator issue: more than one use status indicator appears in the same sentence. For example, "Still off estrogen and started black cohosh because of nightsweats," "He never stopped taking the saw palmetto," "Pt quit taking turmeric – restarted less than a week ago." Under such circumstance, the order of the rules largely impacts the performance of the rule-based classifier. Some errors are due to the indicator word being more than 7 tokens from the supplement mentions. From Table 5 we can see that the largest percentage of error mainly comes from "missing pattern" issue.

Our previous study [13] comparing the rule-based and machine learning-based classifier showed that the rule-based classifier is slightly better when the sample size is much smaller (1300 sentences). However, in the current study, the results indicate that the machine learning-based classifier is more accurate when the sample size (2500) nearly doubles. It should be noted that F-measure of U status of the machine learning-based classifier (F-measure: 0.88) is larger than that of the rule-based classifier (F-measure: 0.86), while in our previous study [13], the rule-based classifier (F-measure: 0.88) performs better in terms of U status than the machine learning-based classifier (F-measure: 0.77). Therefore, the results of the current study show that the performance of the machine learning-based classifier regarding U status not only has been greatly improved, but also outweighs the rule-based classifier.

It is evident that the performance of the rule-based classifier degrades when the sample size increases. The reason might be due to the fact that as the sample size

Table 5 Source of errors for the rule-based classifier

Source of error	Number of sentences	Percentage of errors
Missing pattern	47	6.3%
Indicator words issue	40	5.3%
Distance issue	2	0.3%
Total	89	11.9%

Table 6 The performance of the machine learning-based classifier on the 25 dietary supplements in the test data

Dietary Supplement	Number	Precision	Recall	F-measure
Alfalfa	30	0.904	0.900	0.900
Biotin	30	0.927	0.900	0.904
Black cohosh	30	0.937	0.933	0.933
Coenzyme Q10	30	0.809	0.800	0.799
Cranberry	30	0.945	0.933	0.934
Dandelion	30	0.939	0.933	0.926
Echinacea	30	0.913	0.900	0.902
Fish oil	30	0.938	0.933	0.933
Flax seed	30	0.900	0.900	0.900
Folic acid	30	0.911	0.900	0.900
Garlic	30	0.919	0.900	0.903
Ginger	30	0.893	0.867	0.861
Ginkgo	30	0.943	0.933	0.932
Ginseng	30	0.947	0.933	0.935
Glucosamine	30	0.936	0.933	0.933
Glutamine	30	0.938	0.933	0.934
Kava kava	30	0.913	0.900	0.902
Lecithin	30	0.939	0.933	0.934
Melatonin	30	0.806	0.800	0.801
Milk thistle	30	0.787	0.767	0.751
Saw palmetto	30	0.907	0.900	0.900
St. John's Wort	30	0.910	0.900	0.900
Turmeric	30	0.927	0.900	0.886
Valerian	30	0.944	0.933	0.928
Vitamin E	30	1.000	1.000	1.000

increases, more patterns appear in both training and test datasets and the patterns generated by observing the training data cannot fully represent the test data. Another potential disadvantage of the rule-based classifier is that it is time-consuming and labor-intensive to develop the regular expression rules. In this respect, machine learning-based methods are more scalable and efficient.

Table 7 Comparison between the rule-based and the machine learning-based classifiers regarding four use statuses

Status	Number	TP[a] for RB[a]	TP for ML[a]	RB (+)[a] ML (+)	RB (+) ML (−)	RB (−) ML (+)	RB (−)[a] ML (−)
C	233	212	222	209	3	13	8
D	166	132	148	128	4	20	14
S	178	151	163	147	4	16	12
U	173	166	144	142	24	2	4

[a]TP: true positive; RB: rule-based classifier; ML: machine learning-based classifier; (+): correctly classified; (−): falsely classified

The results of the machine learning-based classifiers (Table 3) show that the features are extremely significant in determining the performance of the supervised text classification algorithms. The performance varies with different feature sets. One limitation of this study is that we only tested 9 types of features. In the future, we will explore more types of feature sets and experiment with combinations of feature sets. Recently, there has been an increasing interest in applying deep learning methods to solve the text classification tasks. One major advantage of deep learning methods is that human-generated features are not required. In the future, we will attempt to try state-of-the-art deep learning methods, such as long short-term memory networks, to detect and classify the use status of dietary supplements from clinical notes. Our future work will also include making use of the specific advantages of both classifiers, such as high precision of the machine learning classifier and high sensitivity of the rule-based classifier to develop a hybrid system.

Conclusions

In this study, both rule-based and machine learning-based classifiers were constructed to detect and categorize the use status of 25 commonly used dietary supplements into 4 use status classes. The performances of rule-based and machine learning-based classifiers were further evaluated and compared in the test data. The comparison results show that the machine learning-based classifier outperforms the rule-based classifier when the sample size increases to 2500 sentences. Future work includes applying deep learning methods and developing a hybrid system for identifying supplement use status in clinical notes.

Abbreviations

C: Continuing; CDC: Centers for disease control and prevention; CDR: Clinical data repository; D: Discontinued; DSHEA: Dietary supplement health and education act; DSIs: Drug-supplement interactions; EHR: Electronic health records; FDA: Food and Drug Administration; IRB: Institutional review board; LVG: Lexical variant generation; NSAIDs: Anticoagulants and nonsteroidal anti-inflammatory drugs; S: Started; SVM: Support vector machine; TF-IDF: Term frequency - inverse document frequency; U: Unclassified

Acknowledgments

The authors thank Fairview Health Services for support of this research. The authors also thank Reed McEwan and Ben Knoll for data extraction, and Lu He for corpus annotation.

Funding

This research and publication cost was supported by the National Institute of Health, National Center for Complementary & Integrative Health Award (R01AT009457) (PI: Zhang) and the University of Minnesota Clinical and Translational Science Award (#8UL1TR000114) (PI: Blazer).
2nd International Workshop on Semantics-Powered Data Analytics. The full contents of the supplement are available online at https://bmcmedinformdecis-mak.biomedcentral.com/articles/supplements/volume-18-supplement-2.

Authors' contributions

RZ and YF conceived the study idea and design. YF retrieved the data and annotated the corpus for the reference standard. Both authors participated in writing and reviewed the manuscript. Both authors read and approved the final manuscript.

Authors' information

Described in the title page.

Competing interests

The authors declare that they have no competing interests.

References

1. Anonymous. NBJ's supplement business report. Nutr Bus J. 2016;2016:13-14
2. Fontanarosa PB, Rennie D, DeAngelis CD. The need for regulation of dietary supplements—lessons from ephedra. JAMA. 2003;289(12):1568–70.
3. Geller AI, Shehab N, Weidle NJ, Lovegrove MC, Wolpert BJ, Timbo BB, Mozersky RP, Budnitz DS. Emergency department visits for adverse events related to dietary supplements. N Engl J Med. 2015;373(16):1531–40.
4. Qato DM, Wilder J, Schumm LP, Gillet V, Alexander GC. Changes in prescription and over-the-counter medication and dietary supplement use among older adults in the United States, 2005 vs 2011. JAMA Intern Med. 2016;176(4):473–82.
5. Sprouse AA, Van Breemen RB. Pharmacokinetic interactions between drugs and botanical dietary supplements. Drug Metab Dispos. 2016;44(2):162–71.
6. Frankos VH, Street DA, O'neill RK. FDA regulation of dietary supplements and requirements regarding adverse event reporting. Clin Pharmacol Ther. 2010;87(2):239–44.
7. Pakhomov SV, Ruggieri A, Chute CG. Maximum entropy modeling for mining patient medication status from free Text Proceedings of the AMIA Symposium; 2002. p. 587. American Medical Informatics Association
8. Sohn S, Murphy SP, Masanz JJ, Kocher JP, Savova GK. Classification of medication status change in clinical narratives. In: AMIA Annual Symposium Proceedings, vol. 2010; 2010. p. 762. American Medical Informatics Association.
9. Meystre SM, Kim Y, Heavirland J, Williams J, Bray BE, Garvin J. Heart failure medications detection and prescription status classification in clinical narrative documents. Stud Health Technol Inform. 2015;216:609.
10. Liu M, Jiang M, Kawai VK, Stein CM, Roden DM, Denny JC, Xu H. Modeling drug exposure data in electronic medical records: an application to warfarin. AMIA annual symposium proceedings, vol. 2011; 2011. p. 815. American Medical Informatics Association
11. Fan Y, He L, Zhang R. Classification of use status for dietary supplements in clinical notes. Bioinformat Biomed. 2016:1054–61. IEEE International Conference on 2016 Dec 15 IEEE
12. Fan Y, He L, Pakhomov SVS, Melton GB, Zhang R. Classifying supplement use status in clinical notes. AMIA Jt Summits Transl Sci Proc. 2017;2017:493–501.
13. Fan Y, He L, Zhang R. Evaluating automatic methods to extract patients' supplement use from clinical reports. In: Proceedings IEEE International Conference on Bioinformatics and Biomedicine, vol. 2017; 2017. p. 1258. NIH Public Access.
14. https://www.fda.gov/food/resourcesforyou/consumers/ucm109760.htm (Accessed on 26 Mar 2018).
15. Abebe W, Herman W, Konzelman J. Herbal supplement use among adult dental patients in a USA dental school clinic: prevalence, patient demographics, and clinical implications. Oral Surg Oral Med Oral Pathol Oral Radiol Endod. 2011;111(3):320–5.
16. Wu CH, Wang CC, Kennedy J. The prevalence of herb and dietary supplement use among children and adolescents in the United States: results from the 2007 National Health Interview Survey. Complement Ther Med. 2013;21(4):358–63.
17. Stys T, Stys A, Kelly P, Lawson W. Use of herbal medicines by elderly patients: A systematic review. Clin Cardiol. 2004;27(2):87–90. Trends in use of herbal and nutritional supplements in cardiovascular patients
18. LVG. https://www.nlm.nih.gov/research/umls/new_users/online_learning/LEX_004.html (Accessed on 26 Mar 2018).

16

A bibliometric analysis of natural language processing in medical research

Xieling Chen[1], Haoran Xie[2], Fu Lee Wang[3], Ziqing Liu[4], Juan Xu[5] and Tianyong Hao[6,7*]

Abstract

Background: Natural language processing (NLP) has become an increasingly significant role in advancing medicine. Rich research achievements of NLP methods and applications for medical information processing are available. It is of great significance to conduct a deep analysis to understand the recent development of NLP-empowered medical research field. However, limited study examining the research status of this field could be found. Therefore, this study aims to quantitatively assess the academic output of NLP in medical research field.

Methods: We conducted a bibliometric analysis on NLP-empowered medical research publications retrieved from PubMed in the period 2007–2016. The analysis focused on three aspects. Firstly, the literature distribution characteristics were obtained with a statistics analysis method. Secondly, a network analysis method was used to reveal scientific collaboration relations. Finally, thematic discovery and evolution was reflected using an affinity propagation clustering method.

Results: There were 1405 NLP-empowered medical research publications published during the 10 years with an average annual growth rate of 18.39%. 10 most productive publication sources together contributed more than 50% of the total publications. The USA had the highest number of publications. A moderately significant correlation between country's publications and GDP per capita was revealed. *Denny, Joshua C* was the most productive author. *Mayo Clinic* was the most productive affiliation. The annual co-affiliation and co-country rates reached 64.04% and 15.79% in 2016, respectively. 10 main great thematic areas were identified including *Computational biology*, *Terminology mining*, *Information extraction*, *Text classification*, *Social medium as data source*, *Information retrieval*, etc.

Conclusions: A bibliometric analysis of NLP-empowered medical research publications for uncovering the recent research status is presented. The results can assist relevant researchers, especially newcomers in understanding the research development systematically, seeking scientific cooperation partners, optimizing research topic choices and monitoring new scientific or technological activities.

Keywords: Natural language processing, Medical, Bibliometrics, Statistical characteristics, Scientific collaboration, Thematic discovery and evolution

* Correspondence: haoty@gdufs.edu.cn
[6]School of Information Science and Technology, Guangdong University of
Foreign Studies, Guangzhou, China
[7]School of Computer, South China Normal University, Guangzhou, China
Full list of author information is available at the end of the article

Background

Natural language processing (NLP) is a theoretically motivated range of computational techniques for the automatic analysis and representation of human language [1]. Its goal is to realize human-like language understanding for a wide range of applications and tasks [2]. As a large and complex domain, medicine is rich in synonymy and semantically similar and related concepts [3]. Most clinical information resources including Electronic Medical Records (EMRs), Electronic Health Records (EHRs) and medical knowledge contain considerable amount of information. However, much of this information comes in unstructured form, also called free-text [4]. NLP is crucial for transforming relevant unstructured information hidden in free-text into structured information and is extremely useful in improving healthcare and advancing medicine [5].

There have been rich research achievements of NLP methods and applications for processing medical information [6]. Emerging interests of medical information processing with NLP methods include speech information recognition [7], semantic labeling [8], syntactic parsing [9], word sense disambiguation [10, 11], negation detection [12], and temporal analysis [13, 14]. Medical practical problems can also gain solutions from NLP-empowered applications including adverse drug reactions detection [15], medication discrepancy detection [16], EMRs or EHRs coding and classification [17], clinical trial computation [18–21], etc. NLP-empowered medical research field grows fast and draws more and more attention [6]. It is of great significance to understand its research status through a systematic analysis on relevant research output.

In the analysis research, bibliometrics is defined as the use of statistical methods for quantitative assessment of academic output [22, 23]. Benefits of bibliometric analysis include evaluating leading scientific researchers or publications [24], studying the structure of the network of a scientific field [25], identifying major topics [26], discovering new developments [27], etc.

This paper thus carries out a thorough bibliometric analysis on NLP-empowered medical publications from PubMed during the year 2007–2016. The descriptive statistics analysis, social network analysis, and Affinity Propagation clustering analysis are used in the analysis. Specifically, the purpose of the analysis is to: 1) identify productive publication sources, authors, affiliations, and countries in NLP-empowered medical research field; 2) visualize the number of countries and scientific collaboration among authors and affiliations; and 3) distinguish major themes and their evolution.

Related work

Applications of bibliometrics are numerous. Many studies focused on publication statistical characteristics evaluation with elements such as publication data, influential journals, productive authors, affiliations, and countries. Based on two separate databases Web of Science (WoS) and Google Scholar, Diem and Stefan [28] investigated the fitness-for-purpose of bibliometric indicators for measuring the research performance of individual researchers in education sciences field in Switzerland. The study results indicated that the indicators for research performance measurement such as quantity of publications and citation impact measure were highly positively correlated. Fan et al. [29] conducted a bibliometric study for the evaluation of the quantity and quality of Chinese publications on burns at both the international and domestic levels with basis of PubMed records during 1985 and 2014. Similar works have also been conducted for medical research output. A study for the determination of whether a correlation existed between bibliometrics and National Institutes of Health (NIH) funding data among academic neurosurgeons was conducted by Venable et al. [30]. Their work revealed that bibliometric indices were higher among neurosurgeons with NIH funding, but only the contemporary h-index was shown to be predictive of NIH funding. By examining the growth of published literature on diabetes in three countries including Nigeria, Argentina and Thailand, Harande and Alhaji [31] showed that the literature of the disease grew and spread very widely. Ramos [32] found that the research output in countries with more estimated cases of tuberculosis was less compared with industrialized countries through a bibliometric analysis of tuberculosis research output. In addition, bibliometric analysis on research publications related with cancer [33], eye disease [34], obesity [35], dental traumatology [36], etc., could also be found. Bibliometric analysis for publication statistical characteristics evaluation was also available for specific journals, e.g., *Journal of Intellectual Property Rights* [37] and *The Electronic Library* [38].

Studies on collaboration relationship among authors, affiliations, or countries were commonly found. Based on researches covering biomedical, physics, and mathematics, Newman [39] compared the scientific co-authorship patterns using network analysis. Radev et al. [40] investigated the publications published by *The Association for Computational Linguistics* using citation and collaboration network analysis to identify the most central papers and authors. A bibliometric and visual study on consumer behavior research publications from 1966 to 2008 was presented by Muñoz-Leiva et al. [41]. Geaney et al. [42] provided a detailed evaluation of type 2 diabetes mellitus research output during the year 1951–2012 with methods of large-scale data analysis, bibliometric indicators, and density-equalizing mapping. They came to the conclusion that the number of research was rising in step with the increasing global burden of the disease. With a chord diagram of the 20 most productive countries, Li et al. [43] confirmed the predominance of the USA in international geo-ontology research collaboration. They also found that the international cooperation of countries such as Sweden, Switzerland, and New Zealand were relatively high although with fewer publications.

There were also a few studies centering on research topic detection of a certain field using bibliometrics. For example, Heo et al. [44] analyzed the field of bioinformatics using a multi-faceted topic modeling method. By combining performance analysis and science mapping, some studies conducted thematic evolution detection and visualization of a given research field, e.g., hydropower [45], neuroscience [46], and social work [47]. Similar works have also been conducted for specific journals such as *Knowledge-Based Systems* [22]. Based on co-word analysis, Cobo et al. [48] proposed an automatic approach with the combination of performance analysis and science mapping to show the conceptual evolution of intelligent transportation systems research field during three consecutive periods. Six main thematic areas were identified out. With the purpose of mapping and analyzing the structure and evolution of the scientific literature on gender differences in higher education and science, Dehdarirad et al. [49] applied co-word analysis to identify main concepts, used hierarchical cluster analysis to cluster the keywords, and created a strategic diagram to analyze trends.

Most relevant studies chose WoS as publication retrieval data source, and therefore, author-defined keywords and ISI keywords plus were usually used as topic candidates [22, 23, 46]. This might lead to information loss without considering title and abstract fields. The key terms in title and abstract fields were extracted and analyzed using VOSviewer with equal importance in the study of Yeung et al. [46]. However, it is more reasonable to bestow weighing for terms from different fields.

To our knowledge, there was no study applying bibliometrics to assess research output of NLP-empowered medical research field. Therefore, giving the deficiencies in existing research, this study uses PubMed as data source. With 1405 NLP-empowered medical research publications retrieved, literature distribution characteristics and scientific collaboration are acquired using a descriptive statistics method and a social network analysis method, respectively. In addition to author defined keywords and PubMed medical subject headings (MeSH), key terms extracted from title and abstract fields using a developed Python program are also included in AP clustering analysis for thematic discovery and evolution.

Methods
Data set
PubMed is an important data source on life sciences and biomedical topics. We used PubMed as data source and

downloaded documents using the following query: (("2007"[Publication Date]: "2016"[Publication Date])) AND (("NLP"[Title] OR "Natural Language Processing"[Title]) OR ("NLP"[Title/Abstract] OR "Natural Language Processing"[Title/Abstract])).

Using the query, we retrieved a total of 1776 documents in XML format. Key elements including title, published year, publication source, author address, author keywords, PubMed MeSH, and abstract were extracted. Due to the issues of information missing and irrelevant documents, manual information supplement and document exclusion were conducted. After that, 1405 NLP-empowered medical research publications between 2007 and 2016 were identified out as dataset.

According to the author addresses information, the corresponding affiliations and countries were manually preprocessed and automated identified. As for the title and abstract fields, a developed Python program was applied to extract key terms (including single words and phrases). According to observation on 50 samples, we found that most of the extracted single words were meaningful, e.g., "influenza", "surveillance", and "misdiagnoses". Furthermore, in order to improve data quality, a de-duplicating process was applied (author defined keywords, PubMed MeSH, and extracted key terms as units of analysis). Some abbreviations were replaced by the corresponding full-names. For example, "EHR" was replaced by "Electronic Health Record". Words representing the same concepts were grouped. In addition, words with a very broad and general meaning, e.g., "natural language processing", "algorithm", were removed. After the above pre-processing, the dataset was analyzed using software R. Some statistical characteristics of the dataset are shown as Table 1.

Statistical analysis
Some publication characteristics are obtained through statistical analysis using a descriptive statistical method, a regression analysis method, and a hypothesis testing method. Descriptive statistics is used for quantitatively summarizing the basic characteristics of a collection of data [50]. It simplifies large amounts of data in a sensible way by presenting quantitative descriptions in a manageable form, generally along with simple graphics analysis. Regression analysis is a set of statistical processes for estimating the relationships between a dependent variable and one or more independent variables. It helps one find out how the dependent variable changes when any one of the independent variables is varied while the other independent variables remain fixed. As a method of statistical inference, statistical hypothesis testing is used to determine whether a hypothesis is a reasonable statement and should not be

Table 1 The statistical characteristics of the dataset

Characteristics	Statistics
Total #pub.	1405
#pub. with author address information	1386
#pub. with abstract	1382
#pub. with author keywords or PubMed MeSH	1277
#unique publication sources	324
#unique countries/first countries	56/45
#unique authors/first authors	4391/1053
#unique affiliations/first affiliations	961/514
Average #words/word characters in title	12.53; 6.50
Average number/standard deviation of character in title	95.43; 29.72
Average #words/word characters in abstract	215.24; 5.62
Average number/standard deviation of character in abstract	1456.95; 536.2
Top 10 frequency words/phrases in author keywords or PubMed MeSH	Electronic health record (363; 25.84%); Data mining (278; 19.79%); Information storage and retrieval (239; 17.01%); Artificial intelligence (179; 12.74%); Female (163; 11.60%); Semantics (156; 11.10%); Male (153; 10.89%); Controlled vocabulary (140; 9.96%); Automatic pattern recognition (127; 9.04%); Medical record system (112; 7.97%)
Top 10 frequency words/phrases extracted from title	Electronic health record (69; 4.91%); Medical record (55; 3.91%); Clinical text (45; 3.20%); Clinical note (41; 2.92%); Patient (37; 2.63%); Text mining (23; 1.64%); Classification (22; 1.57%); Clinical narrative (21; 1.49%); Radiology report (21; 1.49%); Natural language processing method (20; 1.42%)
Top 10 frequency words/phrases extracted from abstract	Patient (322; 22.92%); Precision (217; 15.44%); F-measure (205; 14.59%); Recall (178; 12.67%); Accuracy (164; 11.67%); Electronic health record (161; 11.46%); Natural language processing method (155; 11.03%); Medical record (143; 10.18%); Disease (141; 10.04%); Concept (128; 9.11%)

rejected or if it is an unreasonable statement and should be rejected based on sample statistics and probability theory. A hypothesis is proposed for the statistical relationship between two datasets as an alternative, and is compared with an idealized null hypothesis proposing no relationship between two datasets. The comparison is regarded statistically significant if the null hypothesis is unlikely to realize according to a threshold probability, i.e., a significance level.

In this study, a descriptive statistics method was applied to acquire the distribution characteristics of the dataset, including publication distribution by year, productive publication sources, authors, affiliations, and countries, as well as annual cooperation publication distribution. Based on the number of publications, 3 fitting models including linear model without intercept, linear model with intercept, and non-linear model with quadratic term, were built with *year/ 1000* and *(year/1000)^2* as independent variables. Akaike Information Criterion (AIC) and adjusted R-squared ($\overline{R^2}$) were used to select the optimal fitting model. In order to understand the relationship between number of publications and GDP per capita, a Spearman's rank correlation test was applied to test the hypothesis as:

Hypothesis: There is no significant relationship between publications and GDP per capita

Spearman's rank correlation coefficient is a nonparametric measure of statistical dependence between the rankings of two variables, which is expressed as:

$$r_s = \rho_{rg_X, rg_Y} = \frac{\text{cov}(rg_X, rg_Y)}{\sigma_{rg_X} \sigma_{rg_Y}} \tag{1}$$

where ρ denotes the usual Pearson correlation coefficient, but applies to the rank variables. $\text{cov}(rg_X, rg_Y)$ is the covariance of the rank variables. σ_{rg_X} and σ_{rg_Y} are the standard deviations of rank variables.

Geographic visualization

Geographic visualization is a set of techniques for analyzing spatial data with an emphasis on knowledge construction over knowledge storage or information transmission. Aiming at facilitating the exploration, analysis, synthesis, and presentation of georeferenced information, geographic visualization integrates principles from geographic information systems, exploratory data analysis, cartography, as well as information visualization [51].Techniques such as multimedia, image processing, computer graphics, and virtual reality are combined for presenting information in a way that patterns can be found, and greater understanding can be acquired. In this study, we applied geographic visualization analysis to explore worldwide geographical distribution of NLP-empowered medical research publications in country-level.

Social network analysis

Social network analysis, related to network theory, is a process of investigating social structures based on networks and graph theory in modern sociology [52]. Social network perspective concentrates on relationships among social entities [53] with two main focuses, i.e., the actors and the relationships between them in a specific social context [54]. Networked structures are characterized in terms of nodes with the ties, edges, or links connecting them.

In this study, we applied social network analysis to explore the cooperation relationships for specific authors and affiliations in NLP-empowered medical research field. The cooperation among affiliations and authors were visualized with force directed network graphs, respectively. In the network graphs, the nodes represented specific affiliations or authors, and the lines represented the cooperation relationship. The size of node indicated the number of publications of a specific author or affiliation. The width of link indicated the cooperation frequencies between the two affiliations or authors.

Term importance weighting

In thematic evolution discovery, author defined keywords, PubMed MeSH, and key terms extracted from title and abstract were jointly used as units of analysis. Since the importance of different parts of a publication was different, we conducted a weighting process with the combination of subjective and objective methods. Suppose there were n unique words among author defined keywords, PubMed MeSH, and key terms extracted from title and abstract of a sample of 30 publications ($p = 1,2,...,30$). The objective method was as Eq. (2).

$$
\left\{
\begin{aligned}
& 0 \leq \alpha \leq 1, stepsize = 0.1 \\
& 0 \leq \beta \leq 1-\alpha, stepsize = 0.1 \\
& \gamma = 1-\alpha-\beta \\
& F^O_{w_i,\alpha,\beta,\gamma} = \alpha f_{1w_i} + \beta f_{2w_i} + \gamma f_{3w_i}, i = 1, 2, ..., n \\
& F^O_{\alpha,\beta,\gamma} = \left\{ F^O_{w_i,\alpha,\beta,\gamma}, i = 1, 2, ..., n \right\} \\
& R^O_{\alpha,\beta,\gamma} = rank\left(F^O_{\alpha,\beta,\gamma} \right) \\
& R^O_{\alpha,\beta,\gamma} = \left\{ R^O_{w_i,\alpha,\beta,\gamma}, i = 1, 2, ..., n \right\}
\end{aligned}
\right.
\tag{2}
$$

where α, β, and γ represented weights for author defined keywords and PubMed MeSH, key terms extracted from

title, and key terms extracted from abstract, respectively. f_{1w_i}, f_{2w_i}, and f_{3w_i} represented the frequencies of word w_i in author defined keywords and PubMed MeSH, key terms extracted from title, and key terms extracted from abstract, respectively. $F^O_{w_i,\alpha,\beta,\gamma}$ was the frequency of word w_i weighted by α, β, and γ. $F^O_{\alpha,\beta,\gamma}$ was the mathematical set of $F^O_{w_i,\alpha,\beta,\gamma}$. $R^O_{\alpha,\beta,\gamma}$ was the objective ranking of $F^O_{\alpha,\beta,\gamma}$. $R^O_{w_i,\alpha,\beta,\gamma}$ was the ranking of word w_i, and thus $R^O_{\alpha,\beta,\gamma}$ was the mathematical set of $R^O_{w_i,\alpha,\beta,\gamma}$. According to the equation, the total number of $R^O_{\alpha,\beta,\gamma}$ was 66, with 66 kinds of unique combinations of the three parameters.

The subjective method was expressed as Eq. (3).

$$
R^S_{w_i} = \frac{\sum_{p=1}^{30} R_{p,w_i}}{T_i}
\tag{3}
$$

where R_{p,w_i} represented the importance ranking of word w_i in sample p and was determined according to specific sample content. If word w_i did not appear in sample p, then $R_{p,w_i} = 0$. T_i was the number of sample containing word w_i. $R^S_{w_i}$ was the average importance ranking of word w_i.

The optimized combination of the three parameters was determined as Eq. (4).

$$
\left\{
\begin{aligned}
& delt_{\alpha,\beta,\gamma} = \sum_{i=1}^{n} | R^S_{w_i} - R^O_{w_i,\alpha,\beta,\gamma} | \\
& delt_{best} = \min(delt_{\alpha,\beta,\gamma})
\end{aligned}
\right.
\tag{4}
$$

where $delt_{\alpha,\beta,\gamma}$ was the sum of absolute values of the difference between $R^S_{w_i}$ and $R^O_{w_i,\alpha,\beta,\gamma}$. $delt_{best}$ was the minimum of $delt_{\alpha,\beta,\gamma}$.

Using the above method, we got the best combination with $\alpha=0.4$, $\beta=0.4$, and $\gamma=0.2$.

Affinity propagation clustering analysis

Affinity Propagation (AP) clustering algorithm based on message passing was proposed by Frey and Dueck [55]. Unlike clustering algorithms such as k-means or k-medoids, AP does not require the setting of cluster numbers in advance. Instead, it simultaneously considers all data points as potential exemplars and recursively transmits real-valued messages until a high-quality set of exemplars and corresponding clusters emerges [56]. For each node i and each candidate exemplar k, AP calculates the "responsibility" $r(i, k)$ indicating the suitableness of k as an exemplar for i, and the "availability" $a(i, k)$ reflecting the evidence that i should choose k as an exemplar.

$$
r(i,k) \leftarrow s(i,k) - \max_{k':k' \neq k}\{a(i,k') + s(i,k')\}
\tag{5}
$$

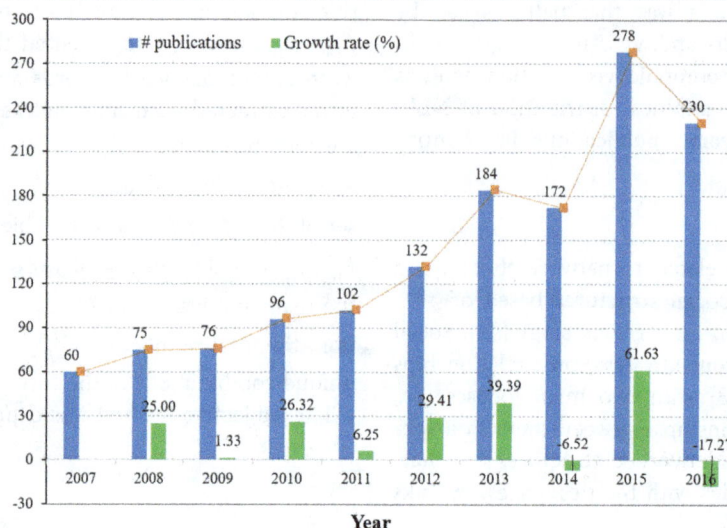

Fig. 1 The number and growth rate of publications by year

$$a(i,k) \leftarrow \min\{0, r(k,k) + \sum_{i':i' \notin \{i,k\}} \max\{0, r(i',k)\}\} \quad (6)$$

where the matrix $s(i, k)$ indicates the similarities (e.g., edge weights) between two nodes i and k, and the diagonal of this matrix contains the preferences for each node. Equations (5) and (6) are iterated until a good set of exemplars emerges. Each node i can then be assigned to the exemplar k which maximizes the sum $a(i, k) + r(i, k)$. If $i = k$, then i is an exemplar. A damping factor between 0 and 1 is used to control numerical oscillations.

As reported in literature, AP achieves considerable improvement over standard clustering methods such as k-means [57], spectral clustering [58] and superparamagnetic clustering [59]. It identifies clusters with lower error rate and lower time consumption [60].

We performed AP clustering using an R package *APCluster* [61] with a key terms correlation matrix as input data. The matrix was generated based on the co-occurrence matrix using Ochiai correlation coefficient calculated as $O_{ij} = A_{ij}/\sqrt{A_i A_j}$. A_i and A_j represent the frequencies of key terms W_i and W_j, respectively. A_{ij} donates the co-occurrence frequencies of W_i and W_j. The Ochiai coefficient is identical to cosine coefficient [62], thus it can express the similarity of two key terms in theme representation. The value range of O_{ij} is [0, 1]. The larger the O_{ij} is between two terms, the more similar the two terms are in theme representation.

Results

Literature distribution characteristics analysis

The number and growth rate of publications by year are shown in Fig. 1. From the figure, the number of NLP-empowered medical research publications was overall showing an increasing trend. Until 2012 the number of publications was around 100 per year. From 2013 to 2015, the number of publications increased to around 200 per year. The annual growth rate reached 18.39% on average, while the rate reached up to 61.63% from 2014 to 2015, witnessing the research upsurge in 2015. According to regression analysis, the non-linear model with the smallest AIC and biggest $\overline{R^2}$ (Table 2) was selected out as $y = 6.422397*10^6 - 6.408129*10^6 x + 1.598485*10^6 x^2$. With this model, the future research output can be estimated.

The 1405 publications were published in 324 unique sources. Table 3 shows the most productive 10 publication sources. These 10 sources together contributed more than 50% of the total publications. Among them, 8 belonged to journals, i.e., *Journal of the American Medical Informatics Association, Journal of Biomedical Informatics, BMC Bioinformatics, PloS ONE, Journal of Biomedical Semantics, Studies in Health Technology and Informatics, BMC Medical Informatics and Decision Making*, and *Biomedical Informatics Insights*. The rest 2 were conferences, i.e., *AMIA Annual Symposium Proceedings* and *AMIA Joint Summits on Translational Science Proceedings*.

There were 1386 publications with author affiliation information. The country distribution for first author

Table 2 AIC and $\overline{R^2}$ of 3 fitting models

Model	AIC	$\overline{R^2}$
$y = 0.06989x$	117.1439	0.7829
$y = -45,270.64 + 22.58x$	98.70681	0.855
$y = 6.422397*10^6 - 6.408129*10^6 x + 1.598485*10^6 x^2$	98.26147	0.8703

Table 3 Top 10 most productive publication sources

Publication sources	# related pub.	Proportion of related pub. against 1405 pub. (%)	Total #pub. of the sources (Proportion of related pub. against total #pub.)
Journal of the American Medical Informatics Association	154	10.96	1689 (9.12%)
AMIA Annual Symposium Proceedings	153	10.89	2283 (6.70%)
Journal of Biomedical Informatics	133	9.47	1378 (9.65%)
Studies in Health Technology and Informatics	91	6.48	7434 (1.22%)
BMC Bioinformatics	61	4.34	6332 (0.96%)
PloS ONE	36	2.56	166,876 (0.02%)
AMIA Joint Summits on Translational Science Proceedings	32	2.28	331 (9.67%)
Journal of Biomedical Semantics	28	1.99	322 (8.70%)
BMC Medical Informatics and Decision Making	27	1.92	1071 (2.52%)
Biomedical Informatics Insights	22	1.57	59 (37.29%)
Total	737	52.46	N/A

affiliation was analyzed based on these publications. Table 4 shows the top 8 countries with the highest number of publications and GDP per capita. The USA and Australia were listed in top 8 for the two metrics. According to the Spearman's rank correlation test applied to explore the relationship between publication numbers and GDP per capita, the testing p-value was 0.003, rejecting the null hypothesis at the significance level of 5%. And the Spearman's rank correlation coefficient was 0.445.

Figure 2 is the Google geomap of country's publications (access via the link [63]). A geomap is a map of a country or continent, with colors and values assigned to specific regions. Values are displayed as a color scale. Here the more publications one country had, the closer the color was to red. For the USA, the red region took a proportion up to 67.17%.

The top productive authors and first authors are presented in Table 5, where *Xu, Hua, Denny, Joshua C* and *Liu, Hongfang* were top 3 productive authors. The top 3 productive first authors were *Denny, Joshua C, Xu, Hua* and *Uzuner, Ozlem*. Three authors *Denny, Joshua C, Xu, Hua* and *Uzuner, Ozlem* appeared in both two ranks. The top productive author affiliations and first author affiliations are shown in Table 6, where *Mayo Clinic, The*

University of Utah, and *Vanderbilt University* ranked top 3 in both ranks.

Scientific collaboration analysis

The result of publication cooperation analysis on the 1386 publications is shown in Table 7. The number of co-author publications was 1318 during the year 2007–2016 with an annual co-author rate around 90%. The co-affiliation rate was generally increasing. Until 2013 the co-affiliation rate was around 45% per year. From 2014 until 2016, the co-affiliation rate increased to above 60%. The annual co-country rate during 2007–2014 was between 6.38% and 13.33%, and the number reached up to around 16% in 2015 and 2016.

We then visualized the cooperation among authors and affiliations. Fig. 3 is a generated network containing 87 authors with publications $> = 8$ (access via the link [64]). Fig. 4 shows a force directed network containing 50 affiliations with publications $> = 10$ (access via the link [65]). Furthermore, cooperation networks containing 204 authors with publications $> = 5$, and 108 affiliations with publications $> = 5$, as well as all authors and affiliations were also visualized (access via the link [66–69]). One can interactively drag and drop any

Table 4 Publications and GDP per capita by country

Country	#pub.	Proportion	Country	GDP per capita (1000 US dollars)
United States	931	67.17%	Norway	897.046
United Kingdom	72	5.19%	Switzerland	780.731
China (including Hong Kong and Macao)	54	3.90%	Denmark	589.324
France	50	3.61%	Ireland	554.754
Canada	29	2.09%	**Australia**	551.685
Germany	28	2.02%	Sweden	545.730
Japan	24	1.73%	**United States**	514.139
Australia	23	1.66%	Netherlands	506.744

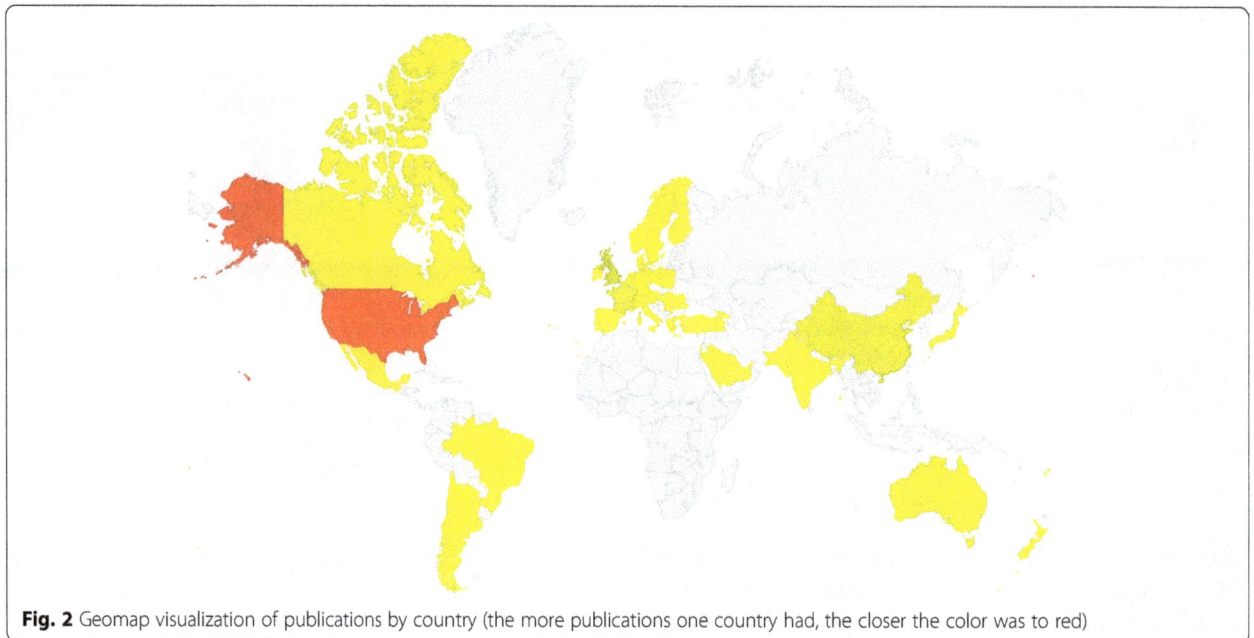

Fig. 2 Geomap visualization of publications by country (the more publications one country had, the closer the color was to red)

node in the networks to view connections for any specific author or affiliation.

Thematic discovery and evolution analysis

Using the optimized weights combination as $\alpha=0.4$, $\beta=0.4$, and $\gamma=0.2$, we finally obtained top 50 key terms with highest frequencies. Based on these key terms, a 50*50 co-occurrence matrix was generated, where the top 10 are shown in Table 8. The values on the main diagonal of the matrix donated the frequencies of terms and the values on the non-main diagonal indicated the numbers of publications that two terms appeared together.

The correlation matrix generated using Ochiai correlation coefficient was then used for AP clustering. The clustering result for the publication during the year 2007–2016 was as Fig. 5 and Table 9. The top 50 key terms were distributed into 10 clusters. We manually labelled each cluster by analyzing the meaning of representative terms and reviewing abstract content.

We further compared theme distribution for periods 2007–2011 and 2012–2016, their AP clustering results is shown in Table 10. As for the two periods, top 50 terms were clustered into 12 clusters. Clusters with same exemplars (i.e., cluster 1–8) were placed in top rows. Terms in bold type donated newly emerging terms for 2012–2016 period comparing with 2007–2011.

Discussion

A bibliometric analysis of NLP-empowered medical research publications from PubMed during the year 2007–2016 has been conducted. The analysis included three aspects: literature distribution characteristics analysis, scientific collaboration analysis, and thematic discovery and evolution analysis. Some findings were as follows:

1) The NLP-empowered medical research field has attracted the interests of scientific research community throughout years, which was observed in the annual growth of publications.
2) 10 most productive publication sources together contributed more than 50% of the 1405 publications. The top 3 were: *Journal of the American Medical Informatics Association*, *AMIA Annual Symposium Proceedings*, and *Journal of Biomedical Informatics*.
3) The USA had the highest number of publications with a proportion up to 67.17%. A moderately

Table 5 Top productive authors and first authors

Rank	Authors	#pub.	Rank	First authors	#pub.
1	Xu, Hua	54	1	Denny, Joshua C	12
2	Denny, Joshua C	50	2	Xu, Hua	9
3	Liu, Hongfang	41	3	Uzuner, Ozlem	8
4	Chute, Christopher G	27	4	Lacson, Ronilda	7
5	Chapman, Wendy W	25	4	Roberts, Kirk	7
6	Friedman, Carol	24	6	Deleger, Louise	6
7	Uzuner, Ozlem	21	6	Doan, Son	6
8	Savova, Guergana K	20	6	Fan, Jung-Wei	6
9	Solti, Imre	19	6	Gundlapalli, Adi V	6
10	Melton, Genevieve B	18	6	Meystre, Stephane M	6
10	Shen, Shuying	18			
10	Sohn, Sunghwan	18			

Table 6 Top productive author affiliations and first author affiliations

Rank	Author affiliations	#pub.	Rank	First author affiliations	#pub.
1	Mayo Clinic	86	1	Mayo Clinic	56
2	The University of Utah	82	2	The University of Utah	54
3	Vanderbilt University	78	3	Vanderbilt University	51
4	National Institutes of Health	64	4	Columbia University	43
5	Columbia University	59	5	National Institutes of Health	41
6	Brigham and Women's Hospital	52	6	Brigham and Women's Hospital	30
7	University of Washington	36	7	University of Minnesota	23
8	University of Pittsburgh	32	7	University of Pittsburgh	23
9	Massachusetts General Hospital	31	9	VA Salt Lake City Health Care System	21
9	Stanford University	31	10	Massachusetts General Hospital	19

significant correlation between country's publications and GDP per capita was revealed by the Spearman's rank correlation coefficient as 0.445.

4) We have identified prominent authors that have made significant contributions to the research field. Top productive authors included *Denny, Joshua C, Xu, Hua, Uzuner, Ozlem*, and *Liu, Hongfang*.

5) The top 3 most productive affiliations including *Mayo Clinic, The University of Utah*, and *Vanderbilt University* have devoted 17.75% of the 1386 publications.

6) The annual co-affiliation rate increased to above 60% from 2014 until 2016, and the annual co-country rate reached up to around 16% in 2015 and 2016. The cooperation among specific authors and affiliations were visualized using network graphs.

7) The NLP-empowered medical research focused on 10 main thematic areas during the year 2007–2016 including *Computational biology, Terminology mining, Information extraction, Text classification, Social medium as data source, Clinical information, Patient characteristics, Performance measurements, Outcome evaluation*, and *Information retrieval*.

8) By observing the newly emerging terms in Table 10, some differences and new research topics can be identified for recent research during the year 2012–2016 compared with 2007–2011. Especially, cluster 1, 2, 8, 9, 10, 11, and 12 were ought to be paid attention to. For example, *Information extraction* and *Named entity recognition* have become more popular in medical research during the year 2012–2016. For Cluster 2, terms related to age, i.e., *Middle aged, Adult*, and *Aged*, indicated that researchers gradually paid more attention to the age characteristic of target population in addition to gender. In cluster 8 for 2012–2016 period, the new term *Social medium* indicated a focus on utilizing social media data for medical analysis [70]. The new term *Machine learning* in cluster 9 for 2012–2016 period witnessed increasing interest in combining *Machine learning* and NLP techniques, e.g., [71, 72].

The findings can potentially benefit relevant researchers, especially newcomers in: understanding the research performance and recent development of NLP-empowered medical research field, selecting scientific cooperation

Table 7 The statistics of author and affiliation cooperation

Year	Total #pub.	#co-author pub.	Co-author rate%	#co-affiliation pub.	Co-affiliation rate%	#co-country pub.	Co-country rate%
2007	58	54	93.10	26	44.83	7	12.07
2008	73	64	87.67	32	43.84	8	10.96
2009	75	70	93.33	36	48.00	9	12.00
2010	94	85	90.43	44	46.81	6	6.38
2011	100	96	96.00	46	46.00	10	10.00
2012	129	121	93.80	63	48.84	13	10.08
2013	180	175	97.22	111	61.67	24	13.33
2014	171	161	94.15	111	64.91	22	12.87
2015	278	273	98.20	170	61.15	46	16.55
2016	228	219	96.05	146	64.04	36	15.79
Total	1386	1318	N/A	785	N/A	181	N/A

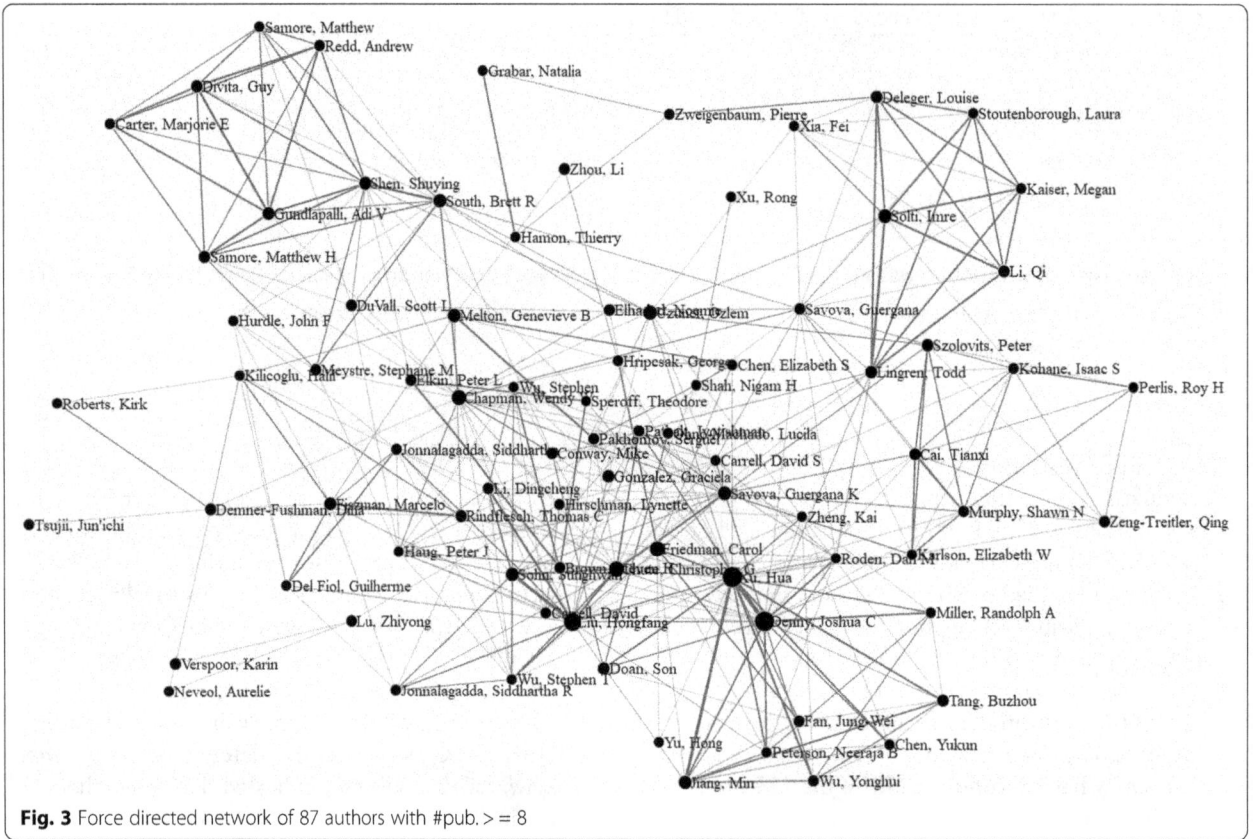

Fig. 3 Force directed network of 87 authors with #pub. >= 8

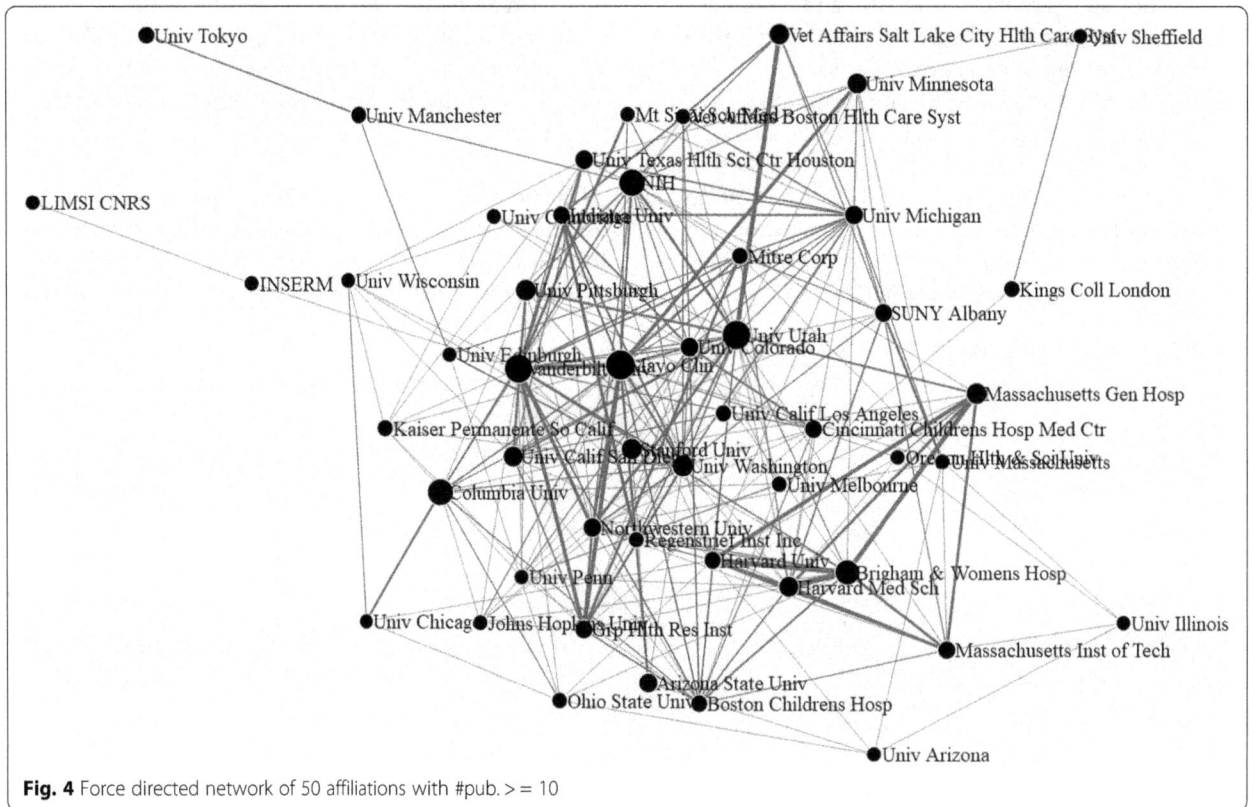

Fig. 4 Force directed network of 50 affiliations with #pub. >= 10

Table 8 The top 10 key terms in the co-occurrence matrix

	Artificial intelligence	Data mining	Electronic health record	Female	Information storage and retrieval	Machine learning	Medical record	Patient	Precision	Semantics
Artificial intelligence	185	52	53	11	56	40	25	33	40	33
Data mining	52	288	122	31	20	53	38	55	46	52
Electronic health record	53	122	420	78	80	60	95	167	77	40
Female	11	31	78	169	15	10	46	82	18	10
Information storage and retrieval	56	20	80	15	239	18	30	42	47	47
Machine learning	40	53	60	10	18	162	25	39	30	22
Medical record	25	38	95	46	30	25	178	77	29	8
Patient	33	55	167	82	42	39	77	326	59	19
Precision	40	46	77	18	47	30	29	59	217	34
Semantics	33	52	40	10	47	22	8	19	34	165

partners with the knowledge of predominant authors, affiliations, and countries, optimizing research topic decision to keep abreast of current research hotspots, and monitoring new scientific or technological activities.

In term importance weighting, the combination of subjective and objective methods was used. The subjective weighing result might vary from person to person due to subjective judgment. Thus, in this paper, we ranked the importance by semantics analysis as well as reviewing text content to keep high consistence with text intention.

In our study, AP clustering method was performed based on top 50 high frequency key terms in order to acquire a moderate number of categories. However, this might result in the ignorance of some sudden terms that are possible for representing research fronts although with low frequencies. Therefore, in our future work, we will make improvement by trying alternative methods such as Latent Dirichlet Allocation to consider every single term.

The AP clustering results were on the whole reasonable and easy-to-understand. However, we still found that terms with similar semantics, i.e., Data mining and Text mining were not clustered into the same cluster in the same context NLP, which might cause confusion. AP clustering was conducted based on the key terms correlation matrix, and the matrix was calculated using Ochiai

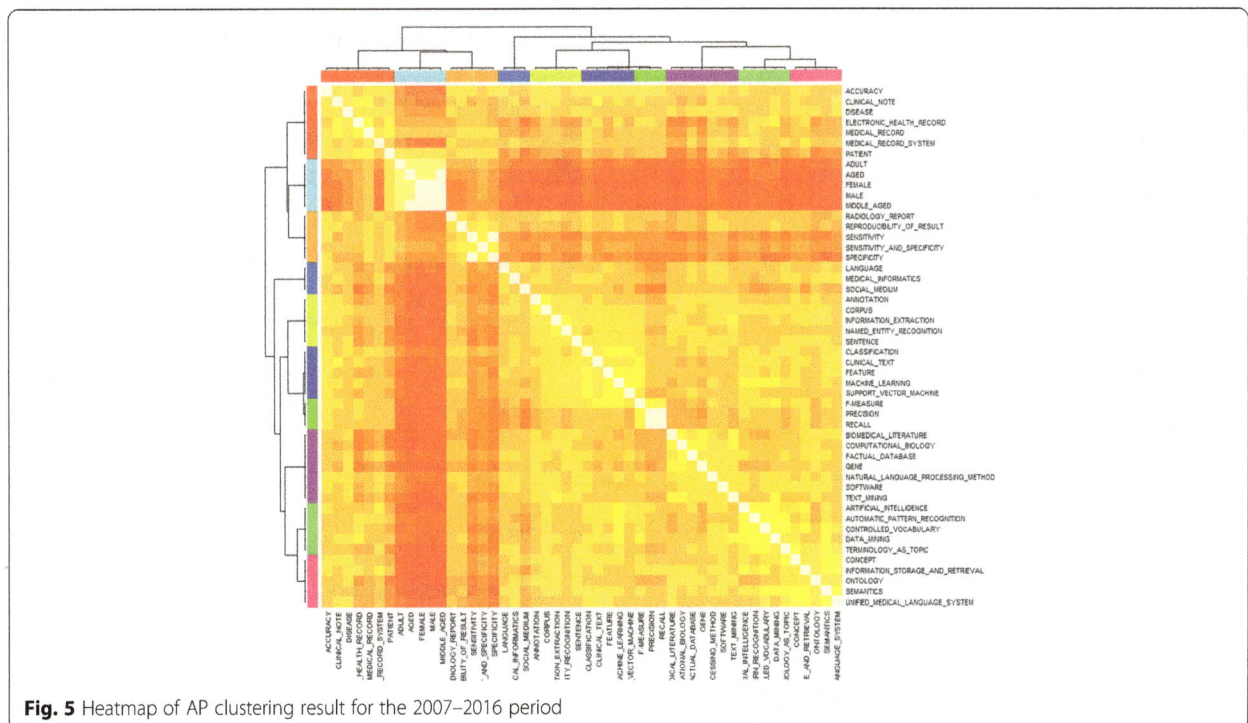

Fig. 5 Heatmap of AP clustering result for the 2007–2016 period

Table 9 AP clustering result for the publication during the year2007–2016

Cluster	Theme	Key terms
1	Computational biology	**Computational biology**; Biomedical literature; Factual database; Gene; Natural language processing method; Software; Text mining
2	Terminology mining	**Controlled vocabulary**; Artificial intelligence; Automatic pattern recognition; Data mining; Terminology as topic
3	Information extraction	**Corpus**; Annotation; Information extraction; Named entity recognition; Sentence
4	Text classification	**Feature**; Classification; Clinical text; Machine learning; Support vector machine
5	Social medium as data source	**Language**; Medical informatics; Social medium
6	Clinical information	**Medical record**; Accuracy; Clinical note; Disease; Electronic health record; Medical record system; Patient
7	Patient characteristics	**Middle aged**; Adult; Aged; Female; Male
8	Performance measurements	**Recall**; F-measure; Precision
9	Outcome evaluation	**Sensitivity and specificity**; Radiology report; Reproducibility of result; Sensitivity; Specificity
10	Information retrieval	**Unified medical language system**; Concept; Information storage and retrieval; Ontology; Semantics

correlation coefficient. Hence, the clustering results might be vulnerable to choices of both calculation method and clustering method. Therefore, in our future work, we will conduct comparison on different calculation methods of correlation matrix as well as different clustering methods for further exploration.

In the study, PubMed as the biggest medical related publication resource was used as data source. However, a minor number of publications might be in NLP-related journals and conferences. Thus, in our future work, we will consider including these journals and conference as additional publication sources.

Conclusions

This paper presents a bibliometric analysis of NLP-empowered medical research publications from PubMed during the year 2007–2016 with the purpose of understanding the research status of the field. Some literature distribution characteristics including productive publication sources, authors, affiliations, and countries are

Table 10 Comparison of AP clustering results for the 2007–2011 and 2012–2016 periods

Cluster	2007–2011	Cluster	2012–2016
1	Text mining; Abstracting and indexing as topic; Annotation; Database management system; Sentence	1	Text mining; **Information extraction**; **Named entity recognition**
2	Female; Male	2	Female; Male; **Middle aged**; **Adult**; **Aged**
3	Recall; Precision; F-measure	3	Recall; Precision; F-measure; Accuracy
4	Artificial intelligence; Information storage and retrieval; Automatic pattern recognition	4	Artificial intelligence; Semantics; Information storage and retrieval; Clinical text; Concept; Language; Sentence; Unified medical language system
5	Computational biology; Factual database; Gene; Protein; Protein-protein interaction	5	Computational biology; Factual database; Software; **Free text**
6	Classification; Feature; Semantics; Data mining; Natural language processing method; Unified medical language system	6	Classification; Feature; Support vector machine; **Classifier**
7	Patient; Disease; Medical record; Medical record system; Patient discharge; Sensitivity and specificity	7	Patient; Medical record; Electronic health record; Clinical note
8	Medical informatics; User-computer interface; Software	8	Medical informatics; Annotation; Corpus; Gene; **Social medium**
9	Clinical text; Accuracy; Clinical decision support system; Clinical note; Electronic health record; Natural language processing system; Support vector machine	9	Automatic pattern recognition; Controlled vocabulary; Data mining; **Machine learning**
10	Word; Corpus; Language	10	**Sensitivity**; **Confidence interval**; **Specificity**
11	Biomedical literature; Knowledge; Medline; Ontology	11	**Reproducibility of result**; **Radiology report**; Sensitivity and specificity
12	Terminology as topic; Concept; Controlled vocabulary	12	Disease; Natural language processing method; **Phenotype**

First term in each cluster donates exemplar. Terms in bold type donate new emergent terms for 2012–2016 period compared with 2007–2011 period

provided with statistics analysis methods. Scientific collaborations among authors and affiliations are visualized with network analysis method. Affinity propagation clustering method is used for thematic discovery and evolution analysis. Some interesting results and findings are presented. To our knowledge, there was no similar study thoroughly examining NLP-empowered medical research publications. Our work can potentially assist relevant researchers, especially newcomers in keeping abreast of the NLP-empowered medical research status, seeking scientific cooperation partners, optimizing research topics choices, and monitoring new scientific or technological activities.

Abbreviations

AIC: Akaike Information Criterion; AP: Affinity Propagation; EHR: Electronic Health Record; EHRs: Electronic Health Records; EMRs: Electronic Medical Records; GDP: Gross Domestic Product; MeSH: Medical subject headings; NIH: National Institutes of Health; NLP: Natural Language Processing; USA: United States; WoS: Web of Science

Funding

Publication of the article is supported by grants from National Natural Science Foundation of China (No.61772146), Research Grants Council of Hong Kong Special Administrative Region, China (UGC/FDS11/E04/16), and Innovative School Project in Higher Education of Guangdong Province (No.YQ2015062).

Authors' contributions

XLC led the method application, experiment conduction and the result analysis. HRX, FLW, ZQL, and JX participated in the design of the research and the revision of the manuscript. TYH provided theoretical guidance, the key term extraction program development and the revision of this paper. All authors read and approved the final manuscript.

Competing interests

The authors declare that they have no competing interests.

Author details

[1]College of Economics, Jinan University, Guangzhou, China. [2]Department of Mathematics and Information Technology, The Education University of Hong Kong, Hong Kong, Hong Kong, Special Administrative Region of China. [3]School of Science and Technology, The Open University of Hong Kong, Hong Kong, Hong Kong, Special Administrative Region of China. [4]The Second Clinical Medical College, Guangzhou University of Chinese Medicine, Guangzhou, China. [5]The Research Institute of National Supervision and Audit Law, Nanjing Audit University, Nanjing, China. [6]School of Information Science and Technology, Guangdong University of Foreign Studies, Guangzhou, China. [7]School of Computer, South China Normal University, Guangzhou, China.

References

1. Cambria E, White B. Jumping NLP curves: a review of natural language processing research. IEEE Comput Intell Mag. 2014;9(2):48–57.
2. Liddy ED. Natural language processing. In: Encyclopedia of Library and Information Science. New York: 2nd ed; 2001. p. 2126–36.
3. Batet M, Sánchez D, Valls A. An ontology-based measure to compute semantic similarity in biomedicine. J Biomed Inform. 2011;44(1):118–25.
4. Meystre S, Automation HPJ. Of a problem list using natural language processing. BMC medical informatics and decision making. 2005;5(1):30.
5. Wang PW, Hao TY, Jin LW, Yan J. Large-Scale Extraction of drug-disease pairs from biomedical literature for drug repurposing. Journal of the Association for Information Science and Technology. 2017;68(11):2649–61.
6. Névéol A, Zweigenbaum P. Clinical natural language processing in 2015: leveraging the variety of texts of clinical interest. IMIA Yearbook. 2016:234–9.
7. Xiao B, Imel ZE, Georgiou PG, Atkins DC, Narayanan SS. "Rate my therapist": automated detection of empathy in drug and alcohol counseling via speech and language processing. PLoS One. 2015;10(12):e0143055.
8. Zhang YY, Tang BZ, Jiang M, Wang JQ, Xu H. Domain adaptation for semantic role labeling of clinical text. J Am Med Inform Assoc. 2015;22(5):967–79.
9. Sidorov G, Velasquez F, Stamatatos E, Gelbukh A, Chanona-Hernández L. Syntactic n-grams as machine learning features for natural language processing. Expert Syst Appl. 2014;41(3):853–60.
10. Chasin R, Rumshisky A, Uzuner O, Szolovits P. Word sense disambiguation in the clinical domain: a comparison of knowledge-rich and knowledge-poor unsupervised methods. J Am Med Inform Assoc. 2014;21(5):842–9.
11. Wang Y, Zheng K, Xu H, Mei QZ. Clinical word sense disambiguation with interactive search and classification. In: Proc. of AMIA annual symposium; 2016. p. 2062–71.
12. Nikfarjam A, Sarker A, O'Connor K, Ginn R, Gonzalez G. Pharmacovigilance from social media: mining adverse drug reaction mentions using sequence labeling with word embedding cluster features. J Am Med Inform Assoc. 2015;22(3):671–81.
13. Sun WY, Rumshisky A, Uzuner O. Normalization of relative and incomplete temporal expressions in clinical narratives. J Am Med Inform Assoc. 2015; 22(5):1001–8.
14. Albers DJ, Elhadad N, Tabak E, Perotte A, Hripcsak G. Dynamical phenotyping: using temporal analysis of clinically collected physiologic data to stratify populations. PLoS One. 2014;9(6):e96443.
15. Lin C, Dligach D, Miller TA, Bethard S, Savova GK. Multilayered temporal modeling for the clinical domain. J Am Med Inform Assoc. 2015;23(2):387–95.
16. Li Q, Spooner SA, Kaiser M, Lingren N, Robbins J, Lingren T, et al. An end-to-end hybrid algorithm for automated medication discrepancy detection. BMC medical informatics and decision making. 2015;15(1):37–49.
17. Zheng L, Wang Y, Hao SY, Shin AY, Jin B, Ngo AD, et al. Web-based real-time case finding for the population health Management of Patients with Diabetes Mellitus: a prospective validation of the natural language processing–based algorithm with statewide electronic medical records. JMIR medical informatics. 2016;4(4):e37.
18. Hao TY, Rusanov A, Boland MR, Weng CH. Clustering clinical trials with similar eligibility criteria features. J Biomed Inform. 2014;52:112–20.
19. Hao TY, Liu HF, Weng CH. Valx: a system for extracting and structuring numeric lab test comparison statements from text. Methods Inf Med. 2016; 55(3):266–75.
20. Hao TY, Weng CH. Adaptive Semantic tag mining from heterogeneous clinical research texts. Methods Inf Med. 2015;54(2):164–70.
21. Hao TY, Chen XL, Huang GM. Discovering commonly shared semantic concepts of eligibility criteria for learning clinical trial design. Lect Notes Comput Sci. 2015;9412:3–13.
22. Cobo MJ, Martínez MA, Gutiérrez-Salcedo M, Fujita H, Herrera-Viedma E. 25 years at knowledge-based systems: a bibliometric analysis. Knowl-Based Syst. 2015;80:3–13.
23. Cobo MJ, López-Herrera AG, Herrera-Viedma E, Herrera F. An approach for detecting, quantifying, and visualizing the evolution of a research field: a practical application to the fuzzy sets theory field. Journal of Informetrics. 2011;5(1):146–66.
24. Chen XL, Chen BY, Zhang CX, Hao TY. Discovering the recent research in natural language processing field based on a statistical approach. Lect Notes Comput Sci. 2017;10676:507–17.
25. Wallace ML, Larivière V, Gingras Y. A small world of citations? The influence of collaboration networks on citation practices. PLoS One. 2012;7(3):e33339.
26. Chen XL, Weng H, Hao TY. A data-driven approach for discovering the recent research status of diabetes in China. Lect Notes Comput Sci. 2017; 10594:89–101.
27. Boudry C, Mouriaux F. Eye neoplasms research: a bibliometric analysis from 1966 to 2012. Eur J Ophthalmol. 2015;25(4):357–65.
28. Diem A, Wolter SC. The use of bibliometrics to measure research performance in education sciences. Res High Educ. 2013;54(1):86–114.

29. Fan XM, Gao Y, Ma B, Xia ZF. Chinese academic contribution to burns: a comprehensive bibliometrics analysis from 1985 to 2014. Burns. 2016;42(7): 1463–70.

30. Venable GT, Khan NR, Taylor DR, Thompson CJ, Michael LM, Klimo P. A correlation between National Institutes of Health funding and bibliometrics in neurosurgery. World neurosurgery. 2014;81(3):468–72.

31. Harande YI, Alhaji IU. Basic Literature of diabetes: a bibliometrics analysis of three countries in different world regions. Journal of Library and Inf Sci. 2014;2(1):49–56.

32. Ramos JM, Padilla S, Masia M, Gutierrez F. A bibliometric analysis of tuberculosis research indexed in PubMed, 1997–2006. The International Journal of Tuberculosis and Lung Disease. 2008;12(12):1461–8.

33. Holliday EB, Ahmed AA, Yoo SK, Jagsi R, Hoffman KE. Does cancer literature reflect multidisciplinary practice? A systematic review of oncology studies in the medical literature over a 20-year period. Int J Radiat Oncol Biol Phys. 2015;92(4):721–31.

34. Boudry C, Denion E, Mortemousque B, Mouriaux F. Trends and topics in eye disease research in PubMed from 2010 to 2014. PeerJ. 2016;4:e1557.

35. Khan A, Choudhury N, Uddin S, Hossain L, Baur LA. Longitudinal trends in global obesity research and collaboration: a review using bibliometric metadata. Obes Rev. 2016;17(4):377–85.

36. Kramer PF, Onetto J, Flores MT, Borges TS, Feldens CA. Traumatic dental injuries in the primary dentition: a 15-year bibliometric analysis of dental traumatology. Dent Traumatol. 2016;32(5):341–6.

37. Velmurugan C. Research trends in journal of intellectual property rights (JIPR): a bibliometric study. Libr Philos Pract. 2013;1043:1–16.

38. Hussain A, Fatima N, Kumar D. Bibliometric analysis of the'Electronic Library'journal (2000-2010). Webology. 2011;8(1):87.

39. Newman ME. Coauthorship networks and patterns of scientific collaboration. Proc Natl Acad Sci. 2004;101(1):5200–5.

40. Radev DR, Joseph MT, Gibson B, Muthukrishnan P. A bibliometric and network analysis of the field of computational linguistics. Journal of the Association for Information Science and Technology. 2016;67(3):683–706.

41. Muñoz-Leiva F, Viedma-del-Jesús MI, Sánchez-Fernández J, López-Herrera AG. An application of co-word analysis and bibliometric maps for detecting the most highlighting themes in the consumer behaviour research from a longitudinal perspective. Quality & Quantity. 2012;46(4):1077–95.

42. Geaney F, Scutaru C, Kelly C, Glynn RW, Perry IJ. Type 2 diabetes research yield, 1951-2012: bibliometrics analysis and density-equalizing mapping. PLoS One. 2015;10(7):e0133009.

43. Li L, Liu Y, Zhu HH, Ying S, Luo QY, Luo H, et al. A bibliometric and visual analysis of global geoontology research. Comput Geosci. 2017;99:1–8.

44. Heo GE, Kang KY, Song M, Lee JH. Analyzing the field of bioinformatics with the multi-faceted topic modeling technique. BMC bioinformatics. 2017;18(7):251.

45. Jiang HC, Qiang MS, Lin P. A topic modeling based bibliometric exploration of hydropower research. Renew Sust Energ Rev. 2016;57:226–37.

46. Yeung AWK, Goto TK, Leung WK. The changing landscape of neuroscience research, 2006–2015: a bibliometric study. Front Neurosci. 2017;11:120.

47. Martínez MA, Cobo MJ, Herrera M, Herrera-Viedma E. Analyzing the scientific evolution of social work using science mapping. Res Soc Work Pract. 2015; 25(2):257–77.

48. Cobo MJ, Chiclana F, Collop A, de Ona J, Herrera-Viedma E. A bibliometric analysis of the intelligent transportation systems research based on science mapping. IEEE Trans Intell Transp Syst. 2014;15(2):901–8.

49. Dehdarirad T, Villarroya A, Barrios M. Research trends in gender differences in higher education and science: a co-word analysis. Scientometrics. 2014; 101(1):273–90.

50. Mann PS. Introductory statistics. New York: John Wiley & Sons; 2007.

51. MacEachren AM, Boscoe FP, Haug D, Pickle LW. Geographic visualization: designing manipulable maps for exploring temporally varying georeferenced statistics. Proc of IEEE Information Visualization Symposium. 1998:87–94.

52. Otte E, Rousseau R. Social network analysis: a powerful strategy, also for the information sciences. J Inf Sci. 2002;28(6):441–53.

53. Wasserman S, Faust K. Social network analysis: methods and applications. Press: Cambridge Univ; 1994.

54. Serrat O. Social network analysis. Singapore: Knowledge solutions. Springer; 2017. p. 39–43.

55. Frey BJ, Dueck D. Clustering by passing messages between data points. Science. 2007;315(5814):972–6.

56. Frey BJ, Dueck D. Response to comment on "clustering by passing messages between data points". Science. 2008;319(5864):726.

57. MacQueen J. Some methods for classification and analysis of multivariate observations. In: Proc of the fifth Berkeley symposium on mathematical statistics and probability. 1967;1(14):281–97.

58. Shi JB, Malik J. Normalized cuts and image segmentation. IEEE Trans Pattern Anal Mach Intell. 2000;22(8):888–905.

59. Shental N, Zomet A, Hertz T, Weiss Y. Pairwise clustering and graphical models. Adv Neural Inf Proces Syst. 2004:185–92.

60. El-Samak AF, Ashour W. Optimization of traveling salesman problem using affinity propagation clustering and genetic algorithm. Journal of Artificial Intelligence and Soft Computing Research. 2015;5(4):239–45.

61. Bodenhofer U, Kothmeier A, Hochreiter S. APCluster: an R package for affinity propagation clustering. Bioinformatics. 2011;27(17):2463–4.

62. Romesburg C. Cluster analysis for researchers: Lulu Press; 2004.

63. Geomap of country publication. http://www.zhukun.org/haoty/resources. asp?id=BMC_publication_map. Accessed 20 Nov 2017.

64. The network of authors (#pub.>= 8). *http://www.zhukun.org/haoty/resources. asp?id=BMC_coauthor_8* (Accessed 20 Nov 2017).

65. The network of affiliations (#pub.>= 10). *http://www.zhukun.org/haoty/ resources.asp?id=BMC_affiliation_10* (Accessed 20 Nov 2017).

66. The network of authors (#pub.>= 5). *http://www.zhukun.org/haoty/resources. asp?id=BMC_coauthor_5* (Accessed 20 Nov 2017).

67. The network of affiliations (#pub.>= 5). *http://www.zhukun.org/haoty/ resources.asp?id=BMC_affiliation_5* (Accessed 20 Nov 2017).

68. The network of all authors. *http://www.zhukun.org/haoty/resources.asp?id= BMC_coauthor_all* (Accessed 20 Nov 2017).

69. The network of all affiliations. *http://www.zhukun.org/haoty/resources.asp?id= BMC_affiliation_all* (Accessed 20 Nov 2017).

70. Demner-Fushman D, ElhadaXd N. Aspiring to unintended consequences of natural language processing: a review of recent developments in clinical and consumer-generated text processing. IMIA Yearbook. 2016:224–33.

71. Osborne JD, Wyatt M, Westfall AO, Willig J, Bethard S, Gordon G. Efficient identification of nationally mandated reportable cancer cases using natural language processing and machine learning. J Am Med Inform Assoc. 2016; 23(6):1077–84.

72. Yadav K, Sarioglu E, Choi H, Cartwright WB, Hinds PS, Chamberlain JM. Automated outcome classification of computed tomography imaging reports for pediatric traumatic brain injury. Acad Emerg Med. 2016;23(2):171–8.

17

Evaluating hospital websites in Kuwait to improve consumer engagement and access to health information

Dari Alhuwail[1,2]* ⓘ, Zainab AlMeraj[1] and Fatima Boujarwah[1] ⓘ

Abstract

Background: Current advances in information and communication technology have made accessing and obtaining health-related information easier than ever before. Today, many hospital websites use a patient-centric approach to promote engagement and encourage learning for better health-related decision making. However, little is known about the current state of hospital websites in the State of Kuwait. This study aims to evaluate hospital websites in Kuwait and offer recommendations to improve patient engagement and access to health information.

Methods: This study employs a cross-sectional analytical approach to evaluate hospital websites in Kuwait in 2017. The websites of hospitals that provide in-patient services were identified through a structured search. Only active websites that were available in either English or Arabic were considered. The evaluation of the websites involved a combination of automated and expert- based evaluation methods and was performed across four dimensions: Accessibility, Usability, Presence, and Content.

Results: Nine hospitals met the inclusion criteria. Most of the websites fell short in all four dimensions. None of the websites passed the accessibility guidelines. The usability of websites varied between hospitals. Overall, the majority of hospitals in Kuwait have rudimentary online presence and their websites require careful reassessment with respect to design, content, and user experience. The websites focus primarily on promoting services provided by the hospital rather than engaging and communicating with patients or providing evidence-based information.

Conclusions: Healthcare organization and website developers should follow best-practices to improve their websites taking into consideration the quality, readability, objectivity, coverage and currency of the information as well as the design of their websites. Hospitals should leverage social media to gain outreach and better engagement with consumers. The websites should be offered in additional languages commonly spoken by people living in Kuwait. Efforts should be made to ensure that health information on hospital websites are evidence-based and checked by healthcare professionals.

Keywords: Website evaluation, Accessibility, Usability, Social media, Consumer health informatics, Patient participation, Patient education

* Correspondence: dari.alhuwail@ku.edu.kw
[1]Department of Information Science, College of Computing Sciences and Engineering, Kuwait University, Adailiya, Kuwait
[2]Health Informatics Unit, Dasman Diabetes Institute, Sharq, Kuwait

Background

In today's connected world, consumers are increasingly using the Internet to seek health-related information [1–4]. This increase is catalyzed by the surge of mobile technologies and affordable access to the World Wide Web [5, 6], thus creating opportunities for healthcare organizations to engage their consumers via informative and educational online platforms. Researchers argue that patients, and their potential role in managing their conditions, have been the least utilized resource in healthcare [7, 8]. Evidence suggests that patients who are more actively involved in their own healthcare experience better outcomes and do not burden the healthcare system with high costs [9]. This is far more feasible as health Information Technology (IT) solutions can facilitate better patient-centered care via improving healthcare processes, clinical outcomes, responsiveness to patients' needs and preferences, shared decision-making, communication between patients and clinicians, and access to medical information [10, 11]. Therefore, many healthcare organizations today are leveraging health IT tools and solutions, such as websites, to better engage, involve, and educate patients [12, 13].

Typically, hospital websites are a good reference for general information about a hospital, its services, and its clinicians [14]. These websites could also serve as a good medium to educate and inform patients, their families, and the general public about diseases, procedures, medications, and healthy lifestyles [15–17]. However, despite the promise of greater information availability, patient-focused healthcare websites have not advanced as quickly as compared to other industries [18]. This is especially true for the Gulf Cooperation Council (GCC)[1] region. Hospital websites in Kuwait, Saudi Arabia and the United Arab Emirates for example, offer limited access to necessary education and support resources for patients' wellbeing and are not tailored to the customs, culture, and language of those living in the region [19–21]. In recent years, Kuwait has had significant movements towards electronic government across its agencies [22]. Yet, little is known about the levels of participation of healthcare facilities, including hospitals, in these initiatives. After all, hospitals are an essential part of successful government interaction with the citizens through the web.

Therefore, it becomes important to understand the current state of hospital websites and evaluate them to improve access to health information as well as patient engagement. This study aims to thoroughly evaluate hospital websites and offer recommendations to improve patient engagement and access to health information. We examine hospital websites in the State of Kuwait as a sample from the GCC region and offer recommendations for healthcare organization and website developers to improve the quality of information, authority and objectivity, coverage and currency, as well as the design of their websites. The countries of the GCC have very similar healthcare systems, face similar challenges, and share a history of cooperation between them [23, 24]. As such, any lessons learned about the status of hospital websites in Kuwait will in turn benefit the entire region.

Healthcare system in Kuwait

Through its constitution, the State of Kuwait is obligated to provide free universal coverage to its citizens while expatriates pay nominal fees for non-emergency health services and government-subsidized medications. In Kuwait, approximately 80% of healthcare services are rendered by the public sector through the Ministry of Health, which acts as the owner, operator, regulator, and financer across the country. The government provides these services through 92 primary care centers, 6 general hospitals, and 13 specialized hospitals and centers [25]. While Kuwait has low rates of infectious and communicable diseases, the non-communicable and chronic diseases account for 73% of total deaths [26]. In 2015, Kuwait's public health expenditure was more than 7% of the total government expenditure [27]. It is clear from the expenditure data that the public healthcare system in Kuwait is heavily reliant on treatment as opposed to preventative services [26]. The alarming rates of non-communicable and chronic diseases pose serious challenges for the government [28] and demand better patient engagement and education via accessible means in todays' connected world (i.e. online health-related websites). Hence this research evaluates the status of hospital websites in Kuwait across multiple dimensions for their consumer engagement and access to health information and services.

Methods

Design and approach

This study employs a cross-sectional analysis approach [29] to evaluate hospital websites in the State of Kuwait. Initially, the list of hospital websites in Kuwait was compiled from the Ranking Web of World Hospitals [30]. An additional manual search was conducted in "Google Search" to locate additional websites of hospitals not listed by the Ranking Web of World Hospitals. For websites to be considered for inclusion, the website must be active, reachable, available in either the Arabic or English language, and associated with a hospital recognized by the Ministry of Health in Kuwait which offers multi-day in-patient admissions and services.

Evaluation

The researchers followed analogous procedures employed by similar studies in analyzing the hospital websites [18, 31–33]. Data collection about the websites began in April 2017 and took approximately 1 week to complete. Data collection was conducted within the week to ensure that information collected across the websites and their pages were not affected by their availability or major modifications. The researchers evaluated English (and Arabic if available) pages of the included websites.

Prior to collecting the data and evaluating the websites, the researchers determined appropriate checklists to evaluate the following dimensions: Accessibility, Usability, Presence, and Content. Similar checklists that were used by other researchers were used as a foundation for the checklists used in this study. The developed checklists were carefully crafted to ensure compatibility with the nature of the healthcare system in Kuwait, the cultural and social norms. For example, the researchers took into account the popular social media platforms used in Kuwait and included them as part of the checklist for Presence.

As shown in Table 1, these checklists involve a set of criteria that could either be checked automatically or by an expert user [18, 31, 32]. The expert-based website evaluations were conducted by two-experts according to the checklists, their scores were compared and in the event that there was disagreement, these differences were discussed and reconciled between them.

Accessibility

This dimension evaluates the website's accessibility according to criteria set by the World Wide Web Consortium (W3C). The Content Accessibility Guidelines (WCAG) [34] at Level AA were chosen for this study. To evaluate the accessibility of the hospital websites, an automated tool named AChecker was used [35]. Three commonly visited web pages were chosen per hospital and evaluated: The home/landing page, the clinicians' directory, and contact page. The resulting dataset included 26 web pages (9*3–1) with one page found to be under construction. For each web page, the automatic tool tests the HTML source code for adherence to the WCAG 2.0 guidelines based on standard principles to ensure the content is: Perceivable,

Operable, Understandable, and Robust. The AChecker tool divides observed problems into three categories:

- (K) Known problems that are identified as obscuring accessibility.
- (L) Likely problems that are identified as probably obscuring accessibility.
- and (P) Potential problems that could not be identified by the tool and requires the help of an expert to determine their nature.

Usability

This dimension is an assessment of the website's ability to present information to its consumers in a useful way. It focuses on the clarity of the information presented, how consistent the website is overall, and whether it offers good functionality or not. The Minervation LIDA Instrument V1.2 [36], an instrument developed specifically to assess healthcare websites, was used to evaluate the websites. The researchers assessed the websites' (a) clarity and appropriateness of language used, (b) consistency of website design and ease of navigation, and (c) functionality of the site in providing users with the right tools to find what they need without overburdening them with unnecessary functions.

Presence

This dimension is an assessment of the website's digital presence and online reach-ability through different channels and mediums. Researchers developed a modified checklist based on prior studies [18]. This checklist considered the presence of the hospital in the most accessed social media channels by people living in Kuwait [37]. The researchers collected information about the number of Facebook page likes, number of Twitter and Instagram followers, the number of YouTube channel subscribers. In instances where the website did not specifically provide a link to its social media accounts, the researchers performed the search manually and directly through the social media websites.

Content

This dimension is an assessment of the website's overall content quality without taking into consideration the technical limitations. The websites' content is assessed using (i) the Health On the Net (HON) Foundation's Site Evaluation checklist [38], which is an overall assessment of the reliability of health-related information available on the Internet, and (ii) the readability scores using the Fletch-Kincaid Reading Ease and Grade Level scales [39].

Table 1 Evaluation methods adopted for the study

Dimension	Criteria	Evaluation mode
Accessibility		
	AChecker [35]	Automated
Usability		
	LIDA [36]	Expert-based
Presence		
	Modified Checklist [18]	Expert-based
Content		
	HON [38]	Expert-based
	Readability [39]	Automated

Results

In total, 15 websites were identified by the researchers. After applying the inclusion/exclusion criteria, four websites were excluded because they were inactive at the time of the data collection and two additional websites were for hospitals that did not offer in-patient admissions. Only nine hospitals with unique website domains were included in the study. This included six private and three government hospitals. Refer to Table 2 for detailed demographic information about the evaluated hospitals [40].

Accessibility

The results of the evaluation indicate that there was no single website that passed the WCAG 2.0 [Level AA] accessibility guidelines.

Table 3 shows the number of identified problems averaged across the set of three pages per hospital according to the four accessibility principles. Notable is the proportion of perceivable errors, which are higher in comparison to others. The tool also identified a total of 3034 Known errors, 35 Likely problems, and 9483 Potential problems across all pages as presented in Table 4. Interestingly, the identified 'Known' problems have the largest impact and are relatively easy to resolve. Descriptions of these problems are summarized in Table 5.

Perceivable

Overall, the majority of the errors found fall under the principle Perceivable. The most common perceptual errors across all tested hospital pages as shown in Table 5 are "image elements missing alternate attributes" (1776 errors), "multiple i (italic) elements used" (142 errors), and "lack of contrast between text and background colors" (69 errors). Additionally, images, plug-ins and embedded media all require alternative text such as captions, sign language, and audio descriptions, with a clear indication of the language used. There are 80 errors pertaining to this problem alone.

Table 2 Hospital demographic information

Hospital ID and type	Outpatient visits	No. of beds	Age (years)	No. of employees
H1 - Private[a]	15,439	117	54	733
H2 - Private[a]	12,255	106	50	529
H3 - Private[a]	17,335	185	9	860
H4 - Private[a]	7481	61	11	267
H5 - Private[a]	6282	105	8	478
H6 - Private[a]	6433	64	19	344
H7 - Government	7723	189	64	650
H8 - Government	20,219	375	52	965
H9 - Government	3525	769	68	716

[a]Full adoption of electronic health records

Table 3 The average known hospital website problems per principle

ID	Perceivable	Operable	Understandable	Robust
H1	317	7	14	1
H2	74	3	2	0
H3	32	32	8	1
H4	612	120	6	1
H5	15	1	0	0
H6	0	0	2	0
H7	6	4	2	0
H8	9	1	2	0
H9	59	0	2	0

Operable

Being able to navigate and find content is very important. Developers are advised to make all functionality, and features added to the websites, available from the keyboard. For example, "mouse over missing event handler" (103 errors) and "scripts not accessible by the keyboard" (61 errors) should be removed to allow users enough time to read and use content. Missing navigation methods to help find content and location on the websites such as "missing titles and anchor texts" (over 100 errors) can be easily overcome.

Understandable and robust

A total of 166 errors were found in relation to understandability. For a website to be readable and understandable, assistive technologies must recognize the document language and the language code. Every hospital website evaluated has at least one missing document language and language code identification (33, 32 errors consecutively), as well as multiple missing labels and label texts (101 errors) that often lead to confusion for webpage visitors.

Usability

The lowest scoring website was that of hospital (H6). This hospital has a fully flash-based website. This made the site completely unusable without a plug-in and reduced the usability scores across all 3 sections of the checklist. The highest scoring hospital overall (H1), did not receive the highest score in all 3 sections, however, it did perform relatively well in all 3 sections. Refer to Fig. 1 for overall usability evaluation scores and Table 6 for the specific scores per website.

Within the Clarity sub-dimension, on average the websites had higher scores for appropriateness of the language, and lower scores for ease of navigation. All websites, except H6, achieved a score of 6 or higher in the Consistency sub-dimension. In the Functionality subdimension, only 3 websites provided an effective search

Table 4 AChecker results[a]

ID	Landing page				Find a clinician				Contact us			
	Result	K	L	P	Result	K	L	P	Result	K	L	P
H1	F	320	10	640	F	316	0	639	F	382	0	506
H2	F	46	0	440	F	149	0	1052	F	42	0	227
H3	F	124	0	1434	F	19	0	240	F	30	0	336
H4	F	143	10	425	F	556	0	682	F	94	1	439
H5	F	21	0	383	F	9	0	282	F	17	0	304
H6	F	2	0	10	F	2	0	20	F	2	0	10
H7	F	30	6	115	F	3	0	44	F	3	0	38
H8	F	14	3	80	F	13	0	88	F	10	0	108
H9	F	8	1	103	F	174	0	148	NA	NA	NA	NA

[a]F Fail, P Pass, K Known, L Likely, P Potential problems

facility. On the other hand, the highest scoring criteria across the sites was the availability of effective browsing facilities.

Presence

The majority of websites had presence on social media platforms, namely Facebook, Twitter, YouTube, and Instagram (Refer to Table 7 for more detailed information). It is worth nothing that government hospital websites did not leverage social media to expand their online presence. Only one government hospital had Twitter and Instagram accounts with less than 700 followers to each account.

Content

Most of the evaluated hospitals (6) had their websites available in both Arabic and English. Overall, the English

Table 5 Top 15 known accessibility issues

List of common *known* problems (Level AA)	Count
Element "img" missing "alt" attribute	1776
Element "i" or italic used	142
On-mouseover event handler missing on-focus event handler	103
Image used as anchor is missing valid "alt" text	80
Insufficient contrast between text color and its background	69
Script not keyboard accessible – on-mouse-out missing on-blur	61
Anchor contains no text	53
Label text is empty	47
Input element type of "text" has no/missing associated label	38
Document language not identified	33
Document has invalid language code	32
Input element type of "text" has no text in label	21
Header nesting error	19
Element selected missing an associated label	18

versions of the websites appeared more comprehensive and contained more information.

Authoritative information

Consistently across all the evaluated websites, some of the health and medical information was not attributed to an author. Only two websites provided information that was not authoritative in nature. Also, there were no clear statement that particular sections of the website contained information from non-medically qualified individuals or organizations.

Complementarity of information

None of the websites declared that the information provided on their sites was designed to support and not replace the relationship that exists between the site visitor and his or her existing healthcare provider.

Statement on privacy

Only one website declared a clear privacy and confidentiality policy regarding the use and storage of e-mail addresses, personal, and medical information via the website. It was not clear whether any of the websites respected the legal requirements, including those concerning medical and personal information privacy, that apply in Kuwait.

Medical information and its sources

While the majority of the websites (7) provided medical information for patients and site visitors in the form of original content, none of the websites provided a modification date, both for the website as a whole or for the pages that contained medical information. Specifically, two of these websites provided medical information from outside source (e.g. information about Diabetes and pregnancy) without properly citing the source. One website offered electronic versions of its printed hospital magazine, which was in the Arabic language. Another

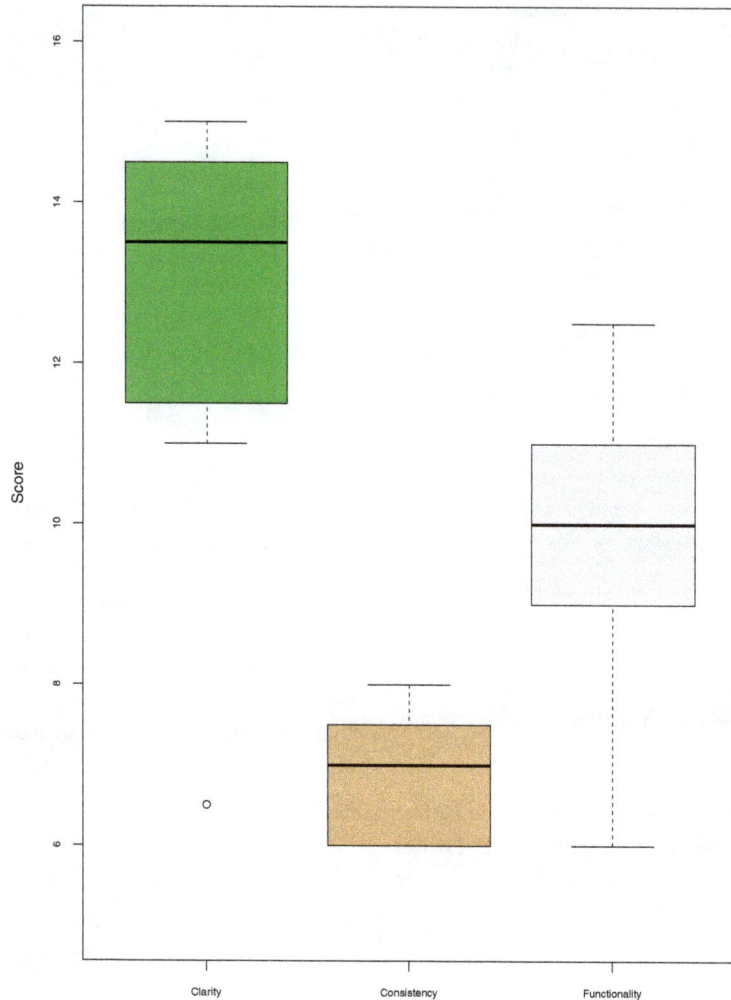

Fig. 1 Boxplot of hospital website usability scores

website offered bilingual (Arabic/English) patient leaflets organized by medical specialties that were available at the hospital. Another website offered only English health education information. Two additional sites embedded health education videos (one website in Arabic and one website in English) from their channels on YouTube.

Table 6 Hospital website usability scores[a]

ID	Clarity (18)	Consistency (9)	Functionality (15)	Overall (42)
H1	13.5	8	12.5	34
H2	14.5	6.5	11	32
H3	15	7	10.5	32.5
H4	14	8	12.5	34.5
H5	11.5	6	9	26.5
H6	13.5	6	10	29.5
H7	11	7.5	9	27.5
H8	14.5	7.5	10	32
H9	6.5	6	6	18.5
Min	6.5	6	6	18.5
Max	15	8	12.5	34.5
Median	13.5	7	10	32

[a]Total score for each usability sub-category is reported in parenthesis

Table 7 Hospitals' presence across social media networks

ID	Facebook	Twitter	YouTube	Instagram
H1	38,872	6971	652	21,700
H2	8743	924	25	21,800
H3	1698	N/A	40	N/A
H4	9111	14,200	3046	24,500
H5	2374	144,000	21	59,500
H6	217	497	0	14,200
H7	N/A	659	10	571
H8	N/A	N/A	N/A	N/A
H9	N/A	N/A	N/A	N/A

Justifiability of the information
Eight websites contained original content and did not make any claims relating to the benefit or performance of a specific medical treatment, commercial product or service. Only two websites made such claims based on personal research or opinions. *Disclosures:* All the websites included in this study did not clearly describe any potential conflicts of interest including funding sources and its advertising policy.

Content readability
The websites' median score for the Flesch-Kincaid Reading Ease test was 41.4. and at the ninth-grade level, exceeding the recommended sixth-grade level. The Flesch-Kincaid readability tests indicates how difficult a passage in English is to understand by specifying the grade level the text is recommended for. As the reading ease score increases, the recommended grade level is lowered. Refer to Table 8 for more detailed scores per website.

Discussion
To the best of our knowledge, no prior study evaluated Kuwaiti hospital websites thoroughly by examining the accessibility, presence, content, and usability dimensions. Overall, the results suggest that the majority of hospitals in Kuwait require careful evaluation of their websites' design and content. Interestingly, while governmental hospitals in Kuwait are older in age and provide care services to a large number of patients, they are behind in adopting and maintaining well-designed websites. This could be attributed to their overall slow adoption of health IT solutions, for example electronic health records, as illustrated in Table 2.

It is interesting to note that despite local residents' extensive reliance on major well-established government hospitals for healthcare, the websites and online presence of these institutions are rudimentary. Our findings also

highlight that the evaluated websites focus primarily on promoting services provided rather than engaging and communicating with patients or providing evidence-based health information. With the growing demand from consumers to locate health information online [41], it becomes essential for hospitals in Kuwait to create and maintain well-designed and engaging websites that adhere to international and national standards [18]. In the remainder of this section we discuss implications for practice and based on our finding offer recommendations relevant to hospital administrators and website developers.

Designing for accessibility
As evident from the results, due to the low level of conformance to the W3C WCAG 2.0 accessibility guidelines, it is necessary for Kuwaiti hospitals to consider the issues highlighted in this evaluation. Failing to adhere to these kinds of standards have recently been considered a form of discrimination against persons with disabilities [42–44]. To improve website accessibility, web developers should:

(a) Experiment with different representations of text whether it be visual, audio, tactile representations or a combination of the three. For example, a blind person can understand a picture if the browser reads out an attached alternative text and analogously a deaf person can understand a picture or audio file if there is a visual alternative on the page.
(b) Provide users the ability to control the contrast between foreground text and background color on the webpages to help users with poor vision read the text on the page.
(c) Avoid the use of bold and italic text as assistive technologies fail to identify these styles. As an alternative, substituting styles with fonts that are easier to read are recommended.
(d) Validate pages and close open tags to help assistive technologies perform parsing will improve robustness of the websites and compatibility across Internet browsers.

Considering the types of errors discussed in the results, it is feasible to consider that the hospital website developers lack awareness of Web accessibility standards and tools such as WGAC 2.0. Therefore, it is important to increase web developers' awareness and knowledge of established accessibility standards and guidelines through appropriate training. Future studies could investigate Web developers' awareness of existing accessibility standards and practices in more detail.

Empowering usability
As demonstrated by the website usability scores (refer to Table 6), it is interesting to note that the government

Table 8 Websites' Flesch-Kincaid readability scores[a]

ID	Reading ease	Grade level
H1	44.2	9
H2	38.2	9
H3	62.7	5.4
H4	35.2	9.1
H5	−6.9	14.9
H6	78.9	4
H7	46.4	8.7
H8	63.4	5.5
H9	33.4	10.1
Median	*41.42*	*9.65*

[a]Scores are reported for only for pages written in English. For reading ease scores, 100–90 = very easy, 30-zeor = very difficult

hospitals scored among the lowest compared to the private hospitals. Our results are consistent with similar studies [45] suggesting the need to improve usability. It is recommended that hospitals conduct usability sessions with patients regularly to enhance usability. Additionally, there is a great opportunity for government hospitals to use their websites to help educate patients as well as provide electronic services such as booking appointments or contacting medical professionals. It is possible that improving website usability could reduce demand for services and help hospitals better manage wait times for services. With well-designed hospital websites, healthcare providers can engage patients and guide them to quality, evidence-based health information [3].

Curating health information

As evident from the findings, across all hospital websites, many webpages that contained health and medical information were not attributed to an author. Therefore, it is important that any medical or health advice provided online should be given by medically-trained and qualified professional only [46]. Clinicians should play a more active role by asking patients what they learned from online resources and where they obtained the information from, including hospital websites [47]. Clinicians can then better assist patients in a shared and collaborative decision-making process that paints a complete picture of for example the risks and benefits of treatment options [48].

All hospital websites can benefit from carefully and thoroughly reviewing the content of their websites and ensuring that it is evidence-based and conforms to the HON principles. The evidence reveals that many hospital webpages that may have contained advertising or promotional health information were indistinguishable from clinical information. As the Internet becomes crowded with biased health and medical information, hospital websites need to clearly label advertisements and promotional information about procedures clearly as to not cloud the judgement of patients [16]. Hospitals need to apply more scrutiny and stricter advertising regulations to eliminate the imbalance between clinical information and the promotional information which can negatively impact the patient decision-making. Additionally, there is a need for authoritative and regulatory bodies (e.g. the Ministry of Health and Public Authority for Food and Nutrition) to take a more active role in certifying health information on hospital websites.

Reaching diverse populations

Despite the fact that nearly 70% of Kuwait's population are expatriates who may not speak Arabic or English [49], the evaluated websites were available in only the Arabic and/or English languages. The hospital websites should be offered in additional languages commonly spoken by people living in Kuwait, such as Hindi, Urdu, and Tagalog [21]. Additionally, the results reveal that the evaluated websites are written at readability levels above the recommended reading levels for the multiethnic, multicultural general public in Kuwait [50]. The website and its content's readability are a concern since many of Kuwait's population are nonnative English (or Arabic) speakers. While the American Medical Association and the National Institutes of Health recommend that the readability of patient education materials should not exceed a sixth-grade reading level [51, 52], no specific reading level recommendation is available for the GCC context [53]. Therefore, hospitals should carefully develop the content on their websites in a manner that is easy to read, understand and comprehend by the general population.

Similar to other findings [54], the results demonstrate the modest presence of hospital websites, especially government hospitals, on social media platforms. Given that most of healthcare services are provisioned by the public sector, it is essential that Kuwaiti government hospitals leverage social media to gain better outreach and engagement with patients. Doing so will also help hospitals increase their market share and improve patient experience and engagement [55, 56].

The results clearly showcase that private hospitals in Kuwait are doing better with regards to having a more professional and engaging website. Perhaps this is due to the fierce nature of competing with other hospitals over funds and to attract more patients with private insurance or those that can pay out-of-pocket. Whereas the government hospitals generally do not compete with any other hospitals, neither private or government.

Comparison with prior work

This study followed similar evaluation approaches to earlier studies conducted in different parts of the world as illustrated in Table 9. The evidence from our study has many similar findings with the evidence from the listed studies and it points out that many hospital websites need careful evaluation and rework to improve the access and quality of information presented on the website as well as improve the website visitors' engagement and the services provided online. Globally, it also appears that many hospitals still have low presence on social media and are not fully leveraging and embracing its power to engage patients. Distinctively, this study focuses on both public and private hospital websites in a specific geographic region, whereas some of the other studies focused on specific diseases. While the Internet and the World Wide Web has no boundaries, the contextual determinants, i.e. the structure of the healthcare systems, culture, and customs, can be different among geographic regions and locations.

Table 9 Summary of similar Studies[a]

Study	Country or region	Website type	Sample size	Year	Major findings
Maifredi et al. [57]	Italy	Italian hospitals	763	2009	High percentage of hospitals do not provide an official website. Very few websites provide information to increase credibility of hospital and user confidence in institution.
Liu et al. [58]	China	Public hospitals	23	2009	Most websites show good performance in content, a normal performance in function and design, but bad performance in website management & usage.
Selig et al. [59]	Germany	Burn centers	44	2010	Websites offer a good overview about institution's online services via numerous multimedia-based elements. However, the quality of specific information for burn patients is relatively poor.
Orlowski et al. [60]	USA	Heart failure websites	5	2011	Websites written at high readability levels (8-9th grade), but easily navigated.
Weber et al. [21]	GCC	General health websites	925	2012	Evaluating HON standards, approximately less than 10% of websites post privacy policy or authorship of information. Over 50% of websites provide a date for information. Only 1.7% report advertising policy and 23.5% disclose sponsorships.
Huerta et al. [32]	USA	Hospital websites	2407	2013	Management of hospitals' online presence is not adequate.
Huerta et al. [18]	USA	Children hospital websites	153	2014	Wide range of websites' score with no perfect website suggesting room for meaningful improvements.
Raj et al. [61]	India	General health websites	32	2014	Most websites have average quality, especially in usability. Many websites written at high readability levels.
Salarvand et al. [33]	Iran	Public hospitals	59	2016	Overall, low level quality of the websites evaluated.

[a]Some studies were focused on general health information and were not specific to hospitals

Study strengths and limitations

Similar to other research, this study has several strengths and limitations. The included nine hospitals in this study represent approximately 40% ($N = 22$) of the healthcare institutions in Kuwait that provide healthcare services beyond primary care. Carefully studying other healthcare organizations, including primary care centers, out-patient clinics, and physician offices will help provide more insights about the overall online presence of healthcare organizations in Kuwait. The researchers performed additional web searches of hospital websites to be included in the study and did not rely solely on the original listing of hospital websites in Kuwait by Ranking Web of World Hospitals. Additionally, while patient perspectives were not in the scope of this study, the researchers, who are informatics experts, recalled their experiences as patients when navigating the websites. Future studies should solicit feedback directly from patients and consumers seeking information from hospital websites. Lastly, the results can be informative for hospitals in Kuwait when evaluating how their current and future websites will support patients' informational needs. However, careful consideration of the specific context is required before directly assuming applicability of the results to all hospitals in the GCC or other Arab countries.

Conclusions

The proliferation of the Internet as a source for health information presents a great opportunity for hospitals to better engage with their patients and improve their care experience. In this study, we provide a comprehensive assessment of nine Kuwaiti in-patient hospitals using automated and expert-based tools and evaluation methods. To the best of our knowledge, no prior study evaluated Kuwaiti hospital websites thoroughly by examining the accessibility, presence, content, and usability dimensions. Most of the websites fell short in all four dimensions. Overall, the majority of hospitals in Kuwait require careful reassessment with respect to design, content, and user experience. The websites focus primarily on promoting services provided by the hospital rather than engaging and communicating with patients or providing evidence-based information. Hospital administrators, public relations managers, and web developers can use the recommendations resulting from this study to improve their hospitals' websites. Future studies can investigate the perceptions and opinions of patients and consumers in the broader GCC areas in terms of accessibility, usability, presence, and content of hospital websites.

Endnotes

[1]GCC countries include Saudi Arabia, Kuwait, the United Arab Emirates, Qatar, Bahrain, and Oman.

Abbreviations
GCC: Gulf Cooperation Council; HON: Health on the Net

Authors' contributions
DA, ZA, FA developed the study design, acquired the data, conducted the analysis and drafted the manuscript. All authors developed the manuscript iteratively and approved the final manuscript.

Competing interests

The authors declare that they have no competing interests.

References

1. Moreno MA. Seeking health information online. JAMA Pediatr. 2017;171:500.
2. Jamal A, Khan SA, AlHumud A, Al-Duhyyim A, Alrashed M, Bin Shabr F, et al. Association of Online Health Information-Seeking Behavior and Self-Care Activities among Type 2 diabetic patients in Saudi Arabia. J Med Internet Res. 2015;17:e196.
3. Lee K, Hoti K, Hughes JD, Emmerton L. Dr Google and the consumer: a qualitative study exploring the navigational needs and online health information-seeking behaviors of consumers with chronic health conditions. J Med Internet Res. 2014;16:e262.
4. Reid P, Borycki EM. Emergence of a new consumer health informatics framework: introducing the healthcare organization. Stud Health Technol Inform. 2011;164:353–7.
5. Ranallo PA, Kilbourne AM, Whatley AS, Pincus HA. Behavioral health information technology: from Chaos to clarity. Health Aff (Millwood). 2016; 35:1106–13.
6. Amante DJ, Hogan TP, Pagoto SL, English TM, Lapane KL. Access to care and use of the internet to search for health information: results from the US National Health Interview Survey. J Med Internet Res. 2015;17(4):e106.
7. Lindblad S, Ernestam S, Van Citters AD, Lind C, Morgan TS, Nelson EC. Creating a culture of health: evolving healthcare systems and patient engagement. QJM Int J Med. 2017;110:125–9.
8. Carman KL, Dardess P, Maurer M, Sofaer S, Adams K, Bechtel C, et al. Patient and family engagement: a framework for understanding the elements and developing interventions and policies. Health Aff (Millwood). 2013;32:223–31.
9. Crawford MJ, Rutter D, Manley C, Weaver T, Bhui K, Fulop N, et al. Systematic review of involving patients in the planning and development of health care. BMJ. 2002;325:1263.
10. Street RL, Liu L, Farber NJ, Chen Y, Calvitti A, Zuest D, et al. Provider interaction with the electronic health record: the effects on patient-centered communication in medical encounters. Patient Educ Couns. 2014;96:315_9.
11. Cipriano PF, Bowles K, Dailey M, Dykes P, Lamb G, Naylor M. The importance of health information technology in care coordination and transitional care. Nurs Outlook. 2013;61:475–89.
12. Coulter A. Patient engagement--what works? J Ambulatory Care Manage. 2012;35:80–9.
13. Snyder CF, Wu AW, Miller RS, Jensen RE, Bantug ET, Wolff AC. The role of informatics in promoting patient-centered care. Cancer J Sudbury Mass. 2011;17:211–8.
14. Snyder K, Ornes LL, Paulson P. Engaging patients through your website. J Healthc Qual Off Publ Natl Assoc Healthc Qual. 2014;36:33–8.
15. Lewis D, Chang BL, Friedman CP. Consumer health informatics. Consum health inform. 1st ed. New York: Springer; 2005. p. 1–7.
16. Schenker Y, London AJ. Risks of imbalanced information on US hospital websites. JAMA Intern Med. 2015;175:441–3.
17. Ow D, Wetherell D, Papa N, Bolton D, Lawrentschuk N. Patients' perspectives of accessibility and digital delivery of factual content provided by official medical and surgical specialty society websites: a qualitative assessment. Interact J Med Res. 2015;4:e7.
18. Huerta TR, Walker DM, Ford EW. An evaluation and ranking of Children's hospital websites in the United States. J Med Internet Res. 2016;18:e228.
19. Househ M, Alsughayar A, Al-Mutairi M. Empowering Saudi patients: how do Saudi health websites compare to international health websites? Stud Health Technol Inform. 2013;183:296–301.
20. Halawa N, Abduo H, Abughefreh A, Dawwas B. The diabetes Kuwait resource Centre: development, implementation, and offered services. Gulf Med J. 2015;4:8–13.
21. Weber AS, Verjee M, Rahman ZH, Ameerudeen F, Al-Baz N. Typology and credibility of internet health websites originating from gulf cooperation council countries. East Mediterr Health J. 2015;20:804–11.
22. AlAwadhi S, Morris A. Factors influencing the adoption of e-government services. J Softw. 2009;4:584–90.
23. Alkhamis A, Hassan A, Cosgrove P. Financing healthcare in gulf cooperation council countries: a focus on Saudi Arabia. Int J Health Plann Manag. 2014; 29:e64–82.
24. Khoja T, Rawaf S, Qidwai W, Rawaf D, Nanji K, Hamad A. Health Care in Gulf Cooperation Council Countries: a review of challenges and opportunities. Cureus. 2017;9:e1586.
25. Kuwait Life Sciences Company. Market Overview 2016, Kuwait. [cited 2018 Mar 15]. Available from: https://www.tfhc.nl/wp-content/uploads/2017/08/KLSC-IMS-Kuwait-Health-Industry-Report-2016-vF2.pdf.
26. World Health Organization. Noncommunicable Diseases (NCD) Country Profiles, Kuwait. [cited 2018 Mar 15]. Available from: http://www.who.int/nmh/countries/kwt_en.pdf
27. Kuwait Life Sciences Company. Kuwait 2015: Health Mega-Projects Report. [cited 2018 Mar 15]. Available from: http://www.internetworldstats.com/stats.htm
28. Asbu EZ, Masri MD, Kaissi A. Health status and health systems financing in the MENA region: roadmap to universal health coverage. Glob Health Res Policy. 2017;2:25.
29. Mann CJ. Observational research methods. Research design II: cohort, cross sectional, and case-control studies. Emerg Med J. 2003;20:54–60.
30. Utrilla Ramírez AM, Fernández M, Ortega JL, Aguillo IF. Ranking the world's web of hospitals: status of the hospitals on the world wide web. Med Clin (Barc). 2009;132:144–53.
31. Aladwani AM, Palvia PC. Developing and validating an instrument for measuring user-perceived web quality. Inf Manag. 2002;39:467–76.
32. Huerta TR, Hefner JL, Ford EW, McAlearney AS, Menachemi N. Hospital website rankings in the United States: expanding benchmarks and standards for effective consumer engagement. J Med Internet Res. 2014;16:e64.
33. Salarvand S, Samadbeik M, Tarrahi MJ, Salarvand H. Quality of public hospitals websites: a cross-sectional analytical study in Iran. Acta Inform Medica AIM J Soc Med Inform Bosnia Herzeg Cas Drustva Za Med Inform BiH. 2016;24:130–3.
34. World Wide Web Consortium (W3C). Web Content Accessibility Guidelines (WCAG). [cited 2018 Mar 15]. Available from: https://www.w3.org/WAI/intro/wcag.php
35. AChecker. Web Accessibility Checker. [cited 2018 Mar 15]. Available from: https://achecker.ca/
36. Küçükdurmaz F, Gomez MM, Secrist E, Parvizi J. Reliability, readability and quality of online information about Femoracetabular impingement. Arch Bone Jt Surg. 2015;3:163–8.
37. Al-Menayes JJ. Dimensions of social media addiction among university students in Kuwait. Psychol Behav Sci. 2015;4:23–8.
38. Boyer C, Selby M, Scherrer J-R, Appel R. The health on the net code of conduct for medical and health websites. Comput Biol Med. 1998;28:603–10.
39. WebpageFX. Readability Test Tool. [cited 2018 Mar 15]. Available from: https://www.webpagefx.com/tools/read-able/
40. National Health Information Center. Kuwait Health, Annual Health Report. Kuwait: Ministry of Health; 2016. Report No.: 52
41. Bhandari N, Shi Y, Jung K. Seeking health information online: does limited healthcare access matter? J Am Med Inform Assoc JAMIA. 2014;21:1113–7.
42. United States Department of Justice - Civil Rights Division. Americans with Disabilities Act. [cited 2018 Mar 15]. Available from: https://www.ada.gov/
43. Office for Disability Issues, HM Government. Equality Act 2010. [cited 2018 Mar 15]. Available from: https://www.gov.uk/government/publications/equality-act-guidance
44. Australia Commonwealth Consolidated Acts. Disability Discrimination Act 1992. [cited 2018 Mar 15]. Available from: http://www.austlii.edu.au/cgi-bin/viewdb/au/legis/cth/consol_act/dda1992264/
45. Lin H-W, Ku C-H, Li J, Tan AC, Chou C-H. A nationwide evaluation on electronic medication-related information provided by hospital websites. J Eval Clin Pract. 2013;19:304–10.
46. Rhebergen MDF, Lenderink AF, van Dijk FJH, Hulshof CTJ. Comparing the use of an online expert health network against common information sources to answer health questions. J Med Internet Res. 2012;14:e9.
47. Fahy E, Hardikar R, Fox A, Mackay S. Quality of patient health information on the internet: reviewing a complex and evolving landscape. Australas Med J. 2014;7:24–8.
48. Ventola CL. Social media and health care professionals: benefits, risks, and best practices. P T Peer Rev J Formul Manag. 2014;39:491–520.
49. Public Authority for Civil Information. Statistics Services System. [cited 2018 Mar 15]. Available from: https://www.paci.gov.kw/stat/.
50. Walsh TM, Volsko TA. Readability assessment of internet-based consumer health information. Respir Care. 2008;53:1310–5.

51. Kher A, Johnson S, Griffith R. Readability assessment of online patient education material on congestive heart failure. Adv Prev Med. 2017;2017: 9780317.

52. Eltorai AEM, Ghanian S, Adams CA, Born CT, Daniels AH. Readability of patient education materials on the american association for surgery of trauma website. Arch Trauma Res. 2014;3:e18161.

53. Nair SC, Ibrahim H, Askar OS. Comparison of good clinical practice compliance and readability ease of the informed consents between observational and interventional clinical studies in the emirates. Perspect Clin Res. 2016;7:123–7.

54. Griffis HM, Kilaru AS, Werner RM, Asch DA, Hershey JC, Hill S, et al. Use of social media across US hospitals: descriptive analysis of adoption and utilization. J Med Internet Res. 2014;16:e264.

55. Thackeray R, Neiger BL, Keller H. Integrating social media and social marketing: a four-step process. Health Promot Pract. 2012;13:165–8.

56. Moorhead SA, Hazlett DE, Harrison L, Carroll JK, Irwin A, Hoving C. A new dimension of health care: systematic review of the uses, benefits, and limitations of social media for health communication. J Med Internet Res. 2013;15:e85.

57. Maifredi G, Orizio G, Bressanelli M, Domenighini S, Gasparotti C, Perini E, et al. Italian hospitals on the web: a cross-sectional analysis of official websites. BMC Med Inform Decis Mak. 2010;10:17.

58. Liu X, Bao Z, Liu H, Wang Z. The quality and characteristics of leading general hospitals' websites in China. J Med Syst. 2011;35:1553–62.

59. Selig HF, Lumenta DB, König C, Andel H, Kamolz LP. Evaluation of the online-presence (homepage) of burn units/burn centers in Germany, Austria and Switzerland. Burns J Int Soc Burn Inj. 2012;38:444–9.

60. Orlowski JL, Oermann MH, Shaw-Kokot J. Evaluation of heart failure websites for patient education. Adv Emerg Nurs J. 2013;35:240–6.

61. Raj S, Sharma VL, Singh AJ, Goel S. Evaluation of quality and readability of health information websites identified through India's major search engines. Adv Prev Med. 2016;2016:4815285.

The QUEST for quality online health information: validation of a short quantitative tool

Julie M. Robillard[1,2,3]* (iD), Jessica H. Jun[1,2], Jen-Ai Lai[1,2] and Tanya L. Feng[1,2]

Abstract

Background: Online health information is unregulated and can be of highly variable quality. There is currently no singular quantitative tool that has undergone a validation process, can be used for a broad range of health information, and strikes a balance between ease of use, concision and comprehensiveness. To address this gap, we developed the QUality Evaluation Scoring Tool (QUEST). Here we report on the analysis of the reliability and validity of the QUEST in assessing the quality of online health information.

Methods: The QUEST and three existing tools designed to measure the quality of online health information were applied to two randomized samples of articles containing information about the treatment ($n = 16$) and prevention ($n = 29$) of Alzheimer disease as a sample health condition. Inter-rater reliability was assessed using a weighted Cohen's kappa (κ) for each item of the QUEST. To compare the quality scores generated by each pair of tools, convergent validity was measured using Kendall's tau (τ) ranked correlation.

Results: The QUEST demonstrated high levels of inter-rater reliability for the seven quality items included in the tool (κ ranging from 0.7387 to 1.0, $P < .05$). The tool was also found to demonstrate high convergent validity. For both treatment- and prevention-related articles, all six pairs of tests exhibited a strong correlation between the tools (τ ranging from 0.41 to 0.65, $P < .05$).

Conclusions: Our findings support the QUEST as a reliable and valid tool to evaluate online articles about health. Results provide evidence that the QUEST integrates the strengths of existing tools and evaluates quality with equal efficacy using a concise, seven-item questionnaire. The QUEST can serve as a rapid, effective, and accessible method of appraising the quality of online health information for researchers and clinicians alike.

Keywords: Online health information, Quality evaluation, eHealth, Instrument validation

Background

The Internet has revolutionized how information is distributed and has led to the rapid expansion of health resources from a wide variety of content providers, ranging from government organizations to for-profit companies. Consulting online health information is an increasingly popular behavior, with 80% of Internet users engaging in this activity [1]. Health information consumers worldwide, particularly those in developing countries and remote areas, may benefit from accessible and immediate retrieval of up-to-date information [2, 3]. This new information gateway also promotes autonomy by allowing patients to be more active in their health [4].

The dynamic nature of the Internet, however, introduces important concerns in parallel with these benefits. Online information is unregulated and can be of highly variable quality [5]. This has critical implications for users as it is estimated that over half of the adult population in the United States and Canada does not possess an adequate level of health literacy [6, 7], and low health literacy is negatively

* Correspondence: jrobilla@mail.ubc.ca
[1]Division of Neurology, Department of Medicine, The University of British Columbia, Vancouver, Canada
[2]BC Children's & Women's Hospital, Vancouver, Canada
Full list of author information is available at the end of the article

correlated with the ability to discriminate between high and low quality eHealth information [8]. Compounding this issue, there is a growing number of individuals who use online information to guide health care decisions, either for themselves or on behalf of another person. It is therefore crucial to develop effective methods to evaluate online health information [9]. To this end, there have been many efforts to develop tools that assess the quality of online health information; while such tools will not solve the issue of regulation, they can assist end-users, health care professionals and researchers in differentiating between high- and low-quality online sources.

A scoping review of the literature on the evaluation of health information was conducted using Arksey and O'Malley's six-stage methodological framework [10]. The scoping review aimed to identify existing health information evaluation tools and information available in the literature on their demonstrated validity and reliability. An iterative team approach was used to determine a search strategy balancing feasibility and comprehensiveness. Data was collected via keyword searches and citation searches on Google Scholar and PubMed. Seven combinations of following keywords were used: online, health information, evaluate, evaluation, tool, quality, validity, testing, validation, and assessment. A total of 49 records were retrieved between January 15, 2016 and February 5, 2016. Thirty-six[1] of these articles were included in the review based on the following inclusion criteria: 1) the article is in the English language; 2) validation of an assessment tool related to quality of health information was the focus of the article. Fifteen tools[2] currently available in the literature were identified in the scoping review. A follow-up search was conducted on September 10, 2018, yielding three additional tools: the Quality Index for health-related Media Reports (QIMR) [11], the "Date, Author, References, Type, and Sponsor" (DARTS) tool [12] and Index of Scientific Quality (ISQ) [13]. The tools identified range from generic assessments, intended for use across multiple domains of online health information, to assessments targeted to a specific: 1) health condition [14, 15]; 2) aspect of a condition such as treatment [12, 16]; 3) audience [17, 18]; or 4) type of media [11, 13]. As such, a disadvantage of existing tools is that they are limited in the scope of their application.

Many of the existing tools identified, with some notable exceptions, are lengthy and potentially arduous to use, out-dated, or no longer available online [3]. Some tools consist of sets of criteria or checklists that do not provide a quantitative result,

making it difficult to compare information from different sources. Finally, while there are many studies evaluating online health information using existing quality evaluation tools, studies assessing the validity, reliability, and efficacy of the tools themselves are lacking in the medical informatics literature.

At present, there is no clear universal standard for evaluating the quality of online health information [3]. Many researchers and regulatory bodies, including the World Health Organization, have called for the establishment of such a standard [9]. Quality criteria across existing tools often overlap and thus may serve as the basis for developing a universalized set of criteria. Aslani et al. distilled a total of 34 criteria from five evaluation tools into 10 general criteria, subdivided into four categories: author, sponsors, and individual(s) responsible for the website; purpose of the website and supporting evidence; design, ease of use, privacy, and interactibility of the website; and date of update [19]. These aggregate criteria largely correspond to groupings of criteria generated in previous reviews of the literature [20, 21]. The criteria also align with the "5 C's" of website quality (credibility, currency, content, construction, and clarity) outlined by Roberts [22].

Of the many criteria-based assessment tools that have been developed, only a fraction have been tested for inter-rater reliability and even fewer have been validated [23]. Of tools that have reported measuring inter-rater reliability, few have consistently achieved acceptable levels of agreement across all criteria [24]. Gagliardi and Jadad [25] found that only five of 51 rating instruments they evaluated provided explicit evaluation criteria and none were validated. In a more recent review of 12 instruments by Breckons et al. [23], only two tools, DISCERN and the LIDA Minervation tool, contained any measure of reliability and validity. The DISCERN tool is the only tool currently available online for which substantive validation data is publicly available. During development of the tool, a questionnaire administered to information providers and self-help organizations was used to establish face and content validity and inter-rater reliability [16]. Additionally, external assessments indicated significant correlation with content coverage and correctness [26], good internal consistency, and significant inter-rater reliability [27]. Past comparisons to other tools, including the Mitretek Information Quality Tool (IQT) [27], Sandvik quality scale [28], EQIP [17], and DARTS [26], found significant convergent validity with DISCERN. However, DISCERN is limited in its scope of application as it is focused on treatment information and as such is not applicable to online content about other aspects of health and illness including prevention and diagnosis.

There is currently no singular quantitative tool that has undergone a validation process, can be used for a broad range of health information, and strikes a balance between ease of use, concision and comprehensiveness (Fig. 1). To address these gaps, we developed the QUality Evaluation Scoring Tool (QUEST). The QUEST quantitatively measures six aspects of the quality of online health information: authorship, attribution, conflict of interest, currency, complementarity, and tone (Fig. 2), yielding an overall quality score between 0 and 28. Attribution is measured through two items, yielding a seven-item evaluation for six measures of health information quality. The criteria were chosen based on a review of existing tools used to evaluate the quality of online information by Chumber et al. [29], Sandvik et al. [28], and Silberg et al. [30]; content analysis was used to capture the overarching categories assessed by these tools [31].

When applying the QUEST, each of the seven quality items is assigned a weighted score. The weighting of each criterion was developed based on two factors: (i) how critical it is to the overall quality of the article, established by a preliminary analysis of a sample

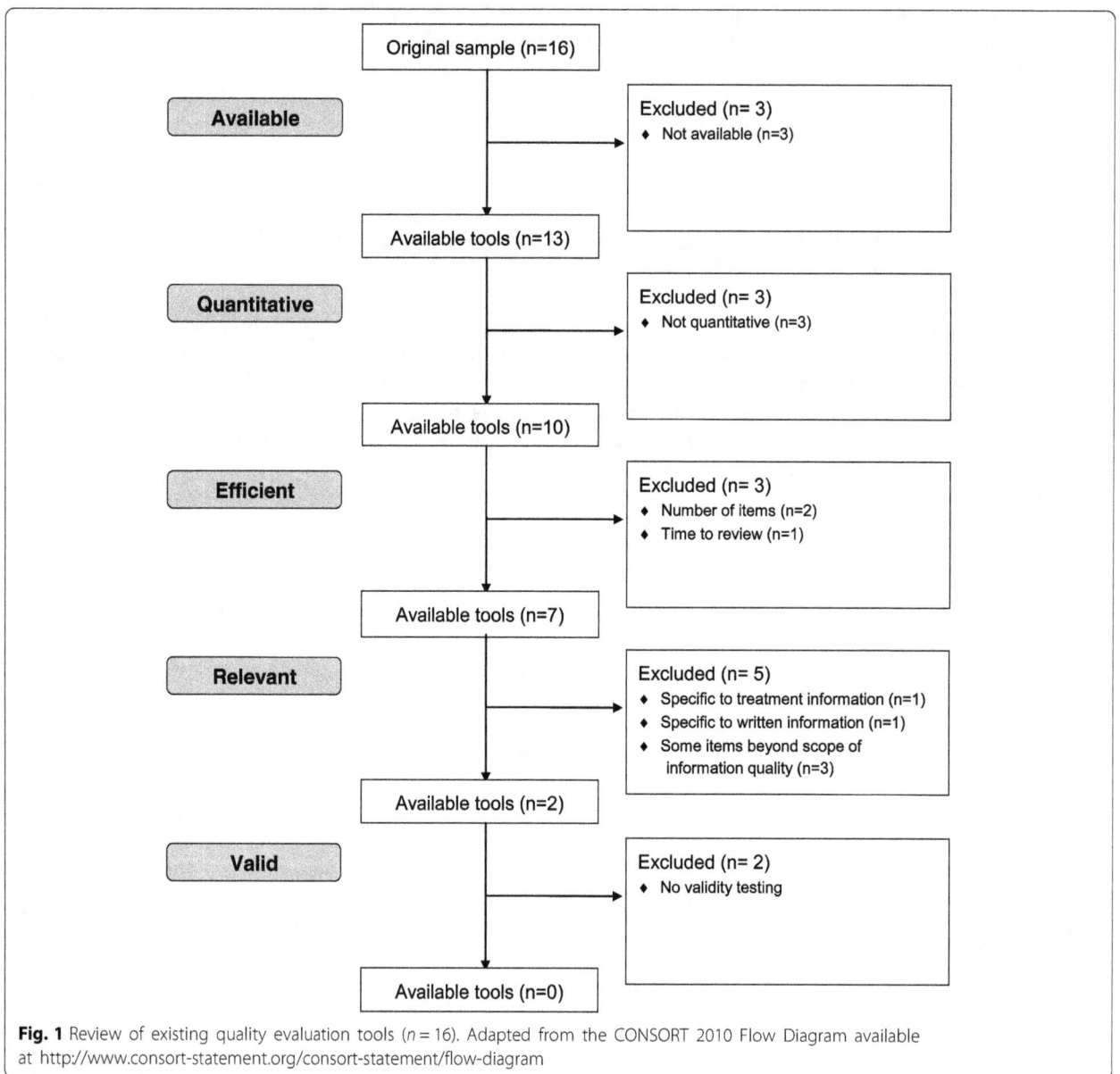

Fig. 1 Review of existing quality evaluation tools (*n* = 16). Adapted from the CONSORT 2010 Flow Diagram available at http://www.consort-statement.org/consort-statement/flow-diagram

Authorship	(Score x 1)
0 – No indication of authorship or username	
1 – All other indications of authorship	
2 – Author's name and qualification clearly stated	

Attribution	(Score x 3)
0 – No sources	
1 – Mention of expert source, research findings (though with insufficient information to identify the specific studies), links to various sites, advocacy body, or other	
2 – Reference to at least one identifiable scientific study, regardless of format (e.g., information in text, reference list)	
3 – Reference to mainly identifiable scientific studies, regardless of format (in >50% of claims)	

For all articles scoring 2 or 3 on Attribution:	(Score x 1)
Type of study	
0 – In vitro, animal models, or editorials	
1 – All observational work	
2 – Meta-analyses, randomized controlled trials, clinical studies	

Conflict of interest	(Score x 3)
0 – Endorsement or promotion of intervention designed to prevent or treat condition (e.g., supplements, brain training games, foods) within the article	
1 – Endorsement or promotion of educational products & services (e.g., books, care home services)	
2 – Unbiased information	

Currency	(Score x 1)
0 – No date present	
1 – Article is dated but 5 years or older	
2 – Article is dated within the last 5 years	

Complementarity	(Score x 1)
0 – No support of the patient-physician relationship	
1 – Support of the patient-physician relationship	

Tone (includes title)	(Score x 3)
0 – Fully supported (authors fully and unequivocally support the claims, strong vocabulary such as "cure", "guarantee", and "easy", mostly use of non-conditional verb tenses ("can", "will"), no discussion of limitations)	
1 – Mainly supported (authors mainly support their claims but with more cautious vocabulary such as "can reduce your risk" or "may help prevent", no discussion of limitations)	
2 – Balanced/cautious support (authors' claims are balanced by caution, includes statements of limitations and/or contrasting findings)	

Fig. 2 Description of the QUEST criteria. Scores in the individual sections are weighted and summed to generate a total score of up to 28

of websites, and (ii) consideration of the criterion's ethical implications. One criterion, attribution, is measured through a two-step process by identifying (1) the presence of references to scientific studies and, (2) the type of studies referenced, if any (e.g., animal models, observational studies, meta-analyses, clinical trials). The second item, which assigns a ranking based on the types of studies included, is in accordance with the GRADE criteria for clinical evidence [32]. This item is scored as a support to the overall quality of the health information presented, not as a judgment of the referenced studies' quality.

The aim of the present study was to evaluate whether the QUEST reliably measures a similar concept of quality to existing tools. Here we present the results of the inter-rater reliability and convergent validity analyses.

Methods

Sample

For the purposes of this study, Alzheimer disease (AD) was used as the reference health condition as there is an abundance of online articles on this topic [33, 34], and there are established methodologies for sampling in this field [31]. Online articles containing AD treatment information were retrieved using a location-disabled search on Google.com/ncr (no country redirect) to avoid localized results. Searches were conducted on an application that prevents the collection of browsing history and cookies during the search and browsing history and cookies were cleared before each search to ensure that search results were not influenced by these factors. Forty-eight different combinations of search terms related to the treatment of AD were used. Articles were extracted from the first three pages of search results, based on analyses of aggregate data on online activity patterns indicating that most Internet users tend not to view past the third page of search results [35]. Each page of search results was comprised of nine articles, totalling 27 articles for each key word combination. Inclusion criteria for the articles were: 1) the article is in the English language; 2) no payment or login is required to access the article; 3) treatment of AD is the main focus of the article as determined by the content of the headline and lead paragraph; and 4) treatment interventions discussed in the article are not solely based on animal experiments. An automatic number generator was used to obtain random 10% samples of articles that met these inclusion criteria in this present study.

In a separate sample, online articles containing information about the prevention of AD were retrieved using similar methods. To retrieve these articles, 105 combinations of search terms related to AD prevention were used. Articles were screened according to criteria 1, 2, and 3 of the inclusion criteria used for treatment articles, with the exception that criterion 3 focused on prevention rather than treatment. As with the treatment-related articles, a random 10% sample of relevant articles was used for validation. In the present study, an article is defined as the heading on a webpage and the text associated with it, excluding links, images and advertising outside of the main body of text. We selected this sampling strategy based on previous investigations of inter-rater reliability and validity of similar tools that have assessed samples of 12 to 40 websites [23, 26, 27, 36, 37].

Reliability analysis

The QUEST was applied to each sample of online articles by two independent raters (JJ and TF for the prevention sample and JJ and JL for the treatment sample). Two of the three raters were naïve to tool development. To evaluate inter-rater agreement between the two reviewers, a weighted Cohen's kappa (κ) was calculated for each item of the tool. Agreement was interpreted according to Landis and Koch, where a κ-value of 0.0 to 0.2 indicates slight agreement, 0.21 to 0.40 indicates fair agreement, 0.41 to 0.60 indicates moderate agreement, 0.61 to 0.80 indicates substantial agreement, and 0.81 to 1.0 indicates almost perfect or perfect agreement [38]. Following initial ratings of the samples, remaining disagreements were resolved by discussion to achieve 100% agreement.

Validity analysis

Three tools were selected for comparison with the QUEST based on availability, ubiquity of use, and relatedness of quality criteria and were applied to both samples. The Health on the Net Foundation's HONcode Code of Conduct and the DISCERN instrument [16] are two of the most widely used and cited quality evaluation tools [5]. The DISCERN instrument is a 16-item questionnaire intended specifically for evaluation of health information on treatment choices, and has been found to demonstrate good inter-rater reliability and face and content validity. The HONcode Code of Conduct is a set of eight criteria used to certify websites containing health information [5]; its creators also developed a Health Website Evaluation Tool, which was used in this analysis due to its closer similarity in purpose and format to the QUEST and other tools. General quality items developed by Sandvik comprised the final tool for comparison [28]. All three tools selected for comparison are criteria-based, can be applied by a non-expert user, and contain quality criteria that, in general, align categorically with each other and the QUEST (Table 1).

The QUEST and the three tools for comparison were applied to the 10% sample of treatment-related articles and the 10% sample of prevention-related articles by one investigator. The numeric scores obtained by each tool were converted to percentage scores to facilitate comparison across tools. The distribution of quality scores generated by the QUEST was plotted as a histogram to determine whether a spectrum of quality was captured by the sample (see Fig. 1, Robillard and Feng 2017 [31]).

For each tool, the articles were ranked based on their scores and rankings were compared across tools in order to measure convergence. To accomplish this, a two-tailed Kendall's tau (τ) ranked correlation [39] was used to measure convergence at $\alpha = .05$. Confidence intervals (CI) of 95% for τ were calculated using $Z_{0.05}$. Six correlational tests, each comparing a unique pair of tools, were performed to compare the results of the QUEST, HONcode, Sandvik, and DISCERN tools. This process was carried out for both the samples of treatment- and prevention-related articles.

Results
Sample

A total of 496 treatment articles were retrieved, with 163 of the articles meeting criteria for inclusion in the analysis and the random 10% sample consisted of 16 articles (Additional file 1). Similarly, a sample of 308 prevention articles were collected, 296 of

Table 1 Comparison of quality items used in the QUEST, HONcode, Sandvik, and DISCERN tools

Quality criteria	QUEST	HONcode	Sandvik	DISCERN
Attribution	X	X	X	X
Currency	X	X	X	X
Authorship	X	X	X	
Balance		X	X	X
Reliability		X		X
Interactivity		X	X	
Tone	X			
Conflict of interest	X			
Complementarity	X			
Mission/target		X		
Audience		X		
Privacy		X		
Overall Reliability		X		
Ownership			X	
Navigability			X	
Quality of information on treatment choices				X
Overall Rating				X

which met inclusion criteria and 29 articles were included in the random 10% sample (Additional file 2). These articles were analyzed using the QUEST in previous quality analysis studies of articles about the prevention of AD [31]. The scores generated by each of the tools for the treatment and prevention samples are included in additional files [see Additional files 1 and 2].

Reliability analysis
Treatment
The level of inter-rater reliability was substantial between the reviewers for Attribution ($\kappa = 0.79$), high to near perfect for authorship, currency, complementarity and tone (κ ranging from 0.86 to 0.91), and perfect for type of study and conflict of interest (Table 2).

Prevention
Inter-rater reliability between the two reviewers ranged from substantial to perfect agreement for each of the

seven items included in the QUEST (κ ranging from 0.74 to 1.0; Table 3).

Validity analysis
Treatment
Scores obtained using HONcode had the widest range, 15–100%. Scores obtained using the Sandvik criteria had a narrower range, 43–100%. The DISCERN instrument returned the narrowest range of scores, 45–86%. The QUEST generated a range of scores (25–100%) wider than those generated by both the DISCERN tool and Sandvik criteria, but narrower than that of HONcode.

The median percentage scores returned by the DISCERN and HONcode tools were 59% and 62% respectively, while the Sandvik criteria generated a median score of 86%. Again, the median score generated by the QUEST, 71%, fell between those of the other instruments.

Quality analysis of the prevention-related articles generated similar results. HONcode generated the widest range of scores (22–100%), while DISCERN returned the narrowest range (30–88%). The range of scores obtained using the Sandvik criteria (29–93%) fell between the ranges generated by the HONcode and DISCERN instruments. The QUEST generated a range of scores (29–96%) wider than those of DISCERN and Sandvik, but narrower than that of HONcode.

On the lower end, the median percentage score obtained using the DISCERN criteria was 54%. On the upper end, the median score generated by HONcode was 68%. Between these values, both the Sandvik criteria and the QUEST returned a median score of 64%.

Of the six correlational tests performed between unique pairs of tools on the articles related to treatment, all six tests demonstrated a significant correlation between the tools (Table 4). Values of τ ranged from 0.47 (QUEST and HONcode) and 0.53 (HONcode and Sandvik) on the lower end to 0.62 (QUEST and Sandvik) and 0.65 (QUEST and DISCERN) on the higher end ($P < .05$ for all tests).

Prevention
Similarly, all six correlational tests performed on the prevention sample demonstrated a significant

Table 2 Weighted Cohen's kappa, standard error and 95% CI for treatment articles ($n = 16$)

	Authorship	Attribution	Type of study	Conflict of interest	Currency	Complementarity	Tone
Observed kappa	0.91	0.79	1	1	0.86	0.86	0.91
SE	0.08	0.10	0	0.24	0.13	0.13	0.08
95% CI	0.75, 1	0.58, 0.99	1, 1	0.32, 1	0.60, 1	0.60, 1	0.75, 1

Table 3 Weighted Cohen's kappa, standard error and 95% CI for prevention articles ($n = 29$)

	Authorship	Attribution	Type of study	Conflict of interest	Currency	Complementarity	Tone
Observed kappa	0.88	0.89	0.89	0.74	1	0.75	0.95
SE	0.09	0.06	0.06	0.16	0	0.14	0.04
95% CI	0.71, 1	0.78, 1	0.77, 1	0.43, 1	1, 1	0.49, 1	0.86, 1

correlation between the tools ($P < .05$; Table 5). The weakest correlations were found between Sandvik and DISCERN, and the QUEST and DISCERN, which produced τ- values of 0.41 and 0.55 respectively. The strongest correlations were found between the QUEST and Sandvik (τ =0.62) and the QUEST and HONcode (τ = 0.64).

Discussion
In the present study to validate a novel tool to assess the quality of health information available on the Internet, we find the QUEST to have high inter-rater reliability and convergent validity when applied to two samples of online articles on AD. The results of the validity analysis of treatment and prevention samples indicate that the rankings of quality scores generated by the QUEST converge with those generated by three other tools – the HONcode Health Website Evaluation tool, the DISCERN instrument, and the Sandvik criteria.

For the sample of articles on AD treatment, the strong correlation between the QUEST and the DISCERN instrument suggests that these tools evaluate a similar concept of quality. As past findings indicate that the DISCERN tool is itself a valid tool for assessing treatment information, its high level of convergence with the QUEST confers promising preliminary evidence for the validity of the QUEST. One limitation of the DISCERN tool is the ambiguity in applying a Likert scale to the data. The QUEST addresses this limitation by providing specific

descriptions of the criteria for each possible score for a given item.

The QUEST's lower level of convergence with the HONcode's evaluation of treatment-related articles may indicate a wider gap between interpretations of the concept of quality evaluated by these two tools. The HONcode tool places emphasis on aspects that are not assessed by the QUEST, such as the website's mission, target audience, privacy policy, and interactivity [40], all of which expand on the concept of quality but increase the time required to apply the tool. However, there may be other factors that account for the discrepancy between the tools' rankings. There exist some ambiguities in scoring websites using HONcode that are intrinsic to the design of the tool. For example, with a few exceptions, the HONcode rates questions on a dichotomous scale (Yes/No). This rating system, unlike the Likert-type scales used by the QUEST, DISCERN, and Sandvik [28], does not allow for an assessment beyond an absence or presence of criteria. Finally, some criteria are only marginally or not applicable to many websites' content. For example, one question asks the responder to evaluate banner content, and website design has moved away from these types of site elements.

Analysis of the scores generated from the sample of prevention-related articles found the strongest correlation between the QUEST and HONcode. Conversely, the QUEST displayed the poorest convergence with the DISCERN instrument. The discrepancy between these findings and those from the treatment sample, which found the strongest

Table 4 Kendall's tau, standard error, 95% CI, and P-value of each test for treatment articles ($n = 16$)

	Kendall's tau (95% CI)	SE	P-value
QUEST vs HONcode	0.47 (0.09–0.85)	0.19	0.015
QUEST vs Sandvik	0.62 (0.23–1.01)	0.20	0.002
QUEST vs DISCERN	0.65 (0.28–1.02)	0.19	< 0.001
HONcode vs Sandvik	0.53 (0.13–0.92)	0.20	0.009
HONcode vs DISCERN	0.58 (0.20–0.96)	0.19	0.003
Sandvik vs DISCERN	0.58 (0.19–0.96)	0.20	0.004

Table 5 Kendall's tau, standard error, 95% CI, and P-value of each test for prevention articles ($n = 29$)

	Kendall's tau (95% CI)	SE	P-value
QUEST vs HONcode	0.64 (0.37–0.99)	0.14	< 0.001
QUEST vs Sandvik	0.62 (0.34–0.90)	0.14	< 0.001
QUEST vs DISCERN	0.55 (0.29–0.82)	0.14	< 0.001
HONcode vs Sandvik	0.61 (0.33–0.89)	0.14	< 0.001
HONcode vs DISCERN	0.57 (0.31–0.84)	0.14	< 0.001
Sandvik vs DISCERN	0.41 (0.13–0.68)	0.14	0.004

convergence between the QUEST and DISCERN and the weakest between the QUEST and HONcode, may reflect intrinsic differences in the purpose of the tools. The DISCERN instrument was developed specifically for the quality evaluation of treatment information, whereas the QUEST, HONcode and Sandvik criteria were developed for health information more broadly.

Overall findings demonstrate a high degree of inter-rater reliability for all seven items of the QUEST. In their evaluation of the DISCERN instrument, Charnock et al. [16] found that lower agreement scores were generally associated with criteria that required more subjective assessment, such as ratings about areas of uncertainty or questions requiring scaled responses. Results from the current study indicate that more subjective items in the QUEST, such as attribution, conflict of interest and tone, achieve about equal or higher levels of inter-reliability as more objective items. Results from the reliability analysis suggest that the QUEST criteria may serve as an effective framework for current as well as future iterations of quality evaluation resources.

The QUEST offers three main advantages over existing tools. Foremost, the QUEST condenses a wide range of quality evaluation criteria into a brief, seven-item questionnaire that evaluates quality with comparable efficacy to established tools. This concise design in conjunction with a weighted criteria approach facilitates the rapid evaluation of health information for a diverse group of users. For example, health care professionals may use the QUEST to evaluate the quality of information brought to them by their patients or to find high-quality articles to recommend. The QUEST may also be of value to the scientific community as it can be used as a research tool to quickly and accurately evaluate quality, facilitating the characterization and comparison of large amounts of information. Additionally, the QUEST may help inform creators of online health content, including government, industry, university, and advocacy groups, during the content development process.

In terms of content, the QUEST tool is differentiated from the three other tools included in the present analysis in its weighted measurement of tone, conflict of interest, and complementarity (see Table 1). These criteria address factors such as potential bias linked to promotion of a product or intervention, whether support of the patient-physician relationship is referenced, and whether the information is presented in a balanced way.

Finally, the QUEST was designed for application to a variety of health topics including information on both treatment and prevention, as well as general health information. Altogether these characteristics, combined with evidence of the QUEST's reliability and validity, are reflective of a versatile tool suited to meet diverse user needs. It is important to note that each individual item provides information about only a single aspect of information quality, and thus the QUEST should be used as a gestalt to provide an overall assessment of quality.

It should be noted that while the QUEST is designed to be a concise and universally applicable tool, there is a range of other evaluation tools in the literature with different and potentially complementary aims to QUEST (please see Appendix 2 for a comparison of currently available tools to QUEST). For example, the QIMR tool released in 2017 may be more suited for evaluating health research reports in the lay media and the AGREE instrument may be best suited to evaluating the quality of clinical practice guidelines. While the versatility of the QUEST tool lies in its applicability to a range of online health information, is not necessarily the only or most suitable tool for all types of health-related media.

The focused area of the samples used in this study addresses an important and growing issue relating to the quality of online health information targeted toward aging populations, who face unique challenges in cognition which can be exacerbated by low health literacy [41]. Additionally, older adults tend to have less experience conducting online searches and critically evaluating the credibility of online information [42, 43]. Due to this combination of factors, this demographic of health consumers may be more susceptible to misinformation online. Beyond the focus on AD used for this validation study, the QUEST will benefit from further testing across a wider range of health conditions.

The study design has several strengths. The correlational method used does not rely on an assumption of normality of the data, and the magnitudes of the correlation coefficients indicate the strength of correlation between the tools being compared [39]. We conducted more than one analysis on the data, comparing the QUEST to three well-established and well-regarded evaluation tools. Careful selection of tools for comparison and use of multiple tools in the analysis both contribute to the rigour of the study.

However, we also recognize the limitations of the study. A sample of convenience of a relatively small number of articles was used, taken from existing collections of AD treatment and prevention articles. Due potentially to the small sample size of articles used, the Kendall's tau scores have substantially overlapping confidence intervals; this indicates a need for further validation studies that include a larger number of articles on other health conditions and on types of health information beyond treatment and prevention, such as descriptions of symptoms and management. Furthermore, our study included only three raters, whereas it may be useful to include more raters in the future when assessing inter-rater reliability. It may also be informative to assess the predictive validity of real-life application of the tool. This may be used to predict whether sustained use of the instrument is associated with higher levels of user knowledge, engagement with care providers on the health topic, or self-efficacy in management of the health condition researched.

Additionally, existing quality evaluation tools generally adopt the perspective of the health care professional in conceptualizing quality [27]. We recognize that the QUEST tool, currently aimed at health care professionals and researchers, falls into this category. Given the time constraints of clinical visits, health care professionals may not be able to assess the quality of online resources during the consultation. To address this issue, attempts have been made to automate tools such as the HONcode and the QUEST [44, 45]. Further, research indicates that the methods used by health consumers to search and appraise online health information differ from the systematic methods used by investigators [46]. As a partially non-academic area of research, a number of health information evaluation tools are not detailed or evaluated in the peer-reviewed literature and may have been excluded from the scoping review presented here. Existing efforts to expand the user base for quality evaluation tools include the HONcode Health Website Evaluation Tool and Provost et al.'s 95-item WebMedQual assessment [47]. This body of work can be expanded upon in the academic space by standardising and ensuring validity of the broad range of heterogeneous tools that exist outside of this space. Future work should continue efforts to develop a more accessible and concise patient-friendly tool that incorporates the values of end-users when assessing online health information, such as privacy and usability factors. To address this need, we are currently in the process of developing a public-friendly adaptation of the existing QUEST criteria that can be easily understood and applied by non-expert users.

Finally, a novel tool aiming to address the issue of misinformation online – whether intended for use by expert or non-expert users – needs to be supplemented by a careful examination of the drivers of public attitudes toward key issues in health care. Studies have shown that social beliefs and attitudes related to a range of health issues (e.g., vaccination uptake [48, 49], health and wellbeing in an ageing population [50], uptake of mental health care [51, 52]) pose significant challenges in obtaining optimal public health outcomes. Tools such as QUEST are designed as downstream interventions that can aid health consumers and providers in differentiating between high- and low-quality information online. It is unlikely that the wide availability of these tools will be effective as a standalone intervention; additional work is required to contextualize the public spaces in which these evaluation tools will be useful and to determine how these tools can best be used in complement to health communication strategies and more upstream, systemic interventions in order to change health behaviours and attitudes.

Conclusions

Developed to address gaps in available quality evaluation tools for online health information, the QUEST is composed of a short set of criteria that can be used by health care professionals and researchers alike. Our findings demonstrate the QUEST's reliability and validity in evaluating online articles on AD treatment and prevention. For example, two similar tools used for comparison, the DISCERN and HONcode Health Website Evaluation tools, are 12–16 questions in length. This study provides evidence that the QUEST builds on the strengths of existing instruments and evaluates quality with similar efficacy using a rapid seven-item questionnaire. As a result, this tool may serve as a more accessible resource that effectively consolidates the quality criteria outlined in previous work. Additionally, due to its simplicity and unique weighting approach, the QUEST reduces the need for users' subjective judgment and indicates potential for future iterations of the tool to be easily tailored to the needs of different users. Based on the current evidence, the QUEST can be used to reliably assess online sources of information on treatment and prevention of AD. Following formal establishment of its reliability and validity across a wide range of health topics, the QUEST may serve as or inform a universal standard for the quality evaluation of online health information.

Endnotes

[1]Please refer to Appendix 1 for characteristics of retrieved articles.

[2]Please refer to Appendix 2 for a complete listing of currently available tools.

Appendix 1

Table 6 Characteristics of articles (n = 36) retrieved between January 15, 2016 and February 5, 2016 using the following search terms on Google Scholar and PubMed: *online, health information, evaluate, evaluation, tool, quality, validity, testing, validation,* and *assessment* and meeting the following inclusion criteria: 1) the article is in the English language; 2) validation of an assessment tool related to quality of health information was the focus of the article

Focus of article	Number of articles	Article title	Author(s)	Date of Publication
Observational or descriptive paper	5	Assessing, controlling, and assuring the quality of medical information on the internet: Caveant lector et viewor—let the reader and viewer beware	Silberg WM, Lundberg GD, and Musacchio RA	1997
		The Health On the Net Code of Conduct for Medical and Health Websites	Boyer, C., M. Selby, J. R. Scherrer, and R. D. Appel	1998
		Emerging Challenges in Using Health Information from the Internet	Theodosiou, Louise, and Jonathan Green	2003
		Health information and the internet: The 5 Cs website evaluation tool	Roberts, Lorraine	2010
		Quality of patient health information on the Internet: reviewing a complex and evolving landscape	Fahy, Eamonn, Rohan Hardikar, Adrian Fox, and Sean Mackay	2014
Evaluation of quality of information using tool(s)	7	Health information and interaction on the internet: a survey of female urinary incontinence	Sandvik, Hogne	1999
		Evaluation of Websites that Provide Information on Alzheimer's Disease	Bouchier, H., and P. A. Bath	2003
		Accuracy of internet recommendations for prehospital care of venomous snake bites	Barker et al	2010
		The quality of online antidepressant drug information: An evaluation of English and Finnish language Web sites	Prusti, Marjo, Susanna Lehtineva, Marika Pohjanoksa-Mäntylä, and J. Simon Bell	2012
		Evaluation of dengue-related health information on the Internet	Rao et al	2012
		A Methodology to Analyze the Quality of Health Information on the Internet The Example of Diabetic Neuropathy	Chumber, Sundeep, Jörg Huber, and Pietro Ghezzi	2014
		Evaluation of Online Health Information on Clubfoot Using the DISCERN Tool	Kumar, Venkatesan S., Suresh Subramani, Senthil Veerapan, and Shah A. Khan	2014
Development of tool	12	DISCERN: an instrument for judging the quality of written consumer health information on treatment choices.	Charnock, D., S. Shepperd, G. Needham, and R. Gann	1999
		Development of a self-assessment method for patients to evaluate health information on the Internet	Jones J.	1999
		Development and Application of a Tool Designed to Evaluate Web Sites Providing Information on Alzheimer's Disease	Bath, P. A., and H. Bouchier	2003
		Development and validation of an international appraisal instrument for assessing the quality of clinical practice guidelines: the AGREE project	Cluzeau et al.	2003
		Design and testing of a tool for evaluating the quality of diabetes consumer-information web sites. Journal of Medical Internet Research	Seidman, Joshua J, Donald Steinwachs, and Haya R Rubin	2003
		The development of QUADAS: a tool for the quality assessment of studies of diagnostic accuracy included in systematic	Whiting, Penny, Anne WS Rutjes, Johannes B. Reitsma, Patrick MM Bossuyt, and Jos Kleijnen	2003

Table 6 Characteristics of articles (*n* = 36) retrieved between January 15, 2016 and February 5, 2016 using the following search terms on Google Scholar and PubMed: *online, health information, evaluate, evaluation, tool, quality, validity, testing, validation,* and *assessment* and meeting the following inclusion criteria: 1) the article is in the English language; 2) validation of an assessment tool related to quality of health information was the focus of the article *(Continued)*

Focus of article	Number of articles	Article title	Author(s)	Date of Publication
		reviews		
		Ensuring Quality Information for Patients: Development and Preliminary Validation of a New Instrument to Improve the Quality of Written Health Care Information	Moult, Beki, Linda S Franck, and Helen Brady	2004
		A model for online consumer health information quality	Stvilia, Besiki, Lorri Mon, and Yong Jeong Yi	2009
		Health Literacy INDEX: Development, Reliability, and Validity of a New Tool for Evaluating the Health Literacy Demands of Health Information Materials	Kaphingst et al.	2012
		Measuring the quality of Patients' goals and action plans: development and validation of a novel tool	Teal, Cayla R., Paul Haidet, Ajay S. Balasubramanyam, Elisa Rodriguez, and Aanand D. Naik	2012
		The Communication AssessmenT Checklist in Health (CATCH): a tool for assessing the quality of printed educational materials for clinicians.	Genova, Juliana, Isaac Nahon-Serfaty, Selma Chipenda Dansokho, Marie-Pierre Gagnon, Jean-Sébastien Renaud, and Anik M. C. Giguère	2014
		Development and Validation of the Guide for Effective Nutrition Interventions and Education (GENIE): A Tool for Assessing the Quality of Proposed Nutrition Education Programs	Hand, Rosa K., Jenica K. Abram, Katie Brown, Paula J. Ziegler, J. Scott Parrott, and Alison L. Steiber	2015
Evaluation of tool(s)	9	Published Criteria for Evaluating Health Related Web Sites: Review	Kim, Paul, Thomas R. Eng, Mary Jo Deering, and Andrew Maxfield	1999
		Examination of instruments used to rate quality of health information on the internet: chronicle of a voyage with an unclear destination	Gagliardi, Anna, and Alejandro R. Jadad	2002
		Evaluating the reliability and validity of three tools to assess the quality of health information on the Internet.	Ademiluyi, Gbogboade, Charlotte E Rees, and Charlotte E Sheard	2003
		The Evaluation Criteria of Internet Health Information	Kang, Nam-Mi, Sukhwa Kim, Seungkuen Hong, Seewon Ryu, Hye-Jung Chang, and Jeongeun Kim	2006
		Assessing the Quality of Websites Providing Information on Multiple Sclerosis: Evaluating Tools and Comparing Sites	Harland, Juliet, and Peter Bath	2007
		What Do Evaluation Instruments Tell Us About the Quality of Complementary Medicine Information on the Internet?	Breckons, Matthew, Ray Jones, Jenny Morris, and Janet Richardson	2008
		Tools Used to Evaluate Written Medicine and Health Information Document and User Perspectives	Luk, Alice, and Parisa Aslani	2011
		Tools for Assessing the Quality and Accessibility of Online Health Information: Initial Testing among Breast Cancer Websites	Whitten, Pamela, Samantha Nazione, and Carolyn Lauckner	2013
		Web-site evaluation tools: a case study in reproductive health information	Aslani, Azam, Omid Pournik, Ameen Abu-Hanna, and Saeid Eslami	2014
Systematic literature review of tools	3	Empirical Studies Assessing the Quality of Health Information for Consumers on the World Wide Web: A Systematic Review	Eysenbach et al.	2002

Table 6 Characteristics of articles (*n* = 36) retrieved between January 15, 2016 and February 5, 2016 using the following search terms on Google Scholar and PubMed: *online, health information, evaluate, evaluation, tool, quality, validity, testing, validation,* and *assessment* and meeting the following inclusion criteria: 1) the article is in the English language; 2) validation of an assessment tool related to quality of health information was the focus of the article *(Continued)*

Focus of article	Number of articles	Article title	Author(s)	Date of Publication
		Online Health Information Tool Effectiveness for Older Patients: A Systematic Review of the Literature	Bolle, Sifra, Julia C. M. van Weert, Joost G. Daams, Eugène F. Loos, Hanneke C. J. M. de Haes, and Ellen M. A. Smets.	2015
		Quality of Health Information for Consumers on the Web: A Systematic Review of Indicators, Criteria, Tools, and Evaluation Results	Zhang, Yan, Yalin Sun, and Bo Xie	2015

Appendix 2

Table 7 Comparison of evaluation tools previously described in the literature and QUEST

	Name of tool	Focus	Criteria	Format
0	QUality Evaluation Scoring Tool (QUEST)	Quality of online health information	Authorship, attribution, conflict of interest, complementarity, currency, tone	6 questions rated on a scale of 0–2 or 0–1 and differentially weighted, yielding an overall quality score between 0 and 28
1	DISCERN	Quality of written information about treatment choices	Reliability, balance, dates, source, quality of information on treatment sources, overall rating	15 questions rated on a scale of 1–5
2	EQIP: Ensuring Quality Information for Patients	Quality of written patient information applicable to all information types	Clarity, patient-oriented design, currency, attributon, conflict of interest, completeness	20 questions rated Y/Partly/N with an equation to generate a % score
3	Jones' Self-Assessment Method	Self-assessment tool for patients to evaluate quality and relevance of health care oriented websites	Content, design, communication, and credibility	9 broad questions based on 4 criteria rated Yes/No/NA
4	Health on the Net Foundation's HONcode Patient Evaluation Tool	Patient evaluation tool for health-related websites	Authorship, attribution, currency, reliability, balance, mission/target audience, privacy, interactivity, overall reliability	16-item interactive questionnaire returning a % score
5	Silberg standards	Standards of quality for online medical information for consumers and professionals	Authorship, attribution, disclosure, currency	Set of core standards; no score is generated
6	Sandvik's General Quality Criteria	General quality measure for online health information	Ownership, authorship, source, currency, interactivity, navigability, balance	7 questions rated on a scale of 0–2
7	Health Information Technology Institute (HITI) Information Quality Tool *No longer available*	Quality measure for health-related websites	Credibility, content, disclosure, links, design, interactivity	*Not available*
8	5 C's website evaluation tool	Structured guide to systematically evaluating websites; specifically developed for nurses to use in patient care and education	Credibility, currency, content, construction, clarity	Series of 36 open-ended and yes/no questions grouped under the "5 C's"; no score is generated
9	Health Literacy INDEX	Tool to evaluate the health literacy demands of health information materials	Plain language, clear purpose, supporting graphics, user involvement, skill-based learning, audience appropriateness, instructions, development details, evaluation methods,	63 indicators/criteria rated yes/ no, yielding criterion-specific scores and an overall % score

Table 7 Comparison of evaluation tools previously described in the literature and QUEST *(Continued)*

	Name of tool	Focus	Criteria	Format
			strength of evidence	
10	Bath and Bouchier's evaluation tool	Tool to evaluate websites providing information on Alzheimer's disease	General details, information for carers, currency, ease of use, general conclusions	47 questions scored from 0 to 2, generating an overall % score
11	Seidman quality evaluation tool	Quality of diabetes consumer-information websites	Explanation of methods, validity of methods, currency, comprehensiveness, accuracy	7 structural measures and 34 performance measures, generating composite scores by section and an overall score
12	Appraisal of Guidelines, REsearch and Evaluation (AGREE) Collaboration instrument	Quality of clinical practice guidelines	Scope and purpose, stakeholder involvement, rigour of development, clarity and presentation, applicability, editorial independence	23 items grouped into six quality domains with a 4 point Likert scale to score each item
13	Communication AssessmenT Checklist in Health (CATCH) tool	Quality of printed educational materials for clinicians	Appearance, layout and typography, clarity of content, language and readability, graphics, risk communication, scientific value, emotional appeal, relevance, social value/source credibility, social value/usefulness for the clinician, social value/usefulness for the health care system (hospital or government)	55 items nested in 12 concepts, each rated yes/no, generating concept-specific and overall scores
14	LIDA Minervation tool	Evaluates the design and content of healthcare websites	Accessibility, usability (clarity, consistency, functionality, engagability), reliability (currency, conflict of interest, content production)	41 questions scored on a scale of 0–3, yielding a total % score
15	Mitretek Information Quality Tool (IQT) *no longer available*	Evaluates information quality of online health information	Authorship, sponsorship, currency, accuracy, confidentiality, navigability	21 questions rated yes/no and weighted according to importance, generating a total score between 0 to 4
16	"Date, Author, References, Type, and Sponsor" (DARTS)	Assists patients in appraising the quality of online medicines information	Currency, authorship, credibility, purpose, conflict of interest	A series of six guiding questions; no score generated
17	Quality Index for health-related Media Reports (QIMR)	Monitors the quality of health research reports in the lay media	Background, sources, results, context, validity	17 items rated on a 0–6 Likert scale with an 18th global rating
18	Index of Scientific Quality (ISQ)	Index of scientific quality for health reports in the lay press	Applicability, opinions vs. facts, validity, magnitude, precision, consistency, consequences	7 items rated on a 1–5 Likert scale with an 8th global rating

Additional files

Additional file 1: Quality scores of treatment articles (*n* = 16). Scores generated by the QUEST, HONcode, Sandvik, and DISCERN tools for the 16 articles containing information on the treatment of AD. (XLSX 57 kb)

Additional file 2: Quality scores of prevention articles (*n* = 29). Scores generated by the QUEST, HONcode, Sandvik, and DISCERN tools for the 29 articles containing information on the prevention of AD. (XLSX 57 kb)

Abbreviations
AD: Alzheimer disease; CI: Confidence interval; QUEST: QUality Evaluation Scoring Tool

Acknowledgements
The authors express appreciation to Kiely Landigran and Emanuel Cabral for their assistance in developing the QUEST.

Funding
This research was supported by the Canadian Consortium on Neurodegeneration in Aging, the Canadian Institutes for Health Research, the British Columbia Knowledge Development Fund, AGE-WELL NCE, the Canadian Foundation for Innovation and the Vancouver Coastal Health Research Institute. The funding bodies had no role in the design of the study and collection, analysis, and interpretation of data and in writing the manuscript.

Authors' contributions
JMR conceptualized the study, took part in data collection and data analysis, and drafted the manuscript. JHJ took part in data collection and data analysis and drafted the manuscript. JL and TLF took part in data collection and data analysis and in manuscript preparation. All authors read and approved the final manuscript.

Competing interests
The authors declare that they have no competing interests.

Author details
[1]Division of Neurology, Department of Medicine, The University of British Columbia, Vancouver, Canada. [2]BC Children's & Women's Hospital, Vancouver, Canada. [3]Djavad Mowafaghian Centre for Brain Health, The University of British Columbia, 2215 Wesbrook Mall, Room 3450D, Vancouver, BC V6T 2B5, Canada.

References

1. Fox S. Health topics: Pew Research Center: Internet, Science & Tech; 2011. http://www.pewinternet.org/2011/02/01/health-topics-2/. Accessed 21 Apr 2016

2. Stvilia B, Mon L, Yi YJ. A model for online consumer health information quality. J Am Soc Inf Sci Technol. 2009;60:1781–91.

3. Theodosiou L, Green J. Emerging challenges in using health information from the internet. Adv Psychiatr Treat. 2003;9:387–96.

4. McCully SN, Don BP, Updegraff JA. Using the internet to help with diet, weight, and physical activity: results from the health information National Trends Survey (HINTS). J Med Internet Res. 2013;15:e148.

5. Fahy E, Hardikar R, Fox A, Mackay S. Quality of patient health information on the internet: reviewing a complex and evolving landscape. Australas Med J. 2014;7:24–8.

6. Rootman I, Gordon-El-Bihbety D. A vision for a health literate Canada: Canadian public health association; 2008. https://www.cpha.ca/vision-health-literate-canada-report-expert-panel-health-literacy. Accessed 22 Aug 2016.

7. Kutner M, Greenberg E, Jin Y, Paulsen C. The health literacy of America's adults: results from the 2003 National Assessment of adult literacy: National Center for Education Statistics; 2006. https://nces.ed.gov/pubsearch/pubsinfo.asp?pubid=2006483. Accessed 22 Aug 2016.

8. Diviani N, van den Putte B, Giani S, van Weert JC. Low health literacy and evaluation of online health information: a systematic review of the literature. J Med Internet Res 2015;17:e112–e112.

9. Devine T, Broderick J, Harris LM, Wu H, Hilfiker SW. Making quality health websites a national public health priority: toward quality standards. J Med Internet Res 2016;18:e211–e211.

10. Arksey H, O'Malley L. Scoping studies: towards a methodological framework. Int J Soc Res Methodol. 2005;8:19–32.

11. Zeraatkar D, Obeda M, Ginsberg JS, Hirsh J. The development and validation of an instrument to measure the quality of health research reports in the lay media. BMC Public Health. 2017;17:343.

12. Närhi U, Pohjanoksa-Mäntylä M, Karjalainen A, Saari JK, Wahlroos H, Airaksinen MS, et al. The DARTS tool for assessing online medicines information. Pharm World Sci. 2008;30:898–906.

13. Oxman AD, Guyatt GH, Cook DJ, Jaeschke R, Heddle N, Keller J. An index of scientific quality for health reports in the lay press. J Clin Epidemiol. 1993;46:987–1001.

14. Hsu W-C, Bath PA. Development of a patient-oriented tool for evaluating the quality of breast cancer information on the internet. Stud Health Technol Inform. 2008;136:297–302.

15. Seidman JJ, Steinwachs D, Rubin HR. Design and testing of a tool for evaluating the quality of diabetes consumer-information web sites. J Med Internet Res. 2003;5:e30.

16. Charnock D, Shepperd S, Needham G, Gann R. DISCERN: an instrument for judging the quality of written consumer health information on treatment choices. J Epidemiol Community Health. 1999;53:105–11.

17. Moult B, Franck LS, Brady H. Ensuring quality information for patients: development and preliminary validation of a new instrument to improve the quality of written health care information. Health Expect Int J Public Particip Health Care Health Policy. 2004;7:165–75.

18. Jones J. Development of a self-assessment method for patients to evaluate health information on the Internet. Proc AMIA Symp. 1999:540–4.

19. Aslani A, Pournik O, Abu-Hanna A, Eslami S. Web-site evaluation tools: a case study in reproductive health information. Stud Health Technol Inform. 2014;205:895–9.

20. Eysenbach G, Powell J, Kuss O, Sa E-R. Empirical studies assessing the quality of health information for consumers on the world wide web: a systematic review. JAMA. 2002;287:2691–700.

21. Kim P, Eng TR, Deering MJ, Maxfield A. Published criteria for evaluating health related web sites: review. BMJ. 1999;318:647–9.

22. Roberts L. Health information and the internet: the 5 Cs website evaluation tool. Br J Nurs. 2010;19:322–5.

23. Breckons M, Jones R, Morris J, Richardson J. What do evaluation instruments tell us about the quality of complementary medicine information on the internet? J Med Internet Res. 2008;10:e3.

24. Bernstam EV, Shelton DM, Walji M, Meric-Bernstam F. Instruments to assess the quality of health information on the world wide web: what can our patients actually use? Int J Med Inf. 2005;74:13–9.

25. Gagliardi A, Jadad AR. Examination of instruments used to rate quality of health information on the internet: chronicle of a voyage with an unclear destination. BMJ. 2002;324:569–73.

26. Prusti M, Lehtineva S, Pohjanoksa-Mäntylä M, Bell JS. The quality of online antidepressant drug information: an evaluation of English and Finnish language web sites. Res Soc Adm Pharm. 2012;8:263–8.

27. Ademiluyi G, Rees CE, Sheard CE. Evaluating the reliability and validity of three tools to assess the quality of health information on the internet. Patient Educ Couns. 2003;50:151–5.

28. Sandvik H. Health information and interaction on the internet: a survey of female urinary incontinence. BMJ. 1999;319:29–32.

29. Chumber S, Huber J, Ghezzi P. A methodology to analyze the quality of health information on the internet: the example of diabetic neuropathy. Diabetes Educ. 2015;41:95–105.

30. Silberg W, Lundberg G, Musacchio R. Assessing, controlling, and assuring the quality of medical information on the internet: caveant lector et viewor—let the reader and viewer beware. JAMA. 1997;277:1244–5.

31. Robillard JM, Feng TL. Health advice in a digital world: quality and content of online information about the prevention of Alzheimer's disease. J Alzheimers Dis. 2017;55:219–29.

32. What is GRADE? BMJ Clinical Evidence. 2012. http://clinicalevidence.bmj.com/x/set/static/ebm/learn/665072.html. Accessed 14 Feb 2017.

33. Robillard JM, Johnson TW, Hennessey C, Beattie BL, Illes J. Aging 2.0: health information about dementia on twitter. PLoS One. 2013;8:1–5.

34. Robillard JM, Illes J, Arcand M, Beattie BL, Hayden S, Lawrence P, et al. Scientific and ethical features of English-language online tests for Alzheimer's disease. Alzheimers Dement Diagn Assess Dis Monit. 2015;1:281–8.

35. Beitzel SM, Jensen EC, Chowdhury A, Frieder O, Grossman D. Temporal analysis of a very large topically categorized web query log. J Am Soc Inf Sci Technol. 2007;58:166–78.

36. Bouchier H, Bath PA. Evaluation of websites that provide information on Alzheimer's disease. Health Informatics J. 2003;9:17–31.

37. Harland J, Bath P. Assessing the quality of websites providing information on multiple sclerosis: evaluating tools and comparing sites. Health Informatics J. 2007;13:207–21.

38. Landis JR, Koch GG. The measurement of observer agreement for categorical data. Biometrics. 1977;33:159–74.

39. Gibbons JD. Nonparametric statistical inference. 2nd ed. New York: Marcel Dekker; 1985.

40. Health Website Evaluation Tool. http://www.hon.ch/HONcode/Patients/HealthEvaluationTool.html. Accessed 11 Apr 2016.

41. Mullen E. Health literacy challenges in the aging population. Nurs Forum (Auckl). 2013;48:248–55.

42. Robertson-Lang L, Major S, Hemming H. An exploration of search patterns and credibility issues among older adults seeking online health information. Can J Aging Rev Can Vieil. 2011;30:631–45.

43. Kruse RL, Koopman RJ, Wakefield BJ, Wakefield DS, Keplinger LE, Canfield SM, et al. Internet use by primary care patients: where is the digital divide? Fam Med. 2012;44:342–7.

44. Boyer C, Dolamic L. Automated detection of HONcode website conformity compared to manual detection: an evaluation. J Med Internet Res. 2015;17:e135.

45. Robillard JM, Alhothali A, Varma S, Hoey J. Intelligent and affectively aligned evaluation of online health information for older adults. In: Workshops at the thirty-first AAAI conference on artificial intelligence; 2017. https://www.aaai.org/ocs/index.php/WS/AAAIW17/paper/view/15078. Accessed 7 Nov 2017.

46. Eysenbach G, Köhler C. How do consumers search for and appraise health information on the world wide web? Qualitative study using focus groups, usability tests, and in-depth interviews. BMJ. 2002;324:573–7.

47. Provost M, Koompalum D, Dong D, Martin BC. The initial development of the WebMedQual scale: domain assessment of the construct of quality of health web sites. Int J Med Inf. 2006;75:42–57.

48. Fournet N, Mollema L, Ruijs WL, Harmsen IA, Keck F, Durand JY, et al. Under-vaccinated groups in Europe and their beliefs, attitudes and reasons for non-vaccination; two systematic reviews. BMC Public Health Lond. 2018; 18. https://doi.org/10.1186/s12889-018-5103-8.

49. Larson HJ, Jarrett C, Schulz WS, Chaudhuri M, Zhou Y, Dube E, et al. Measuring vaccine hesitancy: the development of a survey tool. Vaccine. 2015;33:4165–75.

50. Robertson G. Attitudes towards ageing and their impact on health and wellbeing in later life: an agenda for further analysis. Work Older People. 2016;20:214–8.

51. Prins MA, Verhaak PFM, Bensing JM, van der Meer K. Health beliefs and perceived need for mental health care of anxiety and depression—the patients' perspective explored. Clin Psychol Rev 2008;28:1038–1058.

52. Coates D, Saleeba C, Howe D. Mental health attitudes and beliefs in a community sample on the central coast in Australia: barriers to help seeking. Community Ment Health J. 2018. https://doi.org/10.1007/s10597-018-0270-8.

What maximizes the effectiveness and implementation of technology-based interventions to support healthcare professional practice?

C Keyworth[1]* ⓘ, J Hart[1,2], C J Armitage[1,4,5] and M P Tully[3]

Abstract

Background: Technological support may be crucial in optimizing healthcare professional practice and improving patient outcomes. A focus on electronic health records has left other technological supports relatively neglected. Additionally, there has been no comparison between different types of technology-based interventions, and the importance of delivery setting on the implementation of technology-based interventions to change professional practice. Consequently, there is a need to synthesise and examine intervention characteristics using a methodology suited to identifying important features of effective interventions, and the barriers and facilitators to implementation. Three aims were addressed: to identify interventions with a technological component that are successful at changing professional practice, to determine *if* and *how* such interventions are theory-based, and to examine barriers and facilitators to successful implementation.

Methods: A literature review informed by realist review methods was conducted involving a systematic search of studies reporting either: (1) behavior change interventions that included technology to support professional practice change; or (2) barriers and facilitators to implementation of technological interventions. Extracted data was quantitative and qualitative, and included setting, target professionals, and use of Behaviour Change Techniques (BCTs). The primary outcome was a change in professional practice. A thematic analysis was conducted on studies reporting barriers and facilitators of implementation.

Results: Sixty-nine studies met the inclusion criteria; 48 (27 randomized controlled trials) reported behavior change interventions and 21 reported practicalities of implementation. The most successful technological intervention was decision support providing healthcare professionals with knowledge and/or person-specific information to assist with patient management. Successful technologies were more likely to operationalise BCTs, particularly "instruction on how to perform the behavior". Facilitators of implementation included aligning studies with organisational initiatives, ensuring senior peer endorsement, and integration into clinical workload. Barriers included organisational challenges, and design, content and technical issues of technology-based interventions.

(Continued on next page)

* Correspondence: chris.keyworth@manchester.ac.uk
[1]Manchester Centre for Health Psychology, Division of Psychology and Mental Health, School of Health Sciences, Faculty of Biology, Medicine and Health, University of Manchester, Manchester Academic Health Science Centre, Coupland 1 Building, Oxford Road, Manchester M13 9PL, UK
Full list of author information is available at the end of the article

(Continued from previous page)

Conclusions: Technological interventions must focus on providing decision support for clinical practice using recognized behavior change techniques. Interventions must consider organizational context, clinical workload, and have clearly defined benefits for improving practice and patient outcomes.

Keywords: Healthcare professional behaviour change, Technology, Realist review, Intervention, eHealth

Background

Changing healthcare professional practice is fundamental to the implementation of any health policy, intervention or safety measure intended to deliver best patient care. This is particularly important given the responsibilities that healthcare professionals have with respect to patient management and improving health outcomes [1]. Previously targeted behaviors include prescribing medication [2], conducting screening and health checks [3, 4], providing support and making appropriate referrals [5], and making diagnoses [6]. Optimizing performance of these target behaviors provides an opportunity to influence directly the clinical management of patients and hence accelerate improvement in patient care and/or patient outcomes.

Technology-based interventions can address known barriers in the work environment such as time and workload pressure [7] and provide an opportunity to exert greater impact on patient outcomes by changing professional practice rather than changing the behavior of patients one-by-one. Interventions with a technological component include automated prompts and reminders to support clinical management of patients [8], computer-based skills training [9], and IT-based healthcare professional decision support for clinical decision making [10].

Previous reviews have examined the use of technologies to support healthcare professional practice, such as email to support clinical communication between professionals [11], electronic health information to improve clinical practice (professional behaviors or adherence to clinical practice guidelines) [12], on-screen reminders (such as prompts to conduct a clinical test), and computer-generated reminders delivered on paper [13]. The majority of the preceding literature has tended to focus on effectiveness only, and includes specific interventions, within specific settings, such as electronic health records [14] and computerised provider order entry [15] only. This limits the generalisability of findings to other settings in relation to developing interventions to be delivered at scale.

In addition, it is widely recognized that interventions are most effective when based on behavior change theory and techniques [16, 17]. The use of theory is necessary for explaining and identifying target beliefs involved in clinical practice, and offers a framework for designing and conducting interventions [18, 19]. An important omission from previous reviews is whether technology-based interventions aimed at healthcare professional behaviour change include recognised behaviour change techniques (BCTs), and an understanding of whether such interventions are more or less effective with the inclusion of BCTs. Consequently, there is a need to examine whether interventions with a technological component aimed at changing healthcare professional practice include recognized BCTs, and whether those interventions including BCTs are more effective than interventions without.

There are examples of reviews that focus on implementation of e-health interventions within healthcare settings generally; Ross et al. provide a series of recommendations for implementing e-health interventions across a range of settings [20], however measures of behaviour are not included. Consequently, to build on the previous literature, there is a need to consider the importance of changing healthcare professional practice alongside understanding issues in relation to the implementation of technological interventions. Simply providing healthcare professionals with new technology is unlikely to lead to the transformation in health care that such new technology is proposed to deliver. Specifically, there is a need to conduct an overarching synthesis of diverse technology-based interventions that aim to change healthcare professional behaviour which focuses on three key areas: (1) identifying specific features associated with intervention effectiveness (i.e. what works, for whom interventions for, and under what circumstances interventions work), (2) the BCTs associated with successful interventions, and (3) the barriers and facilitators associated with successful implementation of technology-based interventions. Consequently, there is a need to synthesise and examine intervention characteristics using a methodology suited to identifying important features of effective interventions, and the barriers and facilitators to implementation.

Traditional systematic reviews focus on effectiveness of interventions only. Realist review methods, on the other hand, provide a means of evidence synthesis focused on providing explanations for *how* and *why* interventions may or may not work, and aims to identify features of successful interventions [21]. The advantage of using realist methods over more traditional systematic review methods, is the ability to search for specific explanations regarding implementation of interventions, with no limitations on study design [22–26]. Intervention characteristics (such as study setting, population, and intervention category), as well as the barriers and facilitators of implementation, can be examined using realist review methods to provide a detailed picture of intervention characteristics above and beyond traditional review methods. A realist approach is particularly suited to synthesising evidence about complex interventions [21, 27], including technology-based interventions [28]. This approach determines which interventions work (e.g. computer-based training versus automated reminders), for whom they work (e.g. general practitioners versus nurses), and under what circumstances (e.g. study setting such as primary versus secondary care) they are most effective [29, 30]. This provides rich, detailed and a highly practical understanding of interventions, which is particularly important when planning and implementing interventions on a wider scale [30].

Three specific research questions were addressed:

1. What are the key features of interventions with a technological component that are successful at changing healthcare professional practice?
2. *If* and *how* do such interventions include Behaviour Change Techniques (BCTs) [17] and does the inclusion of BCTs make a difference to practice change?
3. What are the barriers and facilitators to successful implementation of technology-based interventions in practice?

Methods

A literature review informed by realist review methods was conducted using the five-stage approach [21]: (1) establishing the focus of the review; (2) using a purposive and theoretically driven search strategy and appraisal of literature; (3) searching for multiple types of evidence; (4) using an iterative process throughout; and (5) ensuring the findings explain why (or why not) interventions work and how they work, and provide suggestions for future research and practical application of successful interventions.

Inclusion criteria

There were no limitations on study design. Interventions targeting any healthcare profession were included. Technology was defined as any aspect of an intervention that involves information technology used as part of patient management strategies (such as computer-generated reminders or alerts).

Studies must have reported: (a) interventions with at least one healthcare professional outcome relating to a change in behavior/practice. For example, changes in professional behavior, action or performance (such as appropriate prescribing or adherence to clinical guidelines); or

(b) the practicalities of delivering such interventions using technological supports.

Search strategy

Systematic searches were conducted in the following electronic databases (up to December 2016): Medline, Embase, Cumulative Index to Nursing and Allied Health Literature (CINAHL), PsycINFO, ISI Web of Science, and Cochrane Library. The reference lists of key systematic review papers were also included in the hand search of all relevant papers. Conference abstracts/reports identified through the database search were only included if they provided sufficient outcome data relating to changes in healthcare professional practice.

A broad search strategy (Additional file 1) was used to capture the widest possible numbers of studies from a range of categories, which included both intervention studies and studies reporting the practicalities of delivering interventions. Medical Subject Headings (MeSH) terms and key words relating to healthcare professional behavior change and technological supports were used.

Screening

After the initial literature search, two authors (CK and MPT) screened titles and abstracts according to the inclusion criteria. Where abstracts provided insufficient information, full-text review was carried out. Papers meeting the final inclusion criteria were then categorised into two groups; those reporting the results of behavior change interventions aimed at healthcare professionals, and those reporting the practicalities (barriers and facilitators) of delivering such interventions (Additional file 2).

Data extraction and analysis

Data analysis focused on three phases: (1) a quantitative descriptive analysis to identify and evaluate the *characteristics of interventions*, (2) coding interventions for *recognized behavior change techniques (BCTs)*, and (3) a thematic analysis of the *practicalities of designing and implementing technological interventions*.

(1) Characteristics of interventions

Key study characteristics were tabulated using an Excel spreadsheet (including study year, country and healthcare setting). Particular emphasis was given to principles consistent with realist review methodology: the type of intervention used, at whom the intervention was targeted, and the circumstances under which the intervention was described as being effective (target behavior and setting). Specific elements of the intervention were categorised to provide explanations of their effectiveness (a positive change in healthcare professional practice, where $p < .05$, or ineffectiveness, to determine which interventions work) [21]. Study effect sizes were calculated where possible. This included contacting study authors to obtain any missing information. The primary outcome was whether the intervention resulted in a change to healthcare professional clinical practice (both objective and self-reported).

(2) Coding interventions for BCTs

A coding frame was informed by a recognized taxonomy of BCTs [17]. Whilst analysis of behavior change interventions aimed at healthcare professionals has not previously been conducted in the context of technological supports, coding of a similar nature has been conducted in other contexts [31].

Coding was conducted by authors with previous experience of using the BCT taxonomy. One of the study authors (CK) coded the interventions for evidence of BCTs according to the standardised definitions [17], and included both implicit and explicit use of BCTs. A second coder (JH) independently screened a sample selected at random. Disagreements were resolved after discussion, and a third coder (MT) was consulted if agreement could not be reached. An Excel spreadsheet was used to create the coding frame and record intervention descriptions and frequencies of BCTs.

(3) Thematic analysis of the practicalities of designing and implementing technological interventions.

The qualitative software data management tool NVivo was used to sort and categorise the data. Analysis involved coding each study in terms of capturing key ideas and understandings and linking this with the emerging theoretical framework [32]. Thematic analysis was used to provide the best approach to evidence synthesis according to the pre-defined research questions. Findings were summarised under key thematic headings, according to the main findings of each paper, which were used to inform the overall description of the key points [33]. Codes from all identified studies were then compared and cross-referenced, and organised into recurring/higher order themes.

Results

A total of 69 papers were included in the final analysis; 48 studies (of which 27 were randomized controlled trials) were identified in which there was a technological component used to support healthcare professional practice change, and 21 papers reported the practicalities associated with the design and implementation of technology-based interventions (Fig. 1). One paper [34] was included in both parts of the analysis.

Characteristics of interventions
Forty-eight studies (Table 1) met the inclusion criteria to answer review questions 1 (features of effective behavior change interventions with a technological component), and 2 (if and how behavior change theory was used in the interventions). These were conducted in the USA ($n = 25$), United Kingdom ($n = 7$), The Netherlands ($n = 4$), Australia (n = 4) or elsewhere ($n = 8$). One study did not report the country in which the study was conducted.

Types of intervention
Results are presented in Table 2. The use of healthcare professional decision supports, defined as a decision support system providing healthcare professionals with knowledge and/or person-specific information to assist with patient management [35], was the most commonly used technological intervention ($n = 19$ studies); 15 of the 19 (79%) interventions were effective. We were able to extract effect sizes for 12 studies relating to 29 outcomes (small; $n = 19$, medium; n=; 3, large; $n = 7$) according to definitions provided by Cohen [36].

The second most commonly used intervention group was reminders and alerts ($n = 11$ studies), and this also had the second highest percentage of effective interventions (7 of 11 effective; 64%). We were able to extract effect sizes for 3 studies relating to 4 outcomes (small; $n = 2$, medium; $n = 1$, large; $n = 1$).

There were several groups of less frequently used interventions, but that were shown to be effective. One study examined computer-generated feedback, showing positive effects. We were able to extract effect sizes relating to three outcomes (small; $n = 3$). Relating to use of email, 3 of 3 studies showed positive effects. Effect size was calculated for one study relating to one outcome (large; $n = 1$). In the category electronic feedback system, one study showed positive effects, with an effect size relating to six outcomes (small; n = 1, medium; $n = 4$, large; $n = 1$).

Due to the heterogeneity of the studies it was not appropriate to compute summary statistics. In addition due to the varied reporting of study results, we were only able to calculate effect sizes for a sub-sample of papers ($n = 27$), of which there was considerable variation in the size of the effect of reported outcomes (small; $n = 31$, medium; $n = 10$, large; $n = 12$). A forest plot illustrating the range of effect sizes for each outcome of interest is presented in Additional file 3.

Setting of intervention
Whilst the most common intervention setting for technological interventions was primary care ($n = 23$; 48%), studies conducted in hospitals ($n = 14$; 28%) had a higher success rate (12 of 14 described as effective; 86%). Other less frequent settings included interventions

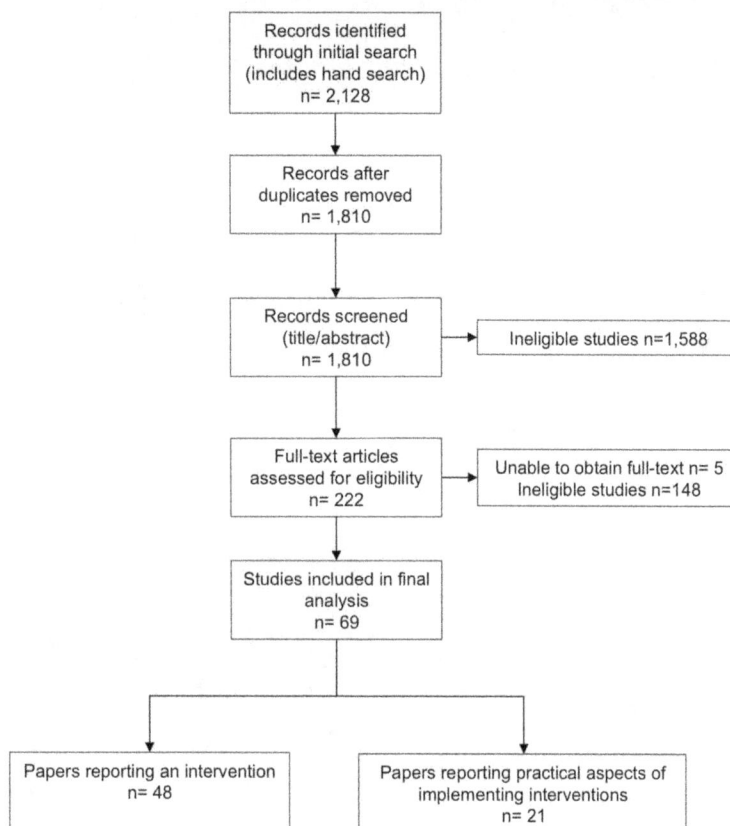

Fig. 1 Flow diagram of search strategy

conducted within both primary and secondary care (1 of 2 effective; 50%).

Target healthcare professional for intervention

Half of the interventions were targeted at General Practitioners ($n = 24$; 50%), with this group also having the highest success rate (18 of 24 studies [75%] resulting in professional behavior change). The second largest group were interventions targeted at two or more types of healthcare professional ($n = 16$; 33%), over half of which resulted in practice change (10 of 19; 61%). There were several other groups of less frequently targeted healthcare professionals among whom technology-based interventions had been tested. These included interventions targeted at mental health therapists (2 of 2 effective; 100%) and pharmacists (1 of 2 effective; 50%).

Target behavior of intervention

Interventions according to target behavior are presented in Table 2. The most common behavior targeted by technological interventions was adherence to clinical guidelines for patient management ($n = 17$; 35%), over half of which were effective in changing practice (10 of 17 studies; 61%).

The second most commonly targeted behavior was prescribing behaviors ($n = 15$; 31%); half of the studies resulted in practice change (9 of the 15 studies; 60%). There were other less frequently targeted behaviors that demonstrated high success rates, including studies targeting increased knowledge or self-efficacy/confidence (4 out of 4 [100%] effective), increasing screening/testing rates (7 out of 8 [88%] effective), and clinical intervention/management (5 out of 6 [83%] effective) all were described as showing positive effects.

Coding interventions for specific BCTs

Of the 48 studies included in the final analysis, 26 (54%) contained evidence of BCTs relating to use of technology or the target behavior (Fig. 2). Seven different BCTs were identified across the 26 studies. The BCT code according to Michie et al. [17] is presented in parentheses, followed by the number of studies using each technique. The most commonly used BCT was *instruction on how to perform the behavior* (BCTTv1 4.1; $n = 22$). This technique was mostly used in the context of healthcare professional decision support interventions ($n = 9$), and reminders and alerts ($n = 9$). Other techniques included *feedback on behavior* (BCTTv1 2.2; $n = 3$), *prompts/cues*

Table 1 Details of included studies ($n = 48$)

Lead author	Year	Setting	Healthcare professional group	Target behavior	Target behavior (category)	Intervention	Participants randomised	Control group	Significant effect[a] found?	Outcomes	Cohens d	Size
Armstrong [56]	2013	Not reported	Nurse practitioners, physician's assistant, physician	Initiation of a recommended therapeutic alternative within 90 days of the fax alert for the 13 PDDIs	Prescribing Behaviors	Faxed alerts	N	N	N	Therapy change	na[d]	
Avery [40]	2012	Primary Care	Doctors	Prescribing errors	Prescribing Behaviors	Computer-generated feedback	Y	Y	Y	Prescription problems / Prescribed B Blocker / Prescribed an NSAID	0.09[b] / 0.08[b] / 0.17[b]	S / S / S
Bahrami [9]	2004	Dentist	Dental practitioners	Guideline implementation for the management of impacted and un-erupted third molars in primary dental care	Adherence to clinical patient management guidelines	Computer-based training	Y	Y	N	Guideline implemented	-0.10[b]	S
Beidas [50]	2012	Community Care	Mental health community therapists	Therapist adherence to CBT for child anxiety, skill in CBT for child anxiety, knowledge about CBT for child anxiety, and satisfaction with training.	Adherence to clinical patient management guidelines	Computer-based training	Y	Y	N	Guideline adherence	-0.15[b]	S
Beeckman [57]	2013	Nursing Home	Nurses, nursing assistants, physiotherapists, occupational therapists	Adherence to recommendations to pressure ulcer prevention	Adherence to clinical patient management guidelines	Healthcare professional decision supports	Y	Y	Y	Guideline adherence	1.26[b]	L
Buising [10]	2008	Tertiary Care	Doctors (senior and junior)	Antibiotic prescribing	Prescribing Behaviors	Healthcare professional decision supports	N	N	Y	Concordant therapy	0.76[b]	M
Carton [58]	2002	Hospital	Junior and senior practitioners	Effects of computer-based guidelines on unnecessary medical imaging	Adherence to clinical patient management guidelines	Reminders/ alerts	N	N	Y	Test requests not confirming to guidelines	0.17[b]	S
Cosgrove [59]	2007	Tertiary Care	Clinicians	Inappropriate antimicrobial therapy	Adherence to clinical patient management guidelines	Text message	N	N	N	Guideline adherence	0.19[b]	S
Curtis [60]	2007	Primary Care & Secondary Care	Physicians	To increase bone mineral density (BMD) testing and osteoporosis medication prescribing among patients receiving long term glucocorticoid therapy	Adherence to clinical patient management guidelines & Prescribing Behaviors	Hyperlinks	Y	Y	N		na[d]	

Table 1 Details of included studies ($n = 48$) (Continued)

Lead author	Year	Setting	Healthcare professional group	Target behavior	Target behavior (category)	Intervention	Participants randomised	Control group	Significant effect[a] found?	Outcomes	Cohens d	Size
Dimeff [61]	2009	Secondary Care	Mental health treatment providers	Increasing knowledge and self-efficacy and application of course content performance-based role plays	Increasing knowledge, or self-efficacy/confidence	Computer-based training	Y	Y	Y	Knowledge	0.52[c]	M
Dykes [62]	2005	Hospital	Nurses, resident physicians, physical therapists, pharmacist, and dieticians	Adherence to practice guidelines for heart failure	Adherence to clinical patient management guidelines	Healthcare professional decision supports	N	Y	Y		na[d]	
Eccles [63]	2002	Primary Care	GPs and practice nurses	Adherence to the guidelines	Adherence to clinical patient management guidelines	Healthcare professional decision supports	Y	Y	N	Blood pressure recorded	0.00[b]	S
										Exercise recorded or advised	-0.16[b]	S
										Weight recorded or advised	-0.11[b]	S
										Smoking status known	-0.28[b]	S
										Smoking education given	0.00[b]	S
										electrocardiogram recorded	0.00[b]	S
										Exercise electrocardiogra m recorded	0.00[b]	S
										Haemoglobin concentration recorded	0.00[b]	S
										Thyroid function recorded	-0.10[b]	S
										Cholesterol or other lipid concentrations recorded	-0.09[b]	S
										Blood glucose or HBA$_{1c}$ concentrations recorded	0.00[b]	S
Edelman [34]	2014	Primary Care	Physicians	Confidence and knowledge	Increasing knowledge, or self-efficacy/confidence	Healthcare professional decision supports	N	N	Y	Confidence discussing sickle cell disease Confidence conducting follow-up	na[d]	

Table 1 Details of included studies (n = 48) (Continued)

Lead author	Year	Setting	Healthcare professional group	Target behavior	Target behavior (category)	Intervention	Participants randomised	Control group	Significant effect[a] found?	Outcomes	Cohens d	Size
Fein [41]	2010	Hospital	Clinical staff	Identification of psychiatric problems/hospital assessments	Increasing screening/testing rates	Healthcare professional decision supports	N	N	Y	Identification of adolescents with psychiatric problems	0.29^b	S
										ED assessments	0.22^b	S
Fifield [64]	2010	Hospital	Primary care physicians	Improving both practitioner adherence to National Asthma Education and Prevention Program Guidelines (NAEPP)	Adherence to clinical patient management guidelines	Reminders/alerts Computer-generated feedback	N	Y	Y	Guideline appropriate prescribing	na^d	
Filippi [65]	2003	Primary Care	GPs	Increasing the use of antiplatelet drugs for diabetic patients at high-risk to develop future CVD	Prescribing Behaviors	Healthcare professional decision supports	Y	Y	Y	Patients treated	0.36^b	S
Fortuna [37]	2009	Hospital	Physicians, nurse practitioners and physician assistants	Reducing prescribing of heavily marketed hypnotic medications in ambulatory care settings	Prescribing Behaviors	Reminders/alerts	Y	Y	Y		na^d	
Gerber [66]	2013	Primary Care	Paediatricians	Decrease inappropriate antibiotic prescribing for common ARTIs over time by primary care paediatricians	Prescribing Behaviors	Email Feedback	Y	Y	Y		na^d	
Goetz [4]	2013	Primary Care	Primary care clinicians	Increasing the rate of risk-based and routine HIV diagnostic tests	Increasing screening/testing rates	Reminders/alerts	Y	Y	Y		na^d	
Goetz [47]	2008	Primary Care & Secondary Care	Academic and non-academic staff physicians, postgraduate medical trainees and mid-level providers	Increasing the rate of HIV diagnostic testing	Increasing screening/testing rates	Reminders/alerts Email Feedback	N	Y	Y		na^d	
Gonzales [67]	2013	Primary Care	Clinicians	Antibiotic treatment of uncomplicated acute bronchitis	Prescribing Behaviors	Healthcare professional decision supports	Y	Y	Y	Unnecessary use of antibiotics	0.46^b	S
Guldberg [68]	2011	Primary Care	GPs	Initiation of treatment	Clinical intervention/management	Electronic Feedback System	Y	Y	Y	Oral antidiabetic treatment initiated (1)	0.71^b	M
										Oral antidiabetic treatment initiated (2)	0.71^b	M
										Insulin treatment initiated (1)	0.55^b	M

Table 1 Details of included studies (n = 48) (Continued)

Lead author	Year	Setting	Healthcare professional group	Target behavior	Target behavior (category)	Intervention	Participants randomised	Control group	Significant effect[a] found?	Outcomes	Cohens d	Size
										Insulin treatment initiated (2)	0.37[b]	S
										Lipid lowering treatment initiated	0.71[b]	M
										Blood-pressure reducing treatment initiated	0.90[b]	L
Gupta [38]	2014	Hospital	Physicians	Appropriate head CT use in patients with mild traumatic brain injury guideline adherence	Adherence to clinical patient management guidelines	Healthcare professional decision supports	N	N	Y		na[d]	
Hibbs [69]	2014	Hospital	Clinicians	Blood transfusion practice of clinicians	Increasing screening/testing rates	Healthcare professional decision supports	N	Y	Y	Transfusion compliance	0.46[b]	S
Hobbs [70]	1996	Primary Care	Primary care practitioners	Prescribing of lipid lowering agents, use of lab tests, and referrals to secondary care for the investigation of hyperlipidaemia	Prescribing Behaviors & Increasing appropriate referrals	Healthcare professional decision supports	Y	Y	N		na[d]	
Hoch [71]	2003	Primary Care	Physicians	Imitating potassium testing	Increasing screening/testing rates	Reminders/alerts	N	N	Y		na[d]	
Kortteisto [72]	2014	Primary Care	Physicians nurses physiotherapists ward nurses a psychologist	Reminders for best practice guidelines/recommendations	Adherence to clinical patient management guidelines	Healthcare professional decision supports	Y	Y	N		na[d]	
Litvin [73]	2013	Primary Care	Physicians, nurse practitioners, physician's assistants	Prescribing behavior - antibiotic prescribing for acute respiratory infections	Prescribing Behaviors	Healthcare professional decision supports	N	N	Y		na[d]	
Lobach [74]	1997	Primary Care	Primary care clinicians: family physicians, general internist, nurse practitioners, physician's assistants, and family medicine residents	Rate of compliance with guideline recommendations for diabetes patient care	Adherence to clinical patient management guidelines	Healthcare professional decision supports	Y	Y	Y	Foot examination	0.62[b]	M
										Complete physical examination	1.07[b]	L
										Chronic glycemia monitoring	0.10[b]	S
										Urine protein determination	2.36[b]	L
										Cholesterol level	0.89[b]	L

Table 1 Details of included studies (*n* = 48) (*Continued*)

Lead author	Year	Setting	Healthcare professional group	Target behavior	Target behavior (category)	Intervention	Participants randomised	Control group	Significant effect[a] found?	Outcomes	Cohens d	Size
Maiburg [39]	2003	Primary Care	GP trainees	Improving knowledge and practice behavior	Increasing knowledge, or self-efficacy/confidence & Clinical intervention/management	Computer-based training	N	Y	Y	Ophthalmologic examination	1.09[b]	L
										Influenza vaccination	0.18[b]	S
										knowledge test	0.44[c]	S
										correct performance in visit	1.59[c]	L
Malone [75]	2012	Pharmacy	Prescribers	Prevention of serious drug-drug interactions (DDI) prescribing patterns of 25 previously identified clinically important potential DDIs	Prescribing Behaviors	Personal Digital Assistant	N	Y	N	Prescribing at least one DDI	0.20[b]	S
Mayne [76]	2014	Hospital	Physician Nurse practitioner	Captured opportunities for HPV vaccination	Increasing screening/testing rates	Reminder within patient electronic health records	Y	Y	Y		na[d]	
Nilasena [77]	1995	Secondary Care	Physicians	Physician compliance with diabetes preventive care guidelines	Adherence to clinical patient management guidelines	Reminders/alerts	Y	Y	N		na[d]	
Patkar [78]	2006	Hospital	Breast clinicians (surgeons)	Adherence to guideline recommendations	Adherence to clinical patient management guidelines	Healthcare professional decision supports	Y	Y	Y	adherence to guidelines	1.03[b]	L
Piening [79]	2013	Hospital	Ophthalmologists and hospital pharmacists	Uptake of drug safety information	Adherence to clinical patient management guidelines	Email Feedback	Y	Y	Y	correctly indicated that a serious increase in intra-ocular pressure could be caused by pegaptanib injections	0.86[b]	L
Reeve [80]	2008	Pharmacy	Pharmacists	Frequency of clinical interventions recorded by community pharmacists/to discuss the suitability of aspirin therapy in eligible patients with diabetes	Clinical intervention/management & Prescribing Behaviors	Healthcare professional decision supports	Y	Y	Y		na[d]	

Table 1 Details of included studies (n = 48) (Continued)

Lead author	Year	Setting	Healthcare professional group	Target behavior	Target behavior (category)	Intervention	Participants randomised	Control group	Significant effect[a] found?	Outcomes	Cohens d	Size
Ribeiro-Vaz [81]	2012	Hospital	Doctor, nurse, pharmacist	To promote spontaneous adverse drug reaction reporting by healthcare professionals	Prescribing Behaviors	Hyperlinks	N	N	Y		na[d]	
Rocha [82]	2001	Tertiary care	Clinicians - staff physicians, physician assistants, nurse practitioners	Practice patterns and consequently improve the detection and management of nosocomial infections.	Clinical intervention/ management	Reminders/ alerts	N	N	N	Patient management recommendations followed		
Ruland [83]	2002	Hospital	Nurses	Clinicians eliciting and integrating patients' preferences into patient care	Clinical intervention/ management	Diagnostic/ risk assessment tool	N	Y	Y	congruence between patient preferences and nurse care priorities	0.67[c]	M
Schwarz [84]	2012	Primary Care	Primary care providers	Provision of family planning services when prescribing potentially teratogenic medications	Clinical intervention/ management	Healthcare professional decision supports	Y	Y	Y	discussion of risk of medication use	0.70[c]	M
Sharifi [85]	2014	Primary Care	Physicians	Tobacco smoke exposure management and quit-line referrals	Increasing appropriate referrals	Reminder within patient electronic health records	N	N	Y	counselling for positive screen	1.36[b]	L
Strayer [86]	2013	Primary Care	Physicians	Smoking cessation counselling behaviors, knowledge and comfort/self-efficacy	Increasing knowledge, or self-efficacy/ confidence & Clinical intervention/ management	Personal Digital Assistant	N	N	Y		na[d]	
Strom [87]	2010	Hospital	Resident physicians and nurse practitioners	Changing prescribing reduce concomitant orders for warfarin and trimethoprim-sulfamethoxazole,	Prescribing Behaviors	Reminders/ alerts	Y	Y	N		na[e]	
Tang [88]	1999	Secondary Care	Clinicians	Influenza vaccination by clinicians Compliance with the guideline: was defined as documentation that a clinician ordered the vaccine, counselled the patient about the vaccine, offered the vaccine to a patient who declined it, or verified that the patient had received the vaccine elsewhere	Adherence to clinical patient management guidelines	Healthcare professional decision supports	N	N	Y	compliance with guidelines	0.88[b]	L

Table 1 Details of included studies (n = 48) (Continued)

Lead author	Year	Setting	Healthcare professional group	Target behavior	Target behavior (category)	Intervention	Participants randomised	Control group	Significant effect[a] found?	Outcomes	Cohens d	Size
Tierney [48]	2003	Primary Care	Physicians and pharmacists	Management of heart disease adherence with care suggestions	Adherence to clinical patient management guidelines	Healthcare professional decision supports	Y	Y	N	Compliance with guidelines	0.04[b]	S
Vagholkar [89]	2014	Primary Care	Family physicians	Prescribing - prescription of antihypertensive and lipid-lowering medication.	Prescribing Behaviors	Diagnostic/ risk assessment tool	Y	Y	N	Prescribing of antihypertensive / Prescribing of lipid-lowering medication	-0.21[b]	S
van Wyk [8]	2008	Primary Care	GPs	Screening and treatment for dyslipidaemia	Increasing screening/ testing rates	Reminders/ alerts	Y	Y	Y	patients screened / patient treated	0.93[b] / 0.68[b]	L / M
Walker [90]	2010	Primary Care	GPs	Increasing opportunistic chlamydia testing	Increasing screening/ testing rates	Reminders/ alerts	Y	Y	N	Testing rates	-0.09[b]	S

[a]A significant change in healthcare professional practice, where $p < .05$
[b]Calculated according to Lipsey and Wilson [91] using n in control/intervention conditions based on whether intervention was successful/unsuccessful (2 X 2 frequency table)
[c]Calculated according to Lipsey and Wilson [91] using means (SDs) and sample sizes
[d]Insufficient data to calculate effect size
[e]Unable to calculate due to incomplete study

Table 2 Details of success of interventions based on type of intervention and target behavior

Domain	Number of interventions in each category	Number of effective interventions[a]	(%) of effective studies
Intervention type			
Computer-generated feedback	1	1	100
Email feedback	3	3	100
Electronic feedback system	1	1	100
Computer-based training	4	2	50
Reminder system within patient electronic health records	2	2	100
Healthcare professional decision support	19	15	79
Hyperlinks	2	1	50
Reminders/alerts	11	7	64
Personal digital assistant	2	1	50
Diagnostic/risk assessment tool	2	1	33
Faxed alerts	1	0	0
Text message	1	0	0
Target behavior			
Adherence to clinical patient management guidelines	17	10	59
Prescribing behaviors	15	9	60
Increasing screening/testing rates	8	7	88
Clinical intervention/management	6	5	83
Increasing knowledge, or self-efficacy/confidence	4	4	100
Increasing appropriate referrals	2	1	50

[a] A statistically significant change in healthcare professional practice, as described by the authors of each study included in this review

(BCTTv1 7.1; $n = 2$), *demonstration of the behavior* (BCTTv1 6.1; $n = 2$), *reducing negative emotions* (BCTTv1 11.2; $n = 1$), *social comparison* (BCTTv1 6.2; $n = 1$), and *problem solving* (BCTTv1 1.2; $n = 1$).

Of the 26 studies containing evidence of BCTs, 16 studies (62%) resulted in practice change (Fig. 2). Of these, five different BCTs were used across the 16

studies. The largest group was *instruction on how to perform the behavior* (BCTTv1 4.1; $n = 15$), such as instructing healthcare professionals which medicines to prescribe [37] or requesting an appropriate clinical test [38]. This second largest group was *demonstration of the behavior* (BCTTv1 6.1; $n = 2$), such as demonstrating effective clinician practice [39].

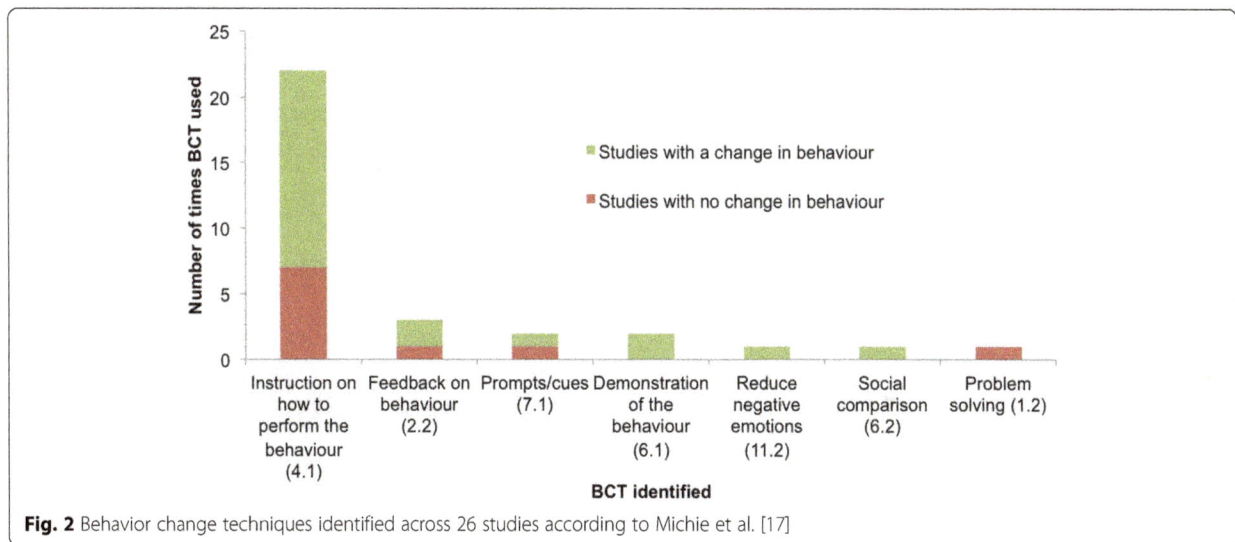

Fig. 2 Behavior change techniques identified across 26 studies according to Michie et al. [17]

Thematic analysis

To answer review question 3 (What are the barriers and facilitators to successful implementation of such technology-based interventions in practice?), a thematic analysis was conducted to address the practicalities of implementing technology in practice. Characteristics of the 21 qualitative ($n = 19$) and quantitative ($n = 2$) studies are presented in Table 3.

Themes identified address the barriers and facilitators of implementing and delivering technology-based interventions aimed at supporting professional practice change. Four major themes were identified (summarised in Fig. 3): (1) *Practice and workload issues,* (2) *Design, content and technical issues,* (3) *Role of the healthcare professional,* and (4) *Usability and impact on the patient care process.* The numbers of papers reporting each finding are reported in parentheses, out of a possible 21 papers.

(1) Practice and workload issues

A number of contextual features (the setting in which the intervention was delivered) were highlighted; practice and workload considerations were perceived as important in the implementation of technology-based interventions. Increased workload was an issue as a result of using technology as part of everyday practice, which may disrupt the workflow of healthcare professionals ($n = 4$; 19%). Time taken to use the system was cited as a barrier to likelihood of healthcare professionals using technology ($n = 5$; 24%), suggesting a need for a more user-friendly design of technology-based interventions. However, technology was seen as a way of improving communication between healthcare professionals ($n = 3$; 14%) and improving the delivery of healthcare in practice ($n = 3$; 14%).

A key factor for the successful implementation of technology into the healthcare environment was whether the intervention met the practice/organizational goals and objectives ($n = 11$; 52%). More specifically, whether the addition of technology met current practice initiatives and could be easily integrated into existing clinical practice, and targeted organizational incentives including patient management approaches and financial incentives.

(2) Design, content and technical issues,

Features of the technology itself were also highlighted. Studies emphasised the importance of pilot testing before wide-scale usage and in particular the need to take an iterative modification approach, such as customising tools

Table 3 Details of practicalities papers ($n = 21$)

Lead author	Year	Country	Data collection method
Ackerman [43]	2013	USA	Qualitative structured telephone surveys
Barnett [92]	2015	UK	Think-aloud and semi-structured interviews
Bokhour [93]	2015	USA	Qualitative semi-structured interviews
Burns [94]	2007	Australia	Semi-structured interviews
Doerr [95]	2014	USA	Semi-structured interviews
Dowding [96]	2009	UK	In-depth semi-structured interviews
Dryden [97]	2012	USA	Qualitative, in-depth semi-structured telephone interviews
Edelman [34]	2014	USA	Semi-structured interviews and quantitative survey data
Guldberg [98]	2010	Denmark	Group and individual semi-structured interviews
Hains [99]	2009	Australia	Semi-structured interviews
Litvin [100]	2012	USA	Semi-structured group interviews
Maguire [101]	2008	UK	Questionnaires and semi-structured interviews
Mandt [102]	2010	Norway	Focus groups
Patterson [42]	2004	USA	Semi-structured interviews
Power [103]	2014	Canada	Surveys
Randell [104]	2010	UK	In-depth semi-structured interviews
Rousseau [105]	2003	UK	Semi-structured interviews
Saleem [106]	2005	USA	Qualitative field observations
Vishwanath [107]	2009	USA	Surveys
Weir [108]	2011	USA	Formative interviews
Zhu [109]	2015	USA	Qualitative Survey

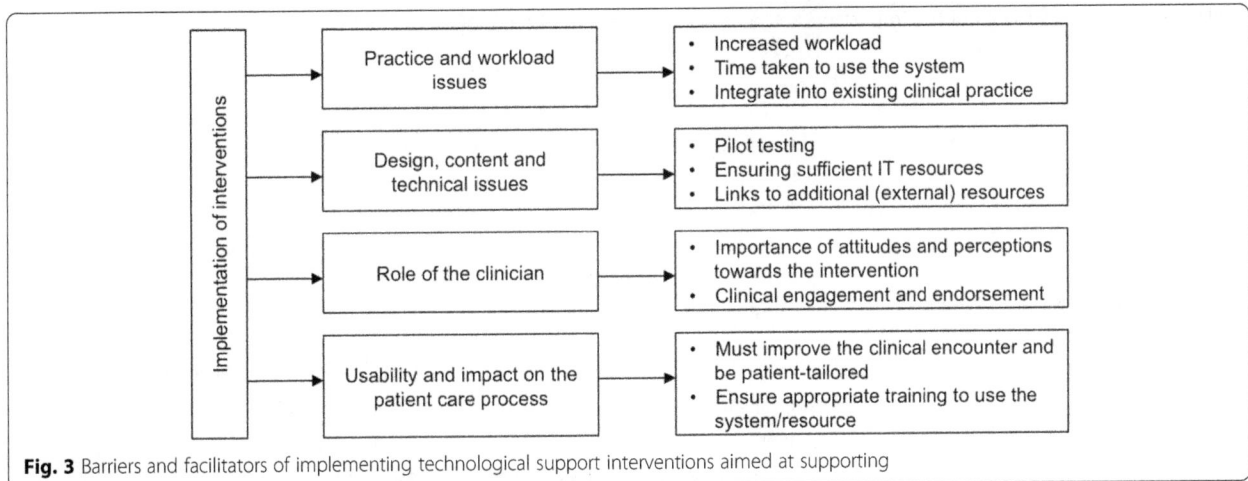

Fig. 3 Barriers and facilitators of implementing technological support interventions aimed at supporting

to the needs of the staff ($n = 5$; 24%). Piloting may identify important technical issues acting as barriers to usage, such as insufficient access to IT resources, software updates and limitations in computer performance ($n = 9$; 43%). Where interventions included patient management guidelines, the need for consistency and reliability was highlighted. Links to external resources such as forums, risk assessment tools or patient information sources, must be used appropriately and in a way to improve the delivery of patient care ($n = 8$; 38%). Guidelines in particular must be relevant to patient management ($n = 4$; 19%).

(3) Usability and benefit for patient care.

Additional important features of the technology included accessibility to important information relevant to the clinical encounter for example medication information, hence making it an important educational resource ($n = 4$; 19%). Technology was also seen as a way of improving other aspects of the clinical encounter such as medication reviews or stimulating provider-patient discussions ($n = 5$; 24%).

An important feature was the ease of use of the technology ($n = 9$; 43%); barriers included system navigation and poor interface issues. A major factor in the uptake and acceptability of technology-based interventions was appropriate training and IT skills ($n = 18$; 86%). Specific considerations include implementing an initial learning/familiarisation period to use the system and providing technical training for users.

(4) Role of the healthcare professional

Technology-based interventions increase healthcare professional confidence in decision making in situations of uncertainty around patient management ($n = 3$; 14%). Attitudes and perceptions of healthcare professionals towards technologies were seen as important in terms of

its usage; positive attitudes were more commonly associated with uptake ($n = 6$; 29%). Two studies emphasised the importance of senior professionals endorsing and driving the use of technology as being key to its success. In particular, healthcare professional engagement with technologies was reported as being key to its implementation, such as assigning one or more groups of healthcare professionals with sole responsibility of using the system, such as practice nurses ($n = 6$; 29%).

Discussion

This review has identified key features of successful interventions with a technological component aimed to improve healthcare professional practice. Results provide insights into the characteristics of successful interventions and provide recommendations for the design and implementation of technologies based on the barriers and facilitators identified.

A summary of the key findings from the present review is presented in Table 4, which outlines successful intervention features and components, effective BCTs used in interventions, and the barriers and facilitators in relation to implementing interventions. The most successful technological intervention was healthcare professional decision support, suggesting this may have an important role to play in clinical practice. The most common intervention *setting* was within primary care; however more practice change occurred in hospitals. This suggests two areas for future research. First, it is necessary to understand how the hospital setting, a key place in which deliver behavior change interventions aimed at supporting healthcare professional practice, such as prescribing practices [40] or screening of health conditions [41] can be utilised to facilitate delivery of technological interventions. Second, research is needed to find ways of overcoming the barriers that exist within primary care settings, particularly those identified by our thematic analysis. For example, organizational/structural

Table 4 Summary of findings of the important factors of implementation of technological interventions aimed at improving professional practice

Construct	Topic	Specific features / recommendations	References	Barrier / facilitator
What works	Type of intervention	Healthcare professional decision support	[10, 34, 38, 41, 57, 62, 65, 67, 69, 73, 74, 78, 80, 84, 88]	
		Reminders and alerts	[4, 8, 37, 47, 58, 64, 71]	
	BCTs	Instruction on how to perform the behaviour (BCTTv1 4.1)	[8, 10, 37–40, 47, 50, 57, 58, 64, 74, 78, 86]	
For whom interventions work for	Target healthcare professional behaviour	Adherence to clinical guidelines for patient management	[38, 57, 58, 62, 64, 74, 78, 79, 88]	
		Prescribing behaviours	[10, 37, 40, 65–67, 73, 80, 81]	
		Increasing knowledge or self-efficacy / confidence	[34, 39, 86, 61]	
		Increasing screening / testing rates	[4, 8, 41, 47, 69, 71, 76]	
		Clinical intervention / management	[68, 80, 83, 84, 86]	
	Target healthcare professional	GPs	[4, 8, 10, 34, 37, 39, 40, 47, 64–68, 71, 73, 74, 84–86]	
		Multiple healthcare professionals (more than two different types of healthcare professional)	[37, 41, 47, 57, 62, 73, 74, 76, 79, 81]	
Under what circumstances	Role of the healthcare professional	Increases confidence in decision making	[43, 96, 103]	Facilitator
		Attitudes and perceptions towards technology important in terms of uptake and usage	[43, 99–102, 107]	Facilitator
		Importance of endorsement from senior peers	[99, 104]	Facilitator
		Engagement important factor for implementation	[95, 100, 104]	Facilitator
		Assigning responsibility to using the system	[34, 100, 106]	Facilitator
				Facilitator
	Design, content and technical issues	Pilot testing - iterative modification to meet staff needs	[100, 101,104, 106, 108]	Facilitator
		Insufficient access to IT resources	[34, 92, 99, 104]	Barrier
		Physical location of computer	[94, 100, 106]	Barrier
		Technical issues such as computer performance and software updates	[94, 95, 98, 100, 102, 104, 105, 108]	Barrier
		Links to external patient information resources important	[92, 95, 99]	Facilitator
		Links to patient guidelines must be readily available, consistent and relevant	[43, 97–100]	Facilitator
	Usability and benefit for patient care	Provides access to important information relevant to the clinical encounter	[98, 99, 103, 109]	Facilitator
		Technology / interface must not be difficult to use	[43, 93, 96, 97, 99, 104–106, 109]	Barrier
		Technical training for staff	[34, 42, 99–101, 103–105, 107, 108]	Facilitator
		Importance of a learning period / time for familiarisation of the technology	[95–98, 108]	Facilitator
		Considers complexities of individual patients (for example patients with specific conditions, or comorbidities)	[42, 43, 97, 105]	Facilitator
		Helps facilitate discussions with patients	[100, 102]	Facilitator
	Practice and workload issues	Use of technology increases workload and may cause disruption	[34, 42, 97, 106]	Barrier
		Time taken to use the system / requirement of additional staff members	[34, 93, 98–100]	Barrier

Table 4 Summary of findings of the important factors of implementation of technological interventions aimed at improving professional practice *(Continued)*

Construct	Topic	Specific features / recommendations	References	Barrier / facilitator
		Improves communication between healthcare professionals	[92, 98, 103]	Facilitator
		Must be easily integrated into day-to-day workload	[34, 43, 97, 106]	Facilitator
		Technology aligns with current practice initiatives, and wider organisational context	[43, 92, 95, 98, 105, 108]	Facilitator

and logistical barriers such as workload and time pressures are often cited as challenges in primary care settings [42, 43], which may consequently influence the effectiveness of interventions. Our review also suggests financial incentives may be a way of engaging healthcare professionals with interventions. Whilst recent evidence suggests financial incentives may not influence long-term practice habits [44], our findings suggest this may be used to engage clinicians in technology-based interventions and therefore focusing on improving uptake.

The barriers and facilitators identified in this review are consistent with theoretical approaches to understanding implementation of interventions. Normalisation Process Theory [45, 46] can be used to understand how technological interventions become embedded in clinical practice. BCTs can be applied to demonstrate how interventions can be delivered in practice to facilitate implementation of technological interventions. Thus, four key recommendations can be made. First, it is necessary to understand how healthcare professionals make sense of the intervention in question. Consequently, technological interventions must have a clear function and meet organizational initiatives (*coherence* domain; e.g. *instruction on how to perform the behaviour* [BCTTv1 4.1]). Second, healthcare professionals must be actively engaged with technological interventions, which must be endorsed by key professionals within organisations, (*cognitive participation* domain; e.g. *social support* [BCTTv1 3.1]). Third, interventions must be easily integrated into clinical practice by: (a) complementing existing workloads of healthcare professionals; and (b) considering the diversity in terms of the setting in which they are delivered, the recipient of the intervention, and the target behaviour (*collective action* domain; e.g. *action planning* [BCTTv1 1.4]). Fourth, ensure that interventions are appraised by the recipients as having a benefit in terms of improving the patient encounter (*reflexive monitoring* domain; e.g. *self-monitoring of outcome(s) of behaviour* [BCTTv1 2.4]).

Our review shows that General Practitioners (GPs) are the most commonly targeted *healthcare professional* for technology-based interventions, and such interventions demonstrate the highest proportion of success in achieving behavior change. The role of the GP may be particularly important in understanding how technological approaches can be used to support professional practice. Of the 24 studies aimed at GPs, eight studies used computerised decision support and a further eight used reminders and alerts. The second largest group involved targeting multiple healthcare professionals, however only half of the studies resulted in behavior change. This is particularly important as part of the healthcare professional role involves referral and signposting to other healthcare professionals, where appropriate, and is recognized in primary care training strategies [5, 6]. One possible application of technological support, suggested by our thematic analysis, is to use technology to improve the communication between multiple healthcare professionals regarding patient management [11].

Use of behaviour change techniques in interventions

Use of recognized behavior change techniques [17] was identified in a number of studies. The most commonly used BCT was *instruction on how to perform the behavior* in the context of instructions from decision support systems, reminders and alerts. This technique may be particularly important for supporting healthcare professional clinical practice in the context of a technological intervention, which often involves tasks related to clinical decision making, such as making referrals and conducting health checks [5, 38, 47, 48].

When using BCTs, there were more studies resulting in healthcare professional behavior change than those showing no change. Given that the BCT framework is still in its infancy, interventions must apply the techniques to important areas of clinical practice (such as increasing appropriate screening and more appropriate medicine prescribing practices). The use of theory offers valuable insights both in terms of understanding and supporting practice change [19, 49], and as a framework to guide interventions. Our review has provided encouraging findings supporting the use of BCTs as part of technology-based interventions supporting healthcare professional practice change. Findings suggest that BCTs can be effective across a range of diverse interventions, target behaviours, and healthcare professionals groups. The BCT *instruction on how to perform the behaviour*, effective in 15 studies, was implemented across prescribing behaviours (e.g.), adherence to patient management guidelines (e.g. [50]), and increasing screening rates (e.g.), and found to be effective when delivered to doctors, therapists [50], nurses, and surgeons. Identifying effective BCTs in this way allows the opportunity to deliver interventions aiming to change healthcare professional practice shown to be effective across a range of diverse contexts. Given that 22 of the 48 studies included in this review did not contain any evidence of BCTs, there is considerable scope for future research to develop interventions that include BCTs. This may involve targeting known psychological constructs involved in behavior change, using established as well as emerging frameworks specifically relating to implementation of interventions [51–53].

Strengths and limitations of this review

Although there are a number of systematic reviews [11–15, 54] that examine the effectiveness of individual types of technology-based interventions aimed at healthcare professionals, this is the first attempt to synthesise evidence across all interventions that include a technological component, and the factors involved in implementation of interventions. We have synthesised the findings from across a diverse range of intervention contexts and settings, and presented a series of barriers and facilitators that are shared across healthcare behaviours and diverse professional groups. The advantage of this approach is this provides a series of recommendations concerning implementation of interventions, and an opportunity for behaviour change interventions to be delivered at scale, targeting multiple healthcare professional groups working in different healthcare settings. This is also an attempt to move beyond the most commonly researched interventions and provide a wider understanding of both intervention function and content. The current review extends the findings of previous reviews by: (1) identifying specific features associated with successful interventions, (2) highlighting opportunities to improve the design of technologies by incorporating known BCTs; and (3) identifying the barriers and facilitators to successful implementation. Future reviews would benefit from including an analysis of patient outcomes, particularly whether changes in healthcare professional practice as a consequence of implementing technological interventions translates into positive patient outcomes.

The realist method of literature review was chosen to guide the present review in order to understand a large and complex literature, with the qualitative findings advancing our quantitative findings by providing an explanatory framework about why and how technological interventions work. This level of detail would not have been possible to identify using the Cochrane style of systematic review methods. Whilst we sought to extract effect sizes for included studies, due to the varied reporting of study results, and in the absence of the relevant statistical information such as p values and sample sizes, it was only possible to calculate effect sizes for a small number of papers. Further, due to the range of outcomes obtained, and often multiple outcomes from individual studies, a direct comparison between groups was not possible.

Conclusions

Technological approaches to improving healthcare professional practice provide opportunities to address challenges in multiple areas of clinical practice [55]. Healthcare professional decision support interventions, when developed using recognized psychological theory such as providing instruction on how to implement interventions, show considerable promise. Interventions must also address known organizational challenges associated with specific settings, as well as focusing on efficiency and user-friendly design content, whilst ensuring interventions complement the day-to-day workload and current knowledge and skillset of the target healthcare professional. Understanding the most important contextual features, and how to apply theoretical insights known to change behavior can all contribute to the design and successful implementation of technologies aiming to directly influence the clinical management of patients.

Abbreviations

BCT: Behaviour change technique; BCTTv1: Behaviour change technique taxonomy version 1; CINAHL: Cumulative index to nursing and allied health literature; GP: General practitioner; IT: Information technology; MeSH: Medical subject heading

Funding

This work was funded through a University Research Institute Pump Priming Programme and supported by the NIHR Manchester Biomedical Research Centre and the NIHR Greater Manchester Patient Safety Translational Research Centre.

Authors' contributions

CK, MPT, JH and CJA designed and conceived the review. CK conducted the search and CK and MPT selected articles for inclusion according to the inclusion/exclusion criteria. CK conducted extraction of the data, CK and MPT conducted analysis. CK drafted the manuscript and revised accordingly based on all co-author comments. All authors approved the final version.

Competing interests

The authors declare that they have no competing interests.

What maximizes the effectiveness and implementation of technology-based interventions to support...

229

Author details

[1]Manchester Centre for Health Psychology, Division of Psychology and Mental Health, School of Health Sciences, Faculty of Biology, Medicine and Health, University of Manchester, Manchester Academic Health Science Centre, Coupland 1 Building, Oxford Road, Manchester M13 9PL, UK. [2]Division of Medical Education, School of Medical Sciences, Faculty of Biology, Medicine and Health, University of Manchester, Manchester Academic Health Science Centre, Oxford Road, Manchester M13 9PL, UK. [3]Division of Pharmacy and Optometry, School of Health Sciences, Faculty of Biology, Medicine and Health, University of Manchester, Manchester Academic Health Science Centre, Stopford Building, Oxford Road, Manchester M13 9PL, UK. [4]NIHR Manchester Biomedical Research Centre, Manchester University NHS Foundation Trust, Manchester Academic Health Science Centre, Manchester M13 9PL, UK. [5]NIHR Greater Manchester Patient Safety Translational Research Centre, Manchester, UK.

References

1. National Institute for Health and Care Excellence. Behaviour change: individual approaches (PH49). London: NICE; 2014.
2. Ashcroft DM, et al. Prevalence, nature, severity and risk factors for prescribing errors in hospital inpatients: prospective study in 20 UK hospitals. Drug Saf. 2015;38(9):833–43.
3. Mant D. Health checks and screening: what works in general practice? Br J Gen Pract. 2014;64(627):493–4.
4. Goetz MB, et al. Central implementation strategies outperform local ones in improving HIV testing in Veterans Healthcare Administration facilities. J Gen Intern Med. 2013;28(10):1311–7.
5. National Health Service (NHS) Yorkshire and the Humber. Prevention and Lifestyle Behaviour Change: A Competence Framework. Yorkshire and the Humber: NHS; 2010.
6. General Medical Council (GMC). Tomorrow's doctors: outcomes and standards for undergraduate medical education: London, GMC; 2009.
7. Ross S, et al. Perceived causes of prescribing errors by junior doctors in hospital inpatients: a study from the PROTECT programme. BMJ Qual Saf. 2013;22(2):97–102.
8. van Wyk JT, et al. Electronic alerts versus on-demand decision support to improve dyslipidemia treatment: a cluster randomized controlled trial. Circulation. 2008;117(3):371–8.
9. Bahrami M, et al. Effectiveness of strategies to disseminate and implement clinical guidelines for the management of impacted and unerupted third molars in primary dental care, a cluster randomised controlled trial. Br Dent J. 2004;197(11):691–6.
10. Buising KL, et al. Improving antibiotic prescribing for adults with community acquired pneumonia: does a computerised decision support system achieve more than academic detailing alone? - A time series analysis. BMC Medical Informatics and Decision Making. 2008;8:35.
11. Goyder C, et al. Email for clinical communication between healthcare professionals. Cochrane Database Syst Rev. 2015;2:CD007979.
12. Fiander M, et al. Interventions to increase the use of electronic health information by healthcare practitioners to improve clinical practice and patient outcomes. Cochrane Database Syst Rev. 2015;3:CD004749.
13. Arditi C, et al. Computer-generated reminders delivered on paper to healthcare professionals; effects on professional practice and health care outcomes. Cochrane Database Syst Rev. 2012;12:CD001175.
14. Campanella P, et al. The impact of electronic health records on healthcare quality: a systematic review and meta-analysis. Eur J Pub Health. 2016;26(1):60–4.
15. Brown CL, et al. A systematic review of the types and causes of prescribing errors generated from using computerized provider order entry systems in primary and secondary care. J Am Med Inform Assoc. 2016.
16. Gardner B, et al. Using theory to synthesise evidence from behaviour change interventions: the example of audit and feedback. Soc Sci Med. 2010;70(10):1618–25.
17. Michie S, et al. The behavior change technique taxonomy (v1) of 93 hierarchically clustered techniques: building an international consensus for the reporting of behavior change interventions. Ann Behav Med. 2013;46(1):81–95.
18. Eccles M, et al. Changing the behaviour of healthcare professionals: the use of theory in promoting the uptake of research findings. J Clin Epidemiol. 2005;58(2):107-12.
19. Eccles MP, et al. Explaining clinical behaviors using multiple theoretical models. Implement Sci. 2012;7(1):1–13.
20. Ross J, et al. Factors that influence the implementation of e-health: a systematic review of systematic reviews (an update). Implement Sci. 2016; 11:146.
21. Rycroft-Malone J, et al. Realist synthesis: illustrating the method for implementation research. Implement Sci. 2012;7:33.
22. Pawson R. The science of evaluation: a realist manifesto. London: SAGE Publication Ltd.; 2013.
23. Mays N, Pope C, Popay J. Systematically reviewing qualitative and quantitative evidence to inform management and policy-making in the health field. J Health Serv Res Policy. 2005;10(Suppl 1):6–20.
24. Tsang JY, et al. Understanding the implementation of interventions to improve the management of chronic kidney disease in primary care: a rapid realist review. Implement Sci. 2016;11:47.
25. Pearson M, et al. Implementing health promotion programmes in schools: a realist systematic review of research and experience in the United Kingdom. Implement Sci. 2015;10:149.
26. Vassilev I, et al. Assessing the implementability of telehealth interventions for self-management support: a realist review. Implement Sci. 2015;10(1):59.
27. Pearson M, et al. Using realist review to inform intervention development: methodological illustration and conceptual platform for collaborative care in offender mental health. Implement Sci. 2015;10:134.
28. Craig P, et al. Developing and evaluating complex interventions: the new Medical Research Council guidance. 2008;337.
29. Greenhalgh T, et al. Protocol—realist and meta-narrative evidence synthesis: evolving standards (RAMESES). BMC Med Res Methodol. 2011;11:115.
30. Pawson R, et al. Realist review—a new method of systematic review designed for complex policy interventions. J Health Serv Res Policy. 2005; 10(Suppl 1):21–34.
31. Michie S, et al. Effective techniques in healthy eating and physical activity interventions: a meta-regression. Health Psychol. 2009;28(6):690–701.
32. Bazeley P, Jackson K. In: Bazeley P, Jackson K, editors. Qualitative data analysis with NVivo, London: Sage Publications Limited.; 2013.
33. Kastner M, et al. What is the most appropriate knowledge synthesis method to conduct a review? Protocol for a scoping review. BMC Med Res Methodol. 2012;12:114.
34. Edelman EA, et al. Evaluation of a novel electronic genetic screening and clinical decision support tool in prenatal clinical settings. Matern Child Health J. 2014;18(5):1233–45.
35. Osheroff JA, et al. A roadmap for national action on clinical decision support. J Am Med Inform Assoc. 2007;14(2):141–5.
36. Cohen J. Statistical power analysis for the behavioural sciences. Hillside: Lawrence Earlbaum Associates; 1988.
37. Fortuna RJ, et al. Reducing the prescribing of heavily marketed medications: a randomized controlled trial. J Gen Intern Med. 2009;24(8):897–903.
38. Gupta A, et al. Effect of clinical decision support on documented guideline adherence for head CT in emergency department patients with mild traumatic brain injury. J Am Med Inform Assoc. 2014;21(e2):e347–51.
39. Maiburg BH, et al. Controlled trial of effect of computer-based nutrition course on knowledge and practice of general practitioner trainees. Am J Clin Nutr. 2003;77(4 Suppl):1019S–24S.
40. Avery AJ, et al. A pharmacist-led information technology intervention for medication errors (PINCER): a multicentre, cluster randomised, controlled trial and cost-effectiveness analysis. Lancet. 2012;379(9823):1310–9.
41. Fein JA, et al. Feasibility and effects of a web-based adolescent psychiatric assessment administered by clinical staff in the pediatric emergency department. Arch Pediatr Adolesc Med. 2010;164(12):1112–7.
42. Patterson ES, et al. Human factors barriers to the effective use of ten HIV clinical reminders. J Am Med Inform Assoc. 2004;11(1):50–9.
43. Ackerman SL, et al. One size does not fit all: evaluating an intervention to reduce antibiotic prescribing for acute bronchitis. BMC Health Serv Res. 2013;13:462.
44. Chauhan BF, et al. Behavior change interventions and policies influencing primary healthcare professionals' practice-an overview of reviews. Implement Sci. 2017;12(1):3.
45. Murray E, et al. Normalisation process theory: a framework for developing, evaluating and implementing complex interventions. BMC Med. 2010;8:63.

46. May CR, et al. Development of a theory of implementation and integration: normalization process theory. Implement Sci. 2009;4:29.

47. Goetz MB, et al. A system-wide intervention to improve HIV testing in the Veterans Health Administration. J Gen Intern Med. 2008;23(8):1200–7.

48. Tierney WM, et al. Effects of computerized guidelines for managing heart disease in primary care. J Gen Intern Med. 2003;18(12):967–76.

49. Johnson MJ, May CR. Promoting professional behaviour change in healthcare: what interventions work, and why? A theory-led overview of systematic reviews. BMJ Open. 2015;5(9):e008592.

50. Beidas RS, et al. Training and consultation to promote implementation of an empirically supported treatment: a randomized trial. Psychiatr Serv. 2012; 63(7):660–5.

51. Michie S, van Stralen MM, West R. The behaviour change wheel: a new method for characterising and designing behaviour change interventions. Implement Sci. 2011;6:42.

52. Hrisos S, et al. An intervention modelling experiment to change GPs' intentions to implement evidence-based practice: using theory-based interventions to promote GP management of upper respiratory tract infection without prescribing antibiotics #2. BMC Health Serv Res. 2008;8:10.

53. Presseau J, et al. Reflective and automatic processes in health care professional behaviour: a dual process model tested across multiple behaviours. Ann Behav Med. 2014;48(3):347–58.

54. Shojania KG, et al. Effect of point-of-care computer reminders on physician behaviour: a systematic review. CMAJ. 2010;182(5):E216–25.

55. Shojania KG, et al. The effects of on-screen, point of care computer reminders on processes and outcomes of care. Cochrane Database Syst Rev. 2009;3:CD001096.

56. Armstrong EP, et al. Evaluation of a drug-drug interaction: fax alert intervention program. BMC Med Inform Decis Mak. 2013;13:32.

57. Beeckman D, et al. A multi-faceted tailored strategy to implement an electronic clinical decision support system for pressure ulcer prevention in nursing homes: a two-armed randomized controlled trial. Int J Nurs Stud. 2013;50(4):475–86.

58. Carton M, et al. Assessment of radiological referral practice and effect of computer-based guidelines on radiological requests in two emergency departments. Clin Radiol. 2002;57(2):123–8.

59. Cosgrove SE, et al. Impact of different methods of feedback to clinicians after postprescription antimicrobial review based on the centers for disease control and prevention's 12 steps to prevent antimicrobial resistance among hospitalized adults. Infect Control Hosp Epidemiol. 2007;28(6):641–6.

60. Curtis JR, et al. Challenges in improving the quality of osteoporosis care for long-term glucocorticoid users: a prospective randomized trial. Arch Intern Med. 2007;167(6):591–6.

61. Dimeff LA, et al. Which training method works best? A randomized controlled trial comparing three methods of training clinicians in dialectical behavior therapy skills. Behav Res Ther. 2009;47(11):921–30.

62. Dykes PC, et al. Clinical practice guideline adherence before and after implementation of the HEARTFELT (HEART Failure Effectiveness & Leadership Team) intervention. J Cardiovasc Nurs. 2005;20(5):306–14.

63. Eccles M, et al. Effect of computerised evidence based guidelines on management of asthma and angina in adults in primary care: cluster randomised controlled trial. BMJ. 2002;325(7370):941.

64. Fifield J, et al. Improving pediatric asthma control among minority children participating in medicaid: providing practice redesign support to deliver a chronic care model. J Asthma. 2010;47(7):718–27.

65. Filippi A, et al. Effects of an automated electronic reminder in changing the antiplatelet drug-prescribing behavior among Italian general practitioners in diabetic patients: an intervention trial. Diabetes Care. 2003;26(5):1497–500.

66. Gerber JS, et al. Effect of an outpatient antimicrobial stewardship intervention on broad-spectrum antibiotic prescribing by primary care pediatricians: a randomized trial. JAMA. 2013;309(22):2345–52.

67. Gonzales R, et al. A cluster randomized trial of decision support strategies for reducing antibiotic use in acute bronchitis. JAMA Intern Med. 2013; 173(4):267–73.

68. Guldberg TL, et al. Improved quality of type 2 diabetes care following electronic feedback of treatment status to general practitioners: a cluster randomized controlled trial. Diabet Med. 2011;28(3):325–32.

69. Hibbs SP, et al. The impact of electronic decision support and electronic remote blood issue on transfusion practice. Transfus Med. 2014;24(5):274–9.

70. Hobbs FD, et al. A prospective controlled trial of computerized decision support for lipid management in primary care. Fam Pract. 1996;13(2):133–7.

71. Hoch I, et al. Countrywide computer alerts to community physicians improve potassium testing in patients receiving diuretics. J Am Med Inform Assoc. 2003;10(6):541–6.

72. Kortteisto T, et al. Patient-specific computer-based decision support in primary healthcare—a randomized trial. Implement Sci. 2014;9:15.

73. Litvin CB, et al. Use of an electronic health record clinical decision support tool to improve antibiotic prescribing for acute respiratory infections: the ABX-TRIP study. J Gen Intern Med. 2013;28(6):810–6.

74. Lobach DF, Hammond WE. Computerized decision support based on a clinical practice guideline improves compliance with care standards. Am J Med. 1997;102(1):89–98.

75. Malone DC, Saverno KR. Evaluation of a wireless handheld medication management device in the prevention of drug-drug interactions in a Medicaid population. J Manag Care Pharm. 2012;18(1):33–45.

76. Mayne SL, et al. Effect of decision support on missed opportunities for human papillomavirus vaccination. Am J Prev Med. 2014;47(6):734–44.

77. Nilasena DS, Lincoln MJ. A computer-generated reminder system improves physician compliance with diabetes preventive care guidelines. Proc Annu Symp Comput Appl Med Care. 1995:640–5.

78. Patkar V, et al. Evidence-based guidelines and decision support services: a discussion and evaluation in triple assessment of suspected breast cancer. Br J Cancer. 2006;95(11):1490–6.

79. Piening S, et al. The additional value of an e-mail to inform healthcare professionals of a drug safety issue: a randomized controlled trial in the Netherlands. Drug Saf. 2013;36(9):723–31.

80. Reeve JF, Tenni PC, Peterson GM. An electronic prompt in dispensing software to promote clinical interventions by community pharmacists: a randomized controlled trial. Br J Clin Pharmacol. 2008;65(3):377–85.

81. Ribeiro-Vaz I, et al. Promoting spontaneous adverse drug reaction reporting in hospitals using a hyperlink to the online reporting form: an ecological study in Portugal. Drug Saf. 2012;35(5):387–94.

82. Rocha BH, et al. Clinicians' response to computerized detection of infections. J Am Med Inform Assoc. 2001;8(2):117–25.

83. Ruland CM. Handheld technology to improve patient care: evaluating a support system for preference-based care planning at the bedside. J Am Med Inform Assoc. 2002;9(2):192–201.

84. Schwarz EB, et al. Clinical decision support to promote safe prescribing to women of reproductive age: a cluster-randomized trial. J Gen Intern Med. 2012;27(7):831–8.

85. Sharifi M, et al. Enhancing the electronic health record to increase counseling and quit-line referral for parents who smoke. Acad Pediatr. 2014;14(5):478–84.

86. Strayer SM, et al. Improving smoking cessation counseling using a point-of-care health intervention tool (IT): from the Virginia Practice Support and Research Network (VaPSRN). J Am Board Fam Med. 2013;26(2):116–25.

87. Strom BL, et al. Unintended effects of a computerized physician order entry nearly hard-stop alert to prevent a drug interaction: a randomized controlled trial. Arch Intern Med. 2010;170(17):1578–83.

88. Tang PC, et al. Measuring the effects of reminders for outpatient influenza immunizations at the point of clinical opportunity. J Am Med Inform Assoc. 1999;6(2):115–21.

89. Vagholkar S, et al. Influence of cardiovascular absolute risk assessment on prescribing of antihypertensive and lipid-lowering medications: a cluster randomized controlled trial. Am Heart J. 2014;167(1):28–35.

90. Walker J, et al. Computer reminders for chlamydia screening in general practice: a randomized controlled trial. Sex Transm Dis. 2010;37(7):445–50.

91. Lipsey MW, Wilson DB. Practical meta-analysis, vol. 49. Thousand Oaks: Sage publications; 2001.

92. Barnett J, et al. myPace: an integrative health platform for supporting weight loss and maintenance behaviors. IEEE J Biomed Health Inform. 2015; 19(1):109–16.

93. Bokhour BG, et al. The role of evidence and context for implementing a multimodal intervention to increase HIV testing. Implement Sci. 2015;10:22.

94. Burns P, et al. The introduction of electronic medication charts and prescribing in aged care facilities: an evaluation. Australas J Ageing. 2007; 26(3):131–4.

95. Doerr M, et al. Formative evaluation of clinician experience with integrating family history-based clinical decision support into clinical practice. J Pers Med. 2014;4(2):115–36.

96. Dowding D, et al. Nurses' use of computerised clinical decision support systems: a case site analysis. J Clin Nurs. 2009;18(8):1159–67.

97. Dryden EM, et al. Provider perspectives on electronic decision supports for obesity prevention. Clin Pediatr (Phila). 2012;51(5):490–7.
98. Guldberg TL, et al. Suboptimal quality of type 2 diabetes care discovered through electronic feedback led to increased nurse-GP cooperation. A qualitative study. Prim Care Diabetes. 2010;4(1):33–9.
99. Hains IM, et al. Standardizing care in medical oncology: are web-based systems the answer? Cancer. 2009;115(23):5579–88.
100. Litvin CB, et al. Adoption of a clinical decision support system to promote judicious use of antibiotics for acute respiratory infections in primary care. Int J Med Inform. 2012;81(8):521–6.
101. Maguire R, et al. Nurse's perceptions and experiences of using of a mobile-phone-based Advanced Symptom Management System (ASyMS©) to monitor and manage chemotherapy-related toxicity. Eur J Oncol Nurs. 2008; 12(4):380–6.
102. Mandt I, Horn AM, Granas AG. [Communication about prescription interventions between pharmacists and general practitioners]. Tidsskr Nor Laegeforen. 2009;129(18):1846–9.
103. Power JMH, et al. Integration of smartphones into clinical pharmacy practice: an evaluation of the impact on pharmacists' efficiency. Health Policy and Technology. 2014;3(4):296–305.
104. Randell R, Dowding D. Organisational influences on nurses' use of clinical decision support systems. Int J Med Inform. 2010;79(6):412–21.
105. Rousseau N, et al. Practice based, longitudinal, qualitative interview study of computerised evidence based guidelines in primary care. BMJ. 2003; 326(7384):314.
106. Saleem JJ, et al. Exploring barriers and facilitators to the use of computerized clinical reminders. J Am Med Inform Assoc. 2005;12(4):438–47.
107. Vishwanath A, et al. Patterns and changes in prescriber attitudes toward PDA prescription-assistive technology. Int J Med Inform. 2009;78(5):330–9.
108. Weir C, et al. The role of information technology in translating educational interventions into practice: an analysis using the PRECEDE/PROCEED model. J Am Med Inform Assoc. 2011;18(6):827–34.
109. Zhu X, Cimino JJ. Clinicians' evaluation of computer-assisted medication summarization of electronic medical records. Comput Biol Med. 2015;59:221–31.

Permissions

All chapters in this book were first published in MI&DM, by BioMed Central; hereby published with permission under the Creative Commons Attribution License or equivalent. Every chapter published in this book has been scrutinized by our experts. Their significance has been extensively debated. The topics covered herein carry significant findings which will fuel the growth of the discipline. They may even be implemented as practical applications or may be referred to as a beginning point for another development.

The contributors of this book come from diverse backgrounds, making this book a truly international effort. This book will bring forth new frontiers with its revolutionizing research information and detailed analysis of the nascent developments around the world.

We would like to thank all the contributing authors for lending their expertise to make the book truly unique. They have played a crucial role in the development of this book. Without their invaluable contributions this book wouldn't have been possible. They have made vital efforts to compile up to date information on the varied aspects of this subject to make this book a valuable addition to the collection of many professionals and students.

This book was conceptualized with the vision of imparting up-to-date information and advanced data in this field. To ensure the same, a matchless editorial board was set up. Every individual on the board went through rigorous rounds of assessment to prove their worth. After which they invested a large part of their time researching and compiling the most relevant data for our readers.

The editorial board has been involved in producing this book since its inception. They have spent rigorous hours researching and exploring the diverse topics which have resulted in the successful publishing of this book. They have passed on their knowledge of decades through this book. To expedite this challenging task, the publisher supported the team at every step. A small team of assistant editors was also appointed to further simplify the editing procedure and attain best results for the readers.

Apart from the editorial board, the designing team has also invested a significant amount of their time in understanding the subject and creating the most relevant covers. They scrutinized every image to scout for the most suitable representation of the subject and create an appropriate cover for the book.

The publishing team has been an ardent support to the editorial, designing and production team. Their endless efforts to recruit the best for this project, has resulted in the accomplishment of this book. They are a veteran in the field of academics and their pool of knowledge is as vast as their experience in printing. Their expertise and guidance has proved useful at every step. Their uncompromising quality standards have made this book an exceptional effort. Their encouragement from time to time has been an inspiration for everyone.

The publisher and the editorial board hope that this book will prove to be a valuable piece of knowledge for researchers, students, practitioners and scholars across the globe.

List of Contributors

Mehmet Saluvan
Center for Applied Pediatric Quality Analytics, Boston Children's Hospital, 300 Longwood Avenue, Boston, MA 02115, USA

Al Ozonoff
Center for Applied Pediatric Quality Analytics, Boston Children's Hospital, 300 Longwood Avenue, Boston, MA 02115, USA
Department of Pediatrics, Harvard Medical School, Boston, MA, USA

Ana Respicio
CMAF-CIO, Faculdade de Ciências, Universidade de Lisboa, Lisbon, Portugal
Departamento de Informática, Faculdade de Ciências, Universidade de Lisboa, Bloco C6, Piso 3, 1749-016 Lisboa, Portugal

Margarida Moz and Margarida Vaz Pato
ISEG and CMAF-CIO, Universidade de Lisboa, Lisbon, Portugal

Rute Somensi
Pavilhão Pereira Filho, Santa Casa de Misericórdia Porto Alegre and Universidade Federal de Ciências da Saúde de Porto Alegre, Hospital São José, Porto Alegre, Brazil

Cecília Dias Flores
Universidade Federal de Ciências da Saúde de Porto Alegre, Porto Alegre, Brazil

Konstantin H. Franke and Benno Kreuels
Division of Tropical Medicine, First Department of Medicine, University Medical Center Hamburg-Eppendorf (UKE), Hamburg, Germany
Infectious Disease Epidemiology, Bernhard Nocht Institute for Tropical Medicine (BNITM), Hamburg, Germany

Ralf Krumkamp and Jürgen May
Infectious Disease Epidemiology, Bernhard Nocht Institute for Tropical Medicine (BNITM), Hamburg, Germany

Aliyu Mohammed, Nimako Sarpong and Ellis Owusu-Dabo
Kumasi Center for Collaborative Research in Tropical Medicine (KCCR), College of Health Sciences, Kwame Nkrumah University of Science and Technology (KNUST), Kumasi, Ghana

Johanna Brinkel
Department of Public Health Medicine, School of Public Health, University of Bielefeld, Bielefeld, Germany

Julius N. Fobil
School of Public Health, University of Ghana, Accra, Ghana

Axel Bonacic Marinovic
National Institute for Public Health and the Environment (RIVM), Bilthoven, The Netherlands.

Philip Asihene and Mark Boots
Viamo, Accra, Ghana

Shamil Haroon and Krishnarajah Nirantharakumar
Institute of Applied Health Research, College of Medical and Dental Sciences, University of Birmingham, Edgbaston, Birmingham B15 2TT, UK

Darren Wooldridge, Jan Hoogewerf and John Williams
Health Informatics Unit, Royal College of Physicians, 11 St Andrews Place, Regent's Park, London NW1 4LE, UK

Lina Martino
Public Health Specialty Registrar, West Midlands, UK

Neeraj Bhala
Queen Elizabeth Hospital Birmingham, Mindelsohn Way, Birmingham B15 2TH, UK

Lingling Zhou, Ping Zhao, Dongdong Wu, Cheng Cheng and Hao Huang
Department of Information, Research Institute of Field Surgery, Daping Hospital of Army Medical University, 10 Changjiang Access Road, Chongqing 400042, China

KS Kylie Lee
University of Sydney, Discipline of Addiction Medicine, Indigenous Health and Substance Use, NHMRC Centre of Research Excellence in Indigenous Health and Alcohol, King George V Building, 83-117 Missenden Road, Camperdown, NSW 2050, Australia
Centre for Alcohol Policy Research, La Trobe University, 215 Franklin Street, Melbourne, VIC 3000, Australia

Robin Room and Sarah Callinan
Centre for Alcohol Policy Research, La Trobe University, 215 Franklin Street, Melbourne, VIC 3000, Australia

Jimmy Perry
Aboriginal Drug and Alcohol Council (ADAC) South Australia, 155 Holbrooks Road Underdale, Adelaide, South Australia 5032, Australia

Scott Wilson
Aboriginal Drug and Alcohol Council (ADAC) South Australia, 155 Holbrooks Road Underdale, Adelaide, South Australia 5032, Australia
University of Sydney, Discipline of Addiction Medicine, Indigenous Health and Substance Use, NHMRC Centre of Research Excellence in Indigenous Health and Alcohol, King George V Building, 83-117 Missenden Road, Camperdown, NSW 2050, Australia

Robert Assan
Alcohol, Tobacco and other Drugs Service, Queensland Health, 190 Palmerston Vincent, Townsville, QLD 4814, Australia

Noel Hayman
Southern Queensland Centre of Excellence in Aboriginal and Torres Strait Islander Primary Health Care, 37 Wirraway Parade, Inala, QLD 4077, Australia
School of Medicine, University of Queensland, Herston Road, Brisbane, QLD 4006, Australia.
School of Medicine, Griffith University, Gold Coast Campus, Gold Coast, Brisbane, QLD 4222, Australia

Tanya Chikritzhs, Dennis Gray and Edward Wilkes
National Drug Research Institute, Curtin University, 10 Selby St, Shenton Park, WA 6008, Australia

Peter Jack
Drug Health Services, Royal Prince Alfred Hospital, Sydney Local Health District, KGV Building, Missenden Road, Camperdown, NSW 2050, Australia

Katherine M. Conigrave
Drug Health Services, Royal Prince Alfred Hospital, Sydney Local Health District, KGV Building, Missenden Road, Camperdown, NSW 2050, Australia
University of Sydney, Discipline of Addiction Medicine, Indigenous Health and Substance Use, NHMRC Centre of Research Excellence in Indigenous Health and Alcohol, King George V Building, 83-117 Missenden Road, Camperdown, NSW 2050, Australia

Erik Joukes, Ronald Cornet, Nicolette F. de Keizer and Ameen Abu-Hanna
Department of Medical Informatics, Amsterdam Public Health research institute, Academic Medical Center, University of Amsterdam, 1100 DE Amsterdam, The Netherlands

Martine C. de Bruijne
Department of Public and Occupational Health, Amsterdam Public Health research institute, VU University Medical Center, Van der Boechorststraat 7, 1081 BT Amsterdam, The Netherlands

Romaric Marcilly and Marie-Catherine Beuscart-Zéphir
Univ. Lille, INSERM, CHU Lille, CIC-IT / Evalab 1403 - Centre d'Investigation clinique, EA 2694, F-59000 Lille, France,
Maison Régionale de la Recherche Clinique, 6 rue du professeur Laguesse, 59000 Lille France

Elske Ammenwerth
Institute of Medical Informatics, UMIT – University for Health Sciences, Medical Informatics and Technology, 6060 Hall in Tirol, Austria

Erin Roehrer
eHealth Services Research Group, School of Engineering and ICT, University of Tasmania, Private Bag 87, Hobart, Tasmania 7001, Australia

Julie Niès
General Electric Healthcare Partners, 92772, Boulogne Billancourt cedex, France

Nooshin J. Fesharaki and Jake Luo
Department of Health Informatics and Administration, Center for Biomedical Data and Language Processing, University of Wisconsin-Milwaukee, 2025 E Newport Ave, NWQ-B Room 6469, Milwaukee, WI 53211, USA

Yiqing Zhao
Department of Health Informatics and Administration, Center for Biomedical Data and Language Processing, University of Wisconsin-Milwaukee, 2025 E Newport Ave, NWQ-B Room 6469, Milwaukee, WI 53211, USA
Division of Biomedical Statistics and Informatics, Mayo Clinic, Rochester, 205 3rd Ave SW, Rochester, MN 55905, USA

Hongfang Liu
Division of Biomedical Statistics and Informatics, Mayo Clinic, Rochester, 205 3rd Ave SW, Rochester, MN 55905, USA

Ronald W. Gimbel, Lu Zhang and Min-Jae Woo
Department of Public Health Sciences, Clemson University, 501 Edwards Hall, Clemson, SC 29634-0745, USA

Zachary Connor
Department of Public Health Sciences, Clemson University, 501 Edwards Hall, Clemson, SC 29634-0745, USA
Department of Radiology, Greenville Health System, Greenville, SC, USA

Ronald G. Pirrallo
Department of Emergency Medicine, Greenville Health System, Greenville, SC, USA

Steven C. Lowe
Department of Radiology, Greenville Health System, Greenville, SC, USA

David W. Wright
Department of Emergency Medicine, Emory University, Atlanta, GA, USA

Paul Fontelo and Fang Liu
Lister Hill National Center for Biomedical Communication, National Library of Medicine, Bethesda, MD, USA

Daniel S. Reuland and Russell P. Harris
Department of General Medicine and Clinical Epidemiology, University of North Carolina School of Medicine, Cecil G Sheps Center for Health Services Research, University of North Carolina at Chapel Hill, 725 Martin Luther King Jr. Blvd, CB 7590, Chapel Hill, NC 27599, USA

Laura Cubillos and Alison T. Brenner
Lineberger Comprehensive Cancer Center, Cecil G Sheps Center for Health Services Research, University of North Carolina at Chapel Hill, 725 Martin Luther King Jr. Blvd, CB 7590, Chapel Hill, NC 27599, USA

Bailey Minish
Department of General Medicine and Clinical Epidemiology, University of North Carolina, School of Medicine, Ambulatory Care Center, University of North Carolina at Chapel Hill, 101 Mason Farm Road, Chapel Hill, NC 27599-7745, USA

Michael P. Pignone
Department of Medicine, Dell Medical School, The University of Texas at Austin, 1912 Speedway, Campus Mail Code D2000, Austin, TX 78712, USA

Stephen Mburu and Robert Oboko
School of Computing and Informatics, University of Nairobi, Nairobi, Kenya

Sunny C. Lin
Department of Health Management and Policy, School of Public Health, University of Michigan, Ann Arbor, MI, USA

Julia Adler-Milstein
Department of Medicine, Center for Clinical Informatics and Improvement Research, University of California, San Francisco, CA, USA

Jung-Ah Lee
Sue and Bill Gross School of Nursing, University of California Irvine, Irvine, CA, USA

Mona Choi
College of Nursing, Mo-Im Kim Nursing Research Institute, Yonsei University, 50 Yonsei-ro, Seodaemun-gu, Seoul, Republic of Korea03722

Sang A Lee
College of Nursing and Health Sciences, University of Massachusetts, Boston, MA, USA.

Natalie Jiang
Program in Public Health, University of California Irvine, Irvine, CA, USA

Yadan Fan
Institute for Health Informatics, University of Minnesota, Minneapolis, MN, USA

Rui Zhang
Institute for Health Informatics, University of Minnesota, Minneapolis, MN, USA
Department of Pharmaceutical Care & Health Systems, College of Pharmacy, University of Minnesota, Minneapolis, MN, USA

Xieling Chen
College of Economics, Jinan University, Guangzhou, China

Haoran Xie
Department of Mathematics and Information Technology, The Education University of Hong Kong, Hong Kong, Hong Kong, Special Administrative Region of China

Fu Lee Wang
School of Science and Technology, The Open University of Hong Kong, Hong Kong, Hong Kong, Special Administrative Region of China

Ziqing Liu
The Second Clinical Medical College, Guangzhou University of Chinese Medicine, Guangzhou, China

Juan Xu
The Research Institute of National Supervision and Audit Law, Nanjing Audit University, Nanjing, China

Tianyong Hao
School of Information Science and Technology, Guangdong University of Foreign Studies, Guangzhou, China
School of Computer, South China Normal University, Guangzhou, China

Zainab AlMeraj and Fatima Boujarwah
Department of Information Science, College of Computing Sciences and Engineering, Kuwait University, Adailiya, Kuwait

Dari Alhuwail
Department of Information Science, College of Computing Sciences and Engineering, Kuwait University, Adailiya, Kuwait
Health Informatics Unit, Dasman Diabetes Institute, Sharq, Kuwait

Jessica H. Jun, Jen-Ai Lai and Tanya L. Feng
Division of Neurology, Department of Medicine, The University of British Columbia, Vancouver, Canada
BC Children's & Women's Hospital, Vancouver, Canada

Julie M. Robillard
Division of Neurology, Department of Medicine, The University of British Columbia, Vancouver, Canada
BC Children's & Women's Hospital, Vancouver, Canada
Djavad Mowafaghian Centre for Brain Health, The University of British Columbia, 2215 Wesbrook Mall, Room 3450D, Vancouver, BC V6T 2B5, Canada

C Keyworth
Manchester Centre for Health Psychology, Division of Psychology and Mental Health, School of Health Sciences, Faculty of Biology, Medicine and Health, University of Manchester, Manchester Academic Health Science Centre, Coupland 1 Building, Oxford Road, Manchester M13 9PL, UK

J Hart
Manchester Centre for Health Psychology, Division of Psychology and Mental Health, School of Health Sciences, Faculty of Biology, Medicine and Health, University of Manchester, Manchester Academic Health Science Centre, Coupland 1 Building, Oxford Road, Manchester M13 9PL, UK
Division of Medical Education, School of Medical Sciences, Faculty of Biology, Medicine and Health, University of Manchester, Manchester Academic Health Science Centre, Oxford Road, Manchester M13 9PL, UK

C J Armitage
Manchester Centre for Health Psychology, Division of Psychology and Mental Health, School of Health Sciences, Faculty of Biology, Medicine and Health, University of Manchester, Manchester Academic Health Science Centre, Coupland 1 Building, Oxford Road, Manchester M13 9PL, UK
NIHR Manchester Biomedical Research Centre, Manchester University NHS Foundation Trust, Manchester Academic Health Science Centre, Manchester M13 9PL, UK

NIHR Greater Manchester Patient Safety Translational Research Centre, Manchester, UK

M P Tully
Division of Pharmacy and Optometry, School of Health Sciences, Faculty of Biology, Medicine and Health, University of Manchester, Manchester Academic Health Science Centre, Stopford Building, Oxford Road, Manchester M13 9PL, UK

Index

A

Aboriginal, 52-54, 56, 59-62

Acute Respiratory Infections, 21, 219, 230-231

Affinity Propagation, 171, 175, 183-184

Alcohol Consumption, 31, 37, 39-40, 52, 54, 56, 58, 61-62

Alcohol Misuse, 30-32, 34-35, 37-39, 62

Alcohol Tracker Applications, 53

Alcohol Use Disorders Identification Test, 30, 39, 54, 56

Alzheimer Disease, 196, 199, 208

Artificial Neural Network, 42, 50

Average Variance Extracted, 66, 72

B

Behaviour Change Techniques, 211-212, 227

Behaviour Science, 121, 123

Bibliometric Analysis, 171-172, 178, 182-184

Bloodstream Infections, 23

C

Cerebrovascular Accident Unit, 14, 20

Chronic Disease Management, 146-147, 157-159, 161-163

Clinical Data Repository, 165

Coding Interventions, 213-214

Cohen's Kappa, 24, 26, 166, 196, 200-202

Communicable Diseases, 186

Computed Tomography, 10, 104-105, 108-112, 119, 184

Consumer Health Informatics, 185, 194

D

Decision Support System, 3, 10, 29, 182, 229-231

Diarrhoeal Disease, 21

Dysentery, 23, 25-26

E

Ehealth, 10-11, 135-136, 147, 196-197, 212

Electronic Health Records, 1, 10-11, 30, 63-64, 72, 113, 137, 164-165, 183, 188, 211, 220-221, 223, 229

Electronic Medical Records, 8, 64, 73, 170, 172, 183, 231

Evidence-based Medicine, 89, 104

Evidence-based Usability Design, 74-75, 88-90

F

Fisher Exact Test, 107-108

G

Gastrointestinal Infection, 23, 26, 28

General Practitioner, 32, 62, 228-229

Gi-infection, 23, 25-26, 28

H

Health Information Exchange, 137, 144-145

Health Information Technology, 1, 10-11, 29, 73, 144-145, 186, 194, 207

Healthcare Professional Behaviour Change, 212

Healthcare Quality, 1-2, 5, 10-11

Herfindahl-hirschman Index, 139, 144

Hospital Information Systems, 1, 10-11, 73

Hybrid Model, 41-42, 46, 50-51

I

Information Extraction, 91, 99, 102-103, 171, 179, 182

Integrated Management of Childhood Illness, 21, 29

Intensive Care Unit, 14

Interactive Voice Response, 21-22, 28-29, 159

L

Lung Cancer, 112-114, 116-120

M

Malaria, 21, 23, 26, 29

Medical Imaging, 91-93, 96, 101, 104-105, 107, 109-110, 216

Medication Alerting Systems, 74-76, 78-79, 87-89

Mhealth, 21-22, 27-29, 121-125, 129-136, 146-149, 153-154, 156-163

Mild Head Trauma, 104

N

Natural Language Processing, 91-92, 101-103, 164, 171-172, 174, 182-184

Neurosurgery, 14-15, 20, 184

New Admission Inpatients, 41-42, 44-46, 48-50

Nonlinear Autoregressive Neural Network, 41, 50

O

Online Health Information, 194, 196-198, 203-209

P

Partial Autocorrelation Function, 42, 50

Pls-sem, 63, 73, 136
Pulmonary Diseases, 112

R
Randomized Controlled Trials, 146-147, 162, 199, 211, 214
Respiratory Distress, 22
Robustness Test, 144
Rule-based Method, 164-165

S
Screening Decision Aid, 112-113, 117-118
Semantic Annotation, 99, 101
Semantic Network, 91-92, 94-96, 99-102
Shared Decision Making, 112, 117, 119-120

Spearman's Rank Correlation Test, 174, 177
Staff Dimensioning, 12-13, 19
Structural Equation Modelling, 63, 72, 136
Syntactic Processing, 92-93, 96, 101
Systems Integration, 137

T
Technology Acceptance Model (TAM), 64, 72, 122-123
Technology-based Interventions, 211-214, 224-225, 227-228
Thematic Analysis, 32, 211, 213-214, 224-225, 227

U
Usability Flaws, 74-78, 85, 87, 89-90